ASIAN MEDICAL SYSTEMS

ASIAN MEDICAL SYSTEMS

Asian Medical Systems: A Comparative Study

Edited by

CHARLES LESLIE

UNIVERSITY OF CALIFORNIA PRESS
BERKELEY, LOS ANGELES, LONDON

UNIVERSITY OF CALIFORNIA PRESS
Berkeley and Los Angeles, California

University of California Press, Ltd.
London, England

Copyright © 1976, by
The Regents of the University of California

ISBN 0-520-02680-2
Library of Congress Catalog Card Number 73-91674

To the Memory of
WILLIAM CAUDILL
1927—1972

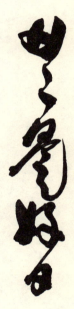

"Every day is a good day."

Contents

Part IV
THE CULTURE OF PLURAL MEDICAL SYSTEMS

Part V
THE ECOLOGY OF INDIGENOUS AND COSMOPOLITAN MEDICAL PRACTICE

Part VI
MEDICAL REVIVALISM

Part VII
PERSPECTIVES

List of Tables

List of Illustrations

List of Contributors

ARTHUR LLEWELLYN BASHAM, Professor and Chairman of the Department of Asian Civilizations, Australian National University, Canberra.

ALAN R. BEALS, Professor and Chairman, Department of Anthropology, University of California at Riverside.

J. CHRISTOPH BÜRGEL, Ordinarius fur Islamwissenschaft in Bern, Switzerland.

WILLIAM CAUDILL at the time of his death in 1972 was Chief, Section on Personality and Environment, Laboratory of Socio-Environmental Studies, National Institute of Mental Health, Bethesda, Maryland.

RALPH C. CROIZIER, Associate Professor of History, Department of History, University of Rochester, New York.

FREDERICK L. DUNN, M.D., Professor of Epidemiology and Anthropology in the Department of International Health and the George Williams Hooper Foundation, University of California, San Francisco.

MARK G. FIELD, Professor of Sociology at Boston University and Associate, Russian Research Center at Harvard University.

RENÉE C. FOX, Professor and Chairman of the Department of Sociology, University of Pennsylvania.

BRAHMANANDA GUPTA, Lecturer in Sanskrit at the Rabindra Bharati University, Calcutta, and Honorary Lecturer in Charaka at the Shymadas Vaidya Sastra Pith, Calcutta.

MERVYN A. JASPAN, at the time of his death in 1975 was Professor of South-East Asian Sociology and Director of the Centre for South-East Asian Studies, The University of Hull, England.

W. T. JONES, Professor of Philosophy at the California Institute of Technology.

CHARLES LESLIE, Professor of Anthropology at New York University, New York City.

EDWARD MONTGOMERY, Assistant Professor of Anthropology at Washington University, St Louis.

GANANATH OBEYESEKERE, Professor of Anthropology, University of California at San Diego.

YASUO OTSUKA, M. D., Instructor in Pharmacology at Yokohama City University Medical School, and Director of the Japanese Society for Oriental Medicine.

IVAN POLUNIN, M.D., Reader, Department of Social Medicine and Public Health, Faculty of Medicine, University of Singapore.

MANFRED PORKERT, Universitatdozent, Philosophische Fakultat II of the University of Munich.

CARL E. TAYLOR, M.D., Professor and Chairman of the Department of International Health, The Johns Hopkins School of Hygiene and Public Health, Baltimore, Maryland.

MARJORIE TOPLEY, Research Fellow of the Centre of Asian Studies, University of Hong Kong.

PAUL U. UNSCHULD, Fellow (1973–74) in the Department of International Medicine, The Johns Hopkins School of Hygiene and Public Health. Dr. Unschuld holds graduate degrees in Sinology and in Pharmaceutical Chemistry, Botany and Physics from the University of Munich.

ASIAN MEDICAL SYSTEMS

Introduction

The health concepts and practices of most people in the world today continue traditions that evolved during antiquity. Ideas about the ways that body processes are thrown off balance by the improper consumption of "hot" or "cold" foods, or the ways that envy, fear, and other strong emotions generate poisonous substances by disturbing the body's equilibrium, are based upon humoral theories that were first elaborated in the classic texts of medical science several thousand years ago. These ideas, and others related to them, are held by the majority of Asians and by large segments of European and African society. Imported to the New World in colonial times, they still play an important role in Latin American communities.

Folk curers throughout the world practice humoral medicine, but in Asia alone educated physicians continue its learned traditions. Most notably in China and India, but also in Japan, Sri Lanka (formerly Ceylon), and other countries, the institutional forms of professional education and practice have been adapted to indigenous medical traditions. Research institutes, colleges, hospitals, professional associations, and pharmaceutical companies for Chinese, Āyurvedic, and Yunānī medicine coexist to a greater or lesser extent with similar institutions for cosmopolitan medicine. Together with folk practitioners, physicians who utilize these institutions provide a major source of medical consultation for all classes of people. Asian medical systems thus provide fascinating opportunities both to observe directly practices that continue ancient scientific modes of thought and to analyze the historical processes that mediate their relationship to modern science and technology.

Three primary traditions of medical science were formulated in what Alfred Louis Kroeber called the *Oikoumenê* of Old World society. The Greeks used the word *Oikoumenê*, the inhabited, to refer to the entire range of mankind, but Kroeber redefined the term to designate the civilizations of Asia, Africa, and Europe that from ancient times to the present day have formed "a great web of cultural growth, areally extensive and rich in content" (Kroeber 1952:392). Ideas and products have been transmitted from one end of this network to the other for thousands of years, and yet stylistically distinctive traditions have continued to exist. The stylistic continuities that distinguish the civilizations of the *Oikoumenê* can be identified in their medical traditions. For example, in the present volume Manfred Porkert and W. T. Jones contrast fundamental styles of thought in Chinese and Western medicine, though they approach the subject from different methodological perspectives. Also, Gananath Obeyesekere and Alan Beals describe long-enduring South Asian forms of thought, in Obeyesekere's case by analyzing the popular

1

culture of Āyurvedic physicians and their patients in urban Sri Lanka, and in Beals' essay by describing the habits of mind of peasant villagers in Mysore State, India, as they decide to use different kinds of therapy.

I will call the three main streams of learned medical practice and theory that originated in the Chinese, South Asian, and Mediterranean civilizations "great-tradition" medicine—a term derived from Robert Redfield's work on the comparative study of civilizations. Observing that the development of civilizations was characterized by the differentiation of great from little traditions, Redfield described this process as "the separation of culture into hierarchic and lay traditions, the appearance of an elite with secular and sacred power and including specialized cultivators of the intellectual life, and the conversion of tribal peoples into peasantry" (Redfield 1956:76). Illustrating the interdependency of great and little traditions, Redfield speculated that "the teaching of Galen about the four humors may have been suggested by ideas current in little communities of simple people becoming but not yet civilized; after development by reflective minds they may have been received by peasantry and reinterpreted in local terms" (*ibid*:71).

The first point that I want to make about the great medical traditions is that they maintained their individual characters although they were in contact with each other. The integrity of the separate traditions needs to be emphasized to avoid the assumption that all significant early medical science originated in Greece (or India or China, for that matter). My second point will be that the three traditions nevertheless share general features of social organization and theory that allow us to describe a generic great-tradition medicine which can be contrasted with cosmopolitan medicine.

The Mediterranean tradition was comprehensively formulated by Galen in the second century. It continued in this form through the Middle Ages in Christian and Islamic societies, and was carried by the spread of Islam to Central Asia, India, and Southeast Asia. The system was called *Yunānī Tibbia* in Arabic, meaning Greek medicine, and it is still practiced under that name in Pakistan, India, Sri Lanka, and other South Asian countries. In his essay for the present volume, J. Christoph Bürgel emphasizes the Galenic character of Arabic medicine: it was not significantly influenced by South Asian theories, although Ali al-Tabari was familiar with Indian medical texts as early as the ninth century. Nor, according to Sir Joseph Needham (1970:14–29), did knowledge of Chinese medicine notably effect the Galenic tradition, though a thirteenth-century Persian physician, Rashid al-din al-Hamadani, directed the preparation of an encyclopedia of Chinese medicine.

Knowledge of the South Asian and Chinese medical traditions was carried through the *Oikoumenê* from the nuclear areas of their development, just as the Mediterranean tradition was carried to distant societies. The South Asian system was called *Āyurveda*, meaning knowledge of life, or longevity. It was known in the Mediterranean region long before the translation of

Greek texts into Arabic. Several Hippocratic authors recommended medications that they attributed to India, and Plato's theory of vision—that a fiery element in the eye joined with the corresponding element in things—resembled that of Āyurveda, as did some details of his conceptions of illness and of anatomy (Filliozat 1964:229–237). The diffusion of Buddhism from India to China was certainly accompanied by exchanges of Āyurvedic and Chinese medical knowledge, yet Chinese medicine had no discernible effect on the development of Āyurveda, and Joseph Needham maintains that the overall influence of Indian on Chinese medicine was minor. Evaluating the relation of Chinese medicine to Greek and Arabic tradition, Needham writes: "It is really hard to find in it any Western influences" (1970:18–19). On the other hand, Chinese medicine strongly affected medical institutions in Korea, Japan, and parts of Southeast Asia, and Āyurveda had a marked influence in Tibet, Burma, and Southeast Asia.

Although the three great medical traditions were relatively independent, they evolved in similar ways. They all became professional branches of scientific learning in the millennium between the fifth century B.C. and the fifth century A.D. Professional standards for education and practice were achieved by appeals to the authority of Galen, Caraka, the *Nei Ching*, and other highly respected texts. Since rational theories and therapeutic formulas were elaborated in the texts far beyond the knowledge of laymen and folk curers, the ability to show acquaintance with them validated claims to a superior social position. Claims to high status were symbolically expressed in special modes of dress and deportment recommended by the texts, and they were rationalized by ethical codes that defined a physician's responsibilities.

Women were not educated in medicine, and the perspective of the classic texts was masculine. Practitioners ranged from physicians who had undergone long periods of training to individuals with little education who practiced a simplified version of the great tradition. Other healers coexisted with these practitioners, their arts falling into special categories: bone-setters, surgeons, midwives, snake-bite curers, shamans, and so on. But the complex and redundant system of learned and humble practitioners, of full-time and part-time practitioners, of generalists and specialists, of naturalist and supernaturalist curers, was ideologically simplified by the distinction elaborated in the texts between quacks and legitimate practitioners. The concern the texts show for this distinction indicates that society assigned learned physicians a lower social status than the one that they aspired to, and that their power to dominate the overall system of medical practice was limited.

The Chinese may have led in rationalizing medical services, for they developed an extensive bureaucratic system to instruct and examine physicians, along with what, according to Joseph Needham and Lu Gwei-djen, "can only be described as a national medical service" (1969:268). But in all of these societies, armies required organized medical services, rulers acted as patrons to medical scholarship, and medical aid was a philanthropic enterprise appropriate to religious institutions and to wealthy individuals. Needham's discussion of Chinese priorities is directed toward correcting the biases that have caused Western writers on the history and philosophy of science to focus on why the Scientific Revolution occurred in Seventeenth-century Europe. The framework in which this question is asked sometimes resembles that of a believer in witchcraft who confronts the death of an old man with the question, "Why did it happen on Tuesday?" The fact that the Scientific Revolution first occurred in Europe is taken by Europeans as *a priori* evidence that the Western tradition possessed a genius for scientific progress lacking in the Chinese and Indian traditions. Thus it is possible to question the orientation—shared by Needham as much as by those he criticizes—that makes temporal priority a predominant issue.

Besides resembling each other in the organization of practice, the great traditions of medicine were formulated from generic physiological and cosmological concepts. All of them were humoral theories: four humors in the Mediterranean tradition (yellow bile, black bile, phlegm, and blood); three humors in the South Asian tradition (*kapha*, *pitta*, and *vayu*, usually translated as phlegm, bile, and wind); and six humors in Chinese medicine (the *chii*, or pneuma, which were held in the sway of *yang* and *yin*). The humors were alignments of opposing qualities: hot-cold, wet-dry, heavy-light, male-female, dark-bright, strong-weak, active-sluggish, and so on. The equilibrium of these qualities maintained health, and their disequilibrium caused illness, whatever the number of humors. Equilibrium was regulated by an individual's age, sex, and temperament in dynamic relationship to climate, season, food consumption, and other activities. Diagnoses required skill in observing and correlating physical symptoms and environment. Therapy utilized physical manipulations, modification of the patient's diet and surroundings, and numerous medications. Some medications required elaborate preparation; others, valuable and esoteric substances such as herbs gathered from distant mountainsides, saffron, gold, precious stones, or parts of rare animals.

Finally, great-tradition medicine conceived human anatomy and physiology to be intimately bound to other physical systems. The arrangement and balance of elements in the human body were microcosmic versions of their arrangement in society at large and throughout the universe. Sir Charles Sherrington's description of the world view of Jean Fernel, a physician in sixteenth-century Paris, applies equally to Chinese or Hindu physicians: "The macrocosm fulfilling its vast circuits and epicycles of meticulous precision, its rising and its settings, its movements within movements, was an immense body fashioned after the likeness of man's body" (1955:61). This conception rationalized the relation of men to their environment by making preventive and curative medicine efforts to maintain or to restore cosmic equilibrium.

At the end of the Middle Ages, scientific research and forms of professional association in Europe began a development which led eventually to the worldwide traditions of cosmopolitan medicine. Mixed with new knowledge, humoral theories and practices continued to be taught through the nineteenth century, and remnants of humoral theory survive in research to the present day. For example, studies that classify people by their body types, and correlate this typology with variations in behavior or in susceptibility to illness, are in the humoral tradition. Practitioners in India who argue that ancient scientific theories can be employed in modern research are correct when they claim that studies of body types by European and American scientists use concepts that resemble fundamental ideas in Āyurvedic medicine.

The scientific theories and social organization of cosmopolitan medicine evolved progressively over several centuries without significant practical consequences for patients. They developed with the expansion of Europe, the rise of modern science, the Industrial Revolution, and other movements that since the Middle Ages have been transforming the *Oikoumenê* of Old World civilizations into a world order. Research on anatomy and physiology during the Renaissance and Reformation generated new methods of scientific work and discovered facts that seemed to invalidate ancient medical authorities (Nef 1967:286–298). Associations of practitioners and government agencies were formed to sponsor and regulate medical services. The institutional network for teaching, research, and publication expanded around the world and became more efficient. But the great advances in therapeutic effectiveness that have become the hallmark of cosmopolitan medicine— the germ theory of disease and new surgical techniques—were not initiated until the late nineteenth century, followed by twentieth-century progress in chemotherapy. These advances, by radically increasing the consequences of medical learning for social welfare, have accelerated the professionalization processes that are creating throughout the world medical systems based upon a standardized university education for physicians. Professionalization also involves special courses of training for dentists, nurses, and numerous paramedical workers; the bureaucratic organization of medical work, dominated by physicians and centered in hospitals; state responsibility for environmental medicine and for organizing or supervising medical services, with the distribution of authority throughout the system enforced by state powers to license and regulate all forms of medical practice.

Another feature of cosmopolitan medicine has been called its "preeminence." Eliot Freidson writes:

If we consider the profession of medicine today, it is clear that its major characteristic is preeminence. Such preeminence is not merely that of prestige but also that of expert authority. This is to say, medicine's knowledge about illness and its treatment is considered to be authoritative and definitive. While there are interesting exceptions like chiropractic and homeopathy, there are no representatives of occupations in

direct competition with medicine who hold official policy-making positions related
to health affairs. Medicine's position today is akin to that of state religious yesterday—
it has an officially approved monopoly of the right to define health and illness and to
treat illness. (1970:5)

The ways in which cosmopolitan medicine progressively subordinates other
forms of practice are major variables for the comparative study of medical
systems. A necessary condition appears to be the respect people in all social
classes have for the recent capacity of this system to generate effective new
therapies, and a necessary means is the use of state power to legitimize and
extend its authority. Among the upper classes everywhere in the world, and
among all social strata in industrial societies, doctors now play a crucial
role in episodes of birth, illness, and death. And in law and popular culture,
the theories and institutions of cosmopolitan medicine define standards
of health and abnormality that shape the ways people think and feel about
themselves and about the norms for social conduct.

Access to medical knowledge and to consultation with specialists is another
critical variable for comparing medical systems. Peasants and tribal peoples
as well as urban dwellers admire the technology of cosmopolitan medicine
and are eager to adopt new medications. At the same time, the abrupt
manners of most physicians and paramedical workers when they deal with
rural and lower-class people are resented, and in communities where these
specialists are outsiders, resistance to their authority usually expresses class
conflict. In this situation, indigenous practitioners adopt whatever seems
useful and is available to them from cosmopolitan medicine. Laymen consult
these eclectic practitioners of traditional and modern therapies, and only
in emergencies risk the possible humiliation, the expense, and the other
difficulties of gaining access to fully trained practitioners of cosmopolitan
medicine. The data, if not always the interpretaions, of earlier studies support
these generalizations, and the essays in Parts IV and V of the present volume,
"The Culture of Plural Medical Systems" and "The Ecology of Indigenous
and Modern Medical Practice," present new ethnographic data consistent
with them.

What I have been calling cosmopolitan medicine is usually called alternatively "modern medicine," or "scientific medicine," or "Western
medicine." Translations of these terms are widely used in Asian languages,
along with other labels: Dutch medicine, English medicine, allopathy,
doctor medicine, and so on. While most authors in this volume follow ordinary
usage, Fred Dunn calls attention in his essay to the biases associated with
this usage and suggests the new designation "cosmopolitan medicine,"
which I have adopted. Dunn's skepticism about current habits of mind
deserves elaboration.

The term "modern medicine," used in contrast to traditional medicine,
encourages the user to confuse inferences from the modernity–traditionalism
dichotomy with reality. For example, the dichotomy opposes the changing

and creative nature of modernity to an assumed stagnant and unchanging traditionalism, but acquaintance with historical documents and with the contemporary medical institutions labeled "traditional" reveals that considerable change has occurred in the last century, and that medicine like everything else has been changing throughout the past. The dichotomy implies that practitioners of traditional medicine are uniformly conservative and reject opportunities to acquire new knowledge, and yet the limited evidence at hand indicates that the opposite situation prevails. Within the resources available to them, many folk practitioners are innovative, and they have certainly been eager to gain new skills. This has also been true among the educated urban practitioners of great-tradition medicine. In Japan the physicians who practice Chinese medicine must be qualified in cosmopolitan medicine. In China the extensive use of traditional medicine in a modern system of health services has attracted worldwide attention. The system of colleges, research institutes, and other facilities for humoral medicine in India has been created by entrepreneural practitioners of traditional medicine, and by their patrons in politics, industry, and other modern occupations (Brass 1972; Leslie 1973). Thus when the term "modern medicine" is used in describing systems that include a large component of traditional medicine, it evokes stereotypes that contradict reality. These stereotypes tempt the advocates of modernity to lapse unconsciously into a self-flattering rhetoric that fights windmills of recalcitrant medical ignorance and superstition.

The term "scientific medicine" is also misleading. It encourages the assumption that all aspects of cosmopolitan medicine are somehow derived from or conducive to science, but by any ordinary criteria many elements in this system are not scientific—for example, the politics of research funding or of professional associations, various routines of hospital administration, or the etiquette of doctor–patient relationships. A second and equally stultifying assumption is that all medicine other than cosmopolitan medicine is unscientific. By commonly recognized criteria, Chinese, Āyurvedic, and Arabic medicine are scientific in substantial degrees. They involve the rational use of naturalistic theories to organize and interpret systematic empirical observations. They have explicit, orderly ways of recording and teaching this knowledge, and they have some efficacious methods for promoting health and for curing illness. Of course, by other criteria, such as the degree of instrumentation and standardization of techniques, or the refinement of experimental methods, these systems are less scientific. In objective comparative research, judgments about the scientific character of medical theories and practices vary because multiple criteria exist for calling them scientific, and because most criteria specify elements that may be more or less well developed. Recognition of the need to evolve conceptual models and to record data for the complex analyses that this subject requires is discouraged by preemptively labeling one set of institutions "scientific medicine."

Finally, the term "Western medicine" is misleading for obvious reasons. The scientific aspects of Western medicine are transcultural. Ethnic interpretations of modern science are the aberrations of nationalistic and totalitarian ideologies or, in this case, a reflex of colonial and neo-colonial thought. Furthermore, the social organization of cosmopolitan medicine as I have described it is as Japanese as it is Western. Because modern science and professionalization processes are intrinsically cosmopolitan, Fred Dunn's phrase "cosmopolitan medicine" is appropriate. Still, in another essay for this volume Ralph Croizier tells us that the Chinese referred to their own tradition simply as medicine, and began self-consciously to call it "Chinese" only in modern times as they adopted the contrasting term "Western medicine." Since ethnographic and historical descriptions benefit by using categories of the cultures they describe, it makes sense to use these terms in writing about modern China. For similar reasons, descriptive accounts of other Asian medical systems may continue to refer to Western medicine. But for comparative purposes another term is needed, and the model that I have outlined in the preceding pages is best referred to as "cosmopolitan medicine."

The picture I have drawn of the great medical traditions formed in the *Oikoumenê* of Old World civilizations, and of the recent full emergence of cosmopolitan medicine, brings the subject of this whole volume in view. Let me restate it briefly. In countries like the United States or Japan, cosmopolitan medicine is preeminent: its representatives dominate medical work and exercise unprecedented legal and cultural authority to define situations and make decisions during birth, illness, and death, as well as to shape norms for sexual conduct, child rearing, or questions of sanity. Although cosmopolitan medical institutions exist in every country, most people alive today continue to depend on humoral theories and practices. In large parts of Asia, educated practitioners still draw upon these traditions and, with folk practitioners, provide a major source of medical care. Thus, great and little medical traditions coexist to various degrees and in various ways with cosmopolitan medicine in China, India, Japan, and other countries. Analyses of these variations are avenues to understanding the role of scientific knowledge and professional organization in transformations of the human condition.

I have defined the subject of our essays in language suited to their scholarly spirit, but my tone has been too cool to indicate the nature of our enterprise. We began in a castle on a mountain in Austria. Ours was the fifty-third Burg Wartenstein Symposium sponsored by the Wenner-Gren Foundation for Anthropological Research. Our aim was to develop new lines of research in medical anthropology, some of which the Foundation had initiated in previous symposia (Galdston 1963 and Poynter 1969). Preliminary drafts of our essays were circulated prior to our discussions, which lasted from July 19 to 27, 1971. Lita Osmundsen, Director of Research for the Founda-

tion, lifted the spirit of the Symposium by participating in it, and by orchestra-
ting arrangements for it to proceed in elegant informality through meals
and intermissions and entertainments. We were honored, too, by Raymond
and Rosemary Firth, who visited the castle briefly during the Symposium.

Had we been members of a single discipline or nationality, our discussions
might have generated more disputes than they did. Most of us arrived at
Burg Wartenstein knowing nothing or very little about most other members
of the Symposium. We had a great deal to learn from and about each other,
and we spent no time at all drawing intellectual boundaries. Initially our
focus was substantive rather than methodological. This will sound dull to
methodologists, and downright anemic to polemicists for whom the good
guys wear white hats and the bad guys wear black. In fact, as the Symposium
progressed we returned continuously to conceptual differences that caused
some of us to think that others of us were naive or dogmatic or fuzzy-minded.
Our guide in clarifying these disagreements was the philosopher W. T. Jones,
whose message was that we did not have to agree on most theoretical issues
so long as we understood how we differed. It worked because he showed
us our commonalities and analyzed our differences with authority and good
humor.

I will describe some of the differences that emerged in our thinking about
the systemic properties of "the medical system." We had not been asked to
develop a particular model for this purpose, though the titles of the Symposium
and of its various sessions and their constituent papers provided guidelines
for our discussions. Mark Field and Edward Montgomery addressed the issue
directly, but all of the papers reasoned from general concepts of the system
that they were reporting. Since they have been revised for publication and
speak for themselves in the following pages, I will describe our conceptual
differences in a schematic manner.

In human affairs, concepts never simply name and describe things without
implying or recommending evaluations of them. The preeminence of cosmopolitan medicine in a country like the United States causes laymen and
specialists alike to identify its professional institutions with *the* medical
system. All other practices are then considered to be irregular, and thus to
be aberrations of the system or altogether outside of it. To some members
of the Symposium, the model of a uniform cosmopolitan medical system with
a monopoly of legitimate practice seemed more scientific and efficient and
therefore truer and more desirable than a pluralistic model, which from
their perspective appeared to legitimize quack medicine, or at least to tolerate
and romanticize medical ignorance.

In fact, medical systems are pluralistic structures of different kinds of
practitioners and institutional norms. Even in the United States, the medical
system is composed of physicians, dentists, druggists, clinical psychologists,
chiropractors, social workers, health food experts, masseurs, yoga teachers,
spirit curers, Chinese herbalists, and so on. The health concepts of a Puerto

Rican worker in New York city, the curers he consults, and the therapies he receives, differ from those of a Chinese laundryman or a Jewish clerk. Their concepts and the practitioners they consult differ in turn from those of middle-class believers in Christian Science or in logical positivism. Yet the institutions of cosmopolitan medicine are so extensive, well organized, and powerful, that the concept of a single, standardized, hieratic medical system administered by university-trained physicians appears to be normative in American popular culture, as well as in law. Since this is not true in Asian countries, where the structures of learned and folk, of humoral and cosmopolitan medicine are coexisting normative institutions, members of the symposium who reasoned from a pluralistic model felt that they were more objective—because less chauvinistic—than those who assumed the norms of a cosmopolitan medical model.

Another disagreement that emerged at our conference is related to different conceptions of cultural organization. Some participants conceived the systemic qualities of "the medical system" by using concepts of standardization and consistency derived from the ideal of mass culture. When Asian respondents differed among themselves in classifying items of food as belonging to "hot" or "cold" categories, or simultaneously used medicines associated with different ways of defining a malady, their ideas and behavior were interpreted as having a low degree of systematization. Other members of the Symposium saw variations of this kind as an essential dimension of the systems under consideration rather than evidence that they were disorganized. They interpreted categories of food and illness, or of the causes of illness and kinds of therapy, as a rhetoric for defining situations, deciding what to do, and justifying one or another course of action. If the categories were fixed and inflexible they could not be used for these purposes.

A third source of disagreement concerned ways of drawing the boundaries of a medical system. Indeed, the format of the Symposium encouraged the use of conceptual models derived from three approaches to this problem, which for convenience can be labeled biological, cultural, and social.

From the point of view of the biological approach, all ideas and behavior that the trained observer finds relevant to interpreting patterns of health and illness are considered to be part of the medical system. Thus behavioral epidemiology, which would analyze such things as the relationships between customary diet or working habits and disease vectors, would be important for developing comparative studies of medical systems. This inclusive conception of the systems under study has the advantage of emphasizing research goals that will be useful to health planners trained in cosmopolitan medicine. By using the best current knowledge in ecology, nutrition, pathology, and other subjects, it provides standards for comparing the health conditions and the utility of health practices in different societies. In contrast, the cultural approach conceives the medical system to be composed of deliberate actions, by members of a society, to maintain or enhance health and to cure illness.

This way of thinking about the system emphasizes categories of thought and traditions within the culture. It excludes many ideas, items of behavior, and ecological relationships that the first approach includes. It emphasizes such things as a mother's self-conscious efforts to promote her child's health by regulating its diet. The social approach to conceiving the medical system would exclude the mother's behavior and conceptions of health and illness until she decided to consult another individual recognized in her community as a specialist. This conception locates the system in the role relationships between people who have reputations as authorities in matters of health and illness, and between these specialists and laymen.

Though our differential preferences for one or another of these approaches did not logically entail disagreements, they did cause us to have different feelings about what was interesting or important in our discussions. But even those who shared a preference for one approach would differ on other grounds. For example, those who used the cultural approach would locate the systemic nature of a medical tradition in the coherence of its theories, and reason that it was the integrity of the theory that held practices together in a medical system. One might argue that Chinese medicine was an integrated system in the past, whereas contemporary physicians who were supposedly working in the tradition did not understand the theories as they were previously understood, or believe in them in the way that they were once believed in. Thus contemporary practices appeared to be an opportunistic or non-systematic set of behaviors. But another student of Chinese tradition would disagree with this conception of history and of the relationship between medical theory and practice; while a third might agree with the general concept but disagree about how to evaluate evidence that the theories of Chinese medicine are now misunderstood or disbelieved.

In general, it is fair to report that those members of the Symposium who focused on the historical continuities in Asian medical systems, and on the systemic qualities of contemporary great and little traditions, appeared "romantic" and "theoretical" to those who emphasized historical discontinuities and who argued that the pluralistic, structurally differentiated Asian medical systems show a low degree of systematization. Of course, the participants who thought that others were "romantic" felt that their own perspective was "realistic" and "pragmatic."

Although I have only briefly described the methodological issues that emerged during our conference, enough has been said to indicate their nature. Our collection of essays as a whole has been designed to show how the comparative study of Asian medical systems opens a new field of scholarship. Such a book required the skills of authors with diverse kinds of training. Those who have contributed to it are trained in history, sociology, anthropology, public health, pharmacology, epidemiology, cosmopolitan medicine, and philosophy. One is a practitioner of Chinese medicine, and two are the sons of Āyurvedic physicians. My task has been to define the subject and to indicate concepts that join our individual essays in a unified dialogue. Our work will have been well done if others find in it both something to correct and something to build upon.

CHARLES LESLIE

Literature Cited

Brass, Paul
  1972 "The Politics of Āyurvedic Education: A Case Study of Revivalism and modernization in India," in Lloyd and Susanne Rudolph, eds., *Politics and Education in India*. Cambridge: Harvard University Press.
Filliozat, Jean
  1964 *The Classical Doctrine of Indian Medicine*. Delhi: Munshi Manoharlal.
Freidson, Eliot
  1970 *The Profession of Medicine: A Study of the Sociology of Applied Knowledge*. New York: Dodd, Mead.
Galdston, Iago
  1963 *Man's Image in Medicine and Anthropology*. New York: International Universities Press.
Kroeber, Alfred Louis
  1952 *The Nature of Culture*. Chicago: University of Chicago Press.
Leslie, Charles
  1973 "The Professionalizing Ideology of Medical Revivalism," in Milton Singer, ed., *Entrepreneurship and Modernization of Occupational Cultures in South Asia*. Durham: Duke University Press.
Needham, Joseph
  1970 *Clerks and Craftsmen in China and the West*. Cambridge: Cambridge University Press.
Needham, Joseph, and Lu Gwei-djen
  1969 "Chinese Medicine," in F.N.L. Poynter, ed., *Medicine and Culture*. London: Wellcome Institute of the History of Medicine.
Nef, John U.
  1967 *The Conquest of the Material World*. Cleveland: World.
Poynter, F. N. L.
  1969 *Medicine and Culture*. London: Wellcome Institute of the History of Medicine.
Redfield, Robert
  1956 *Peasant Society and Culture*. Chicago: University of Chicago Press.
Sherrington, Charles
  1955 *Man on His Nature*. Garden City: Doubleday (Anchor).

PART I

The Great Traditions of
Hindu, Arabic, and Chinese Medicine

COMPARATIVE STUDIES describe historical cases so that we can analyze the similarities and differences between them. Our purpose is to reveal the processes that shaped the character of contemporary Asian medical systems, and for this purpose we must adopt a long-term perspective. R. G. Collingwood wrote:

How the world of nature appears to us depends on how long we take to observe it. . . . To a person who took a view of it extending over a thousand years it would appear in one way, to a person who took a view of it extending over a thousandth of a second it would appear in a different way. . . . That is because when we observe it for a certain length of time we observe the processes which require that length of time in order to occur. . . . If two historians gave each his own answer to the question: "What kinds of events happen, or can or might happen, in history?" their answers would be extremely different if one habitually thought of an event as something that takes an hour and the other as something that takes ten years; and a third who conceived an event as taking anything up to 1,000 years would give a different answer again. (1945:24–25)

Our questions about Asian medicine are special applications of questions asked by all studies which seek to understand comprehensive patterns of historical change. We want to analyze processes of cultural evolution, of scientific creativity, professionalization, and so on. Although these processes occur in different frameworks of time and space, the student who takes a long view is in a better position than others to consider the various elements relevant to a particular historical configuration.

We want to study the social organization of the great medical traditions; their theoretical structure and the relationships between theory and practice; the extent and nature of their contacts with each other; the manner in which they emerged from preceding civilizations; and their course of change to the present day. About social organization we ask: How many learned physicians were there at any one time? How were they educated? How did they communicate with each other and with other learned men? What were their relations with other kinds of curers, and with laymen of different statuses?

15

About theoretical structure we ask: What organization of ideas and sentiments characterized these traditions? How did the world-views of physicians compare to those of other members of their societies? Did they share a mental style? Were their traditions cumulative, so that medical learning was more advanced in the first century A.D. than in the fourth century B.C., and progressively more advanced in the fifth and tenth centuries A.D.?

Of course the evidence will not be available to answer all of these questions, and the evidence that does exist will not speak for itself. Our answers will vary with our conceptions of the nature of science, of causality in human affairs, and so forth. But from the dialogue of individual research and theoretical perspectives, a realm of discourse will emerge for the comparative study of medical systems.

The essays in this section contain data on common topics, but they emphasize different questions. A. L. Basham writes primarily about the social organization of Āyurvedic practice, while Manfred Porkert emphasizes the theoretical structure and chronology of Chinese medicine. Other less explicit differences characterize their work. Although Basham approves the notion that the "intuitive genius" and environmental command of Indian medicine "made it more effective than other systems of antiquity," he writes about it as an obsolete science that was rational, enlightened, and empirical, but never quite free in theory or practice from religious considerations. He tells us, for example, that Āyurvedic physiology was "by all modern standards thoroughly inaccurate," and that an upper-caste religious taboo "prevented the development of anatomical knowledge."

Porkert, on the other hand, appears to write an apologia for Chinese medical theory vis-a-vis Western medicine. He distinguishes a synthetic/inductive approach to knowledge from one that is analytic and causal, and claims that these cognitive modes are suited to apprehend different aspects of reality. The synthetic/inductive approach of Chinese medicine best describes "functions," and the analytic/causal approach of Western medicine best describes "substratum." He asserts an "epistemological complementarity" of these two traditions in which one is not "basically inferior to the other." Even so, he claims that until the late nineteenth century, Chinese medicine was more coherent and theoretically stringent than Western medicine, and that Chinese theories "led to a sensibly better ratio between therapeutic efforts and curative effects than could ever be achieved by the causal Western medicine." Yet Porkert maintains that the very success of this tradition prevented it from continuing to evolve into a "full-fledged science in the narrow sense of the term."

J. Christoph Bürgel analyzes the conflict in Islam between the alien, secular, and rational Galenic tradition and the indigenous, irrational tradition of Prophetic medicine. No one could doubt which side he is on, for he writes of the "dethronment (of Galen) in favor of Bedouin quackery and superstition sanctified by religion," and he defines the social conditions essential for science in order to analyze the "spiritual forces (that) were most potent in paralyzing the scientific impetus of the golden age" of Arabic medicine. While Basham writes in an even-handed encyclopedic manner, and Porkert devotes part of his essay to an argument about the differences and peculiar virtues of Chinese and Western medicine, Bürgel organizes his entire essay to present a thesis about the decline of Arabic medical science and the low symbolic potential of that tradition for modern Islamic revivalism. And so the dialogue begins.

CHARLES LESLIE

Literature Cited

Collingwood, R. G.
  1945 *The Idea of Nature*. London: Clarendon Press, Oxford University.

The Practice of Medicine in Ancient and Medieval India

A. L. BASHAM

MEDICINE IN PROTOHISTORIC TIMES

Since even the most primitive of men have some rudimentary system of medicine, we may assume that in the protohistoric Harappā Culture, which dominated the northwestern part of the Indian subcontinent for several centuries before and after 2000 B.C., there was a system of medicine with professional healers. Though this culture reached a high level of urban civilization, its surviving written records are brief and unintelligible, and therefore our knowledge of it is deficient in many particulars. We know nothing about its medical lore, though it may be suggested that, as in many other features of Indian life, the Harappā Culture contained the seeds of much that was characteristic of later Indian medicine.

A few intimations of a more definite nature are to be found in the earliest literature of India, the *Ṛg Veda*, the data of which may mostly be referred to the latter part of the second millennium B.C. Here we meet the *bhiṣaj*, a word which later became more or less synonymous with *vaidya*, still the standard Indian term for a doctor of the traditional type. The *bhiṣaj* is referred to in one passage (*R.V.*: ix.112.1) as desiring a break, a fracture (*rutam*), in order to gain wealth, and this has been interpreted as indicating that he was originally a bone-setter (Filliozat 1964:86–87). The *bhiṣaj*, however, was definitely a healer of disease generally, for in another hymn he is referred to as conversant with healing herbs *R.V.*: x.97.6). The same verse mentions the *bhiṣaj* as a *vipra*, a term usually applied to members of the emergent priestly class of brahmans, and verse 4 refers to his obtaining a horse, a cow, and a garment as a result of his knowledge of herbal mysteries. Later in the hymn he is identified as a brahman (verse 22; cf. *A.V.*: viii.7).

At this period disease was believed to be largely due to the visitation of punishing gods or to the evil work of demons. The god Varuṇa, particularly associated with moral ideas, punished those who transgressed his commands with disease, especially dropsy (*A.V.*: iv.16.7). Rudra, a god of ambivalent character, might arbitrarily inflict disease on men (*R.V.*: i.114.8; ii.33.11,14;

18

etc.), but was also the guardian of healing herbs (*R.V.*:ii.33.4,13). A class of holy men or witch doctors, called *munis* (a term later taken over by the Jains, but also sometimes used by Hindus and Buddhists with the meaning of "ascetic"), were adepts in the lore of Rudra and knew the magic of his herbs (*R.V.*:x.136).

The idea of healing is particularly associated with the divine twin gods, the *Aśvins* (meaning "horsemen"), who may have some remote connection with the Dioscuri of classical Europe. They are prayed to for healing in several hymns, and some of their miraculous cures are recorded. They were believed to have performed remarkable feats of rejuvenation (*R.V.*:i. 116–118; v.74; vii.68, 71; x. 39; etc.). They gave a bronze leg to a hero who had lost a leg in battle (*R.V.*:i. 112,116–118; x.39). They cured blindness, lameness, and leprosy (*R.V.*:i.112,116–117,120; x.39–40; etc.). Soma, the divine king of plants, is also referred to as a healing deity (*R.V.*:vi.74).

Demons as causes of disease loom large in the later collection of hymns known as the *Atharva Veda*. Most of the hymns of this text are in fact spells, intended to achieve such aims as success in trade, longevity, skill in debate, satisfaction in love, and the curing of disease. These show that it was generally believed that illness was caused by evil spirits, who could be expelled by the utterance of the right formulae by qualified practitioners, often aided by the administration of herbal remedies and other treatments.

At this stage in the evolution of Indian medicine, the *bhiṣaj* was evidently already developing away from the witch-doctor, thaumaturge, and magician, and was in the process of becoming a true physician. He was already a professional man of considerable repute in his society, and gained a competent living from his services to the sick and injured.

THE EVOLUTION OF THE CLASSICAL SYSTEM—TEXTS

In the centuries succeeding the compilation of the *Atharva Veda*—that is, the last five or six centuries before Christ—the traditional Indian medical system evolved into something like its surviving form. Its development can be traced rather inadequately from passing references in the many texts, Hindu, Buddhist, and Jain, composed during that period. Simultaneously, legends and traditions arose among the class of healers, which gave dignity to their profession by connecting them with the gods and divine sages of the mythical past.

During the same period there evolved the strict system of socio-religious taboos controlling the contacts and dietary habits of the Hindus. It is hardly likely that any consciousness of promoting health or avoiding disease was involved in these rules, but it is surprising how many of the instructions in the texts would tend to minimize the dangers of infection and food poisoning. Indian society seems unconsciously to have found a means of remaining healthy as far as possible in a subtropical climate, in its efforts to preserve its ritual purity (Chattopadhyay 1967,1968b, and 1969).

The archetypal physician was the divine sage (*ṛṣi*) Dhanvantari, later looked on as the ancestor of the *vaidya* caste (Mukhopadhyaya 1926: i.312–315). His origin was miraculous, for when the cosmic ocean was churned by the gods and demons to save the world from destruction, he was one of the fourteen precious things produced from the flood. He appeared last of all, bearing in his hands the bowl of *amṛta*, the wonderful potion which conferred immortality upon the gods (Mukhopadhyaya 1926:ii.315–316; Zimmer 1948:36–37). This legend seems to be a comparatively late one, for the earlier medical texts do not refer to it.

A line of sages was believed to have carried the original lore of the *āyurveda*, in various recensions, down to historical times. The traditions about the transmission of medical learning vary from text to text. Numerous sages are mentioned, and in particular the founders of six schools of medicine, all disciples of the sage Punarvasu Ātreya. Of these schools, four have left no trace in literature. That of Bhela survives in one rather jejune manuscript. All other existing texts belong in theory to the school of Agnivesa (Zimmer 1948:48–49). Perhaps we are justified in questioning whether the six schools really existed, for the number may have been artificially made up in order to match the six orthodox schools of Hindu philosophy. But no doubt these traditions do represent the steady development of Indian medicine as knowledge was transmitted, modified, and amplified from one generation of teachers to another. Some of the names mentioned may well be those of actual teachers in the first millennium B.C.

The science of medicine became known as *āyurveda*, "the science of (living to a ripe) age." The term is significant from the semantic point of view, since its first component (*āyur*) implies that the ancient Indian doctor was concerned not only with curing disease but also with promoting positive health and longevity, while the second (*veda*) has religious overtones, being the term used for the most sacred texts of Hinduism. The seventh-century Chinese traveler Hsüan Tsang mistakenly believed that *āyurveda* was one of the four Vedas (Beal 1957:136). *Āyurveda* was in fact linked with sacred lore as an *upāṅga* or secondary science associated with the *Atharva Veda* (*Su.*:i.i.6). It was traditionally divided into eight branches, which, in Caraka's classification, may be paraphrased as: (1) general principles of medicine (*sūtra-sthāna*), (2) pathology (*nidāna-sthāna*), (3) diagnostics (*vimāna-sthāna*), (4) physiology and anatomy (*śarīra-sthāna*), (5) prognosis (*indriya-sthāna*), (6) therapeutics (*cikitsā–sthāna*), (7) pharmaceutics (*kalpa-sthāna*), and (8) means of assuring success in treatment (*siddhi-sthāna*). Several later medical texts are divided into eight sections according to this scheme, but others include sections on surgery and other topics.

The dating of the existing texts is vague. According to a tradition preserved by Chinese sources (Jolly 1901:11), Caraka, the author of the earliest surviving Sanskrit medical manual, was contemporary with the Kusāna king Kaniska, who ruled at the end of the first century A.D. or in the first half of the second century. An early Arabic medical compendium, Abul Ḥasan ʿAlī bin Rabbāni Tabarī's *Firdaus al-Ḥikmat*, compiled in A.D. 856, mentions the texts of Caraka, Suśruta, Mādhava, and Vāgbhaṭa (Askari, 1957:8). Thus the four chief classical medical texts were in circulation and were known beyond India by the ninth century. A medical manuscript in fourth-century characters discovered in Chinese Turkestan in 1890, known as the Bower Manuscript, indicates that the science was well developed at the time of its composition (Zimmer 1948:51). Internal and other evidence suggests that of the four texts mentioned by Tabarī, Caraka is the oldest, and the chronological order of the others may be Suśruta, Vāgbhaṭa, Mādhava. Indian medicine thus reached its classical form in the early centuries of the Christian era, the period crowned by the dynasty of the imperial Guptas, when the level of Indian culture was at its highest.

The authenticity of these documents is not beyond suspicion. According to the text itself (*Caraka*:viii.12,37–39), part of the original version of the *Caraka Saṃhitā* was lost, and was restored by a Kashmiri named Dṛḍhabala, who added seventeen chapters to the sixth section and the whole of the eighth section as well as editing what remained of the original text. It is clearly a compilation in which much disconnected material has been brought together with little alteration (Zimmer 1948:52–53). The *Suśruta Saṃhitā* is noteworthy for its full treatment of surgery, which is virtually ignored by Caraka. Its origins are obscure, and it has links with the Bower Manuscript. Its author (whose name is unusual and may be a kind of title, since it means merely "famous") is referred to occasionally in other medical texts, but not in the context of surgery (Müller 1951:19–21). Vāgbhaṭa, who may be fairly safely dated in the middle of the seventh century (Vogel 1965:8–9), was a Buddhist, and his works were translated into Tibetan.

There are many later texts. As well as general compendia, specialized handbooks were composed on pharmacy, medical botany, and veterinary science, especially applied to elephants and horses. Noteworthy among medical literature is Ānandarāya's *Jīvānanda*, a seventeenth-century allegorical drama in which a host of personified diseases besiege King Jīva ("Life") in the fortress of the body; the enemy is defeated by the joint efforts of medicine, religious devotion (*bhakti*), and yoga, after many hard-fought engagements (Zimmer 1948:62–75). The later texts are marked by the introduction of new drugs such as mercury and opium, learned from the Arabs, and new diseases such as syphilis, acquired directly or indirectly from the Europeans.

PRINCIPLES OF INDIAN MEDICINE

The word *āyurveda*, discussed above, gives a clear idea of the purpose of classical Indian medicine—to prolong life. The *vaidya*'s help was called for especially in time of sickness, but his aims were not only curative but also preventive. Suśruta concisely states the purpose of his book in the first chapter: "To cure the diseases of the sick, to protect the healthy, to prolong life" (*Su.*:i.1.1; cf. *Caraka*:vi.1.4).

Thus Indian medicine was a system of so managing the whole life as to prolong it, and to preserve health and vitality as far as possible. The life and health of man were controlled partly by his *karma*, the effect of good and evil deeds done in former lives or in this life, but also by his efforts and conduct in this life. Caraka (iii.3.29–30) strongly emphasizes this, and goes on to show that health and disease are not predetermined and that life may be lengthened by human effort.

Health was believed to be conditioned by the balance of three primary fluids (*doṣas*, literally "defects") in the body: wind (*vāta*), gall (*pitta*), and mucus (*kapha*). There were five separate "breaths" or "winds" which controlled the main bodily functions. When these vital factors were operating harmoniously, the body—inhabited by the *jīva*, the vital soul, as distinct from the inmost soul, or *ātman*—enjoyed health. "Discord ... is disease, concord ... is health" (*Caraka*:i.9.4). Similar ideas concerning vital humors and vital breaths were known to classical and medieval European physicians, and it is a matter of speculation whether there was influence in one direction or another (Filliozat 1964:198–279; Kutumbiah 1962:xxxvii–xliv; Müller 1958:31–32,76–78).

Ideas of physiology were by all modern standards thoroughly inaccurate. This was probably largely due to the very strong taboo on the handling or dissection of corpses, which we refer to below. The *vaidya* of older days had no clear idea of the functions of the brain or the lungs (Zimmer 1948:161–163), and believed that consciousness resided in the heart, not in the brain. The fantastic neurology associated with *haṭha yoga*, which developed in the latter centuries of the first millennium A.D., implied some recognition that the backbone was not a mere means of holding the body upright. Knowledge of the abdominal organs was somewhat clearer than of the brain and lungs, but even in the case of these there is little evidence of direct observation.

There was, however, a clear realization that the functioning of the body was controlled by natural law, and that diseases were not normally caused by the gods or demons. Man afflicted himself (*Caraka*:ii.7.19). Man was the microcosm of the universe (*Caraka*:iv.5); and just as the universe was subject to laws of cause and effect, and functioned according to a regular rhythm, so was the case with man. The medical texts have transcended the crude superstitions of the *Atharva Veda*. Caraka and Suśruta would never have approved the popular ideas which affect the masses in many parts of India down to the present day, attributing smallpox to the visitation of a special tutelary goddess. Indian medicine had "an intuitive genius and actual command of the details of its environment," which made it more effective than other systems of antiquity (Zimmer 1948:183). That intuitive genius expressed itself particularly in efficient surgical techniques and a deep understanding of the pharmacopoeia provided by the abundant flora and fauna of India.

The concept of medicine as a means of preserving health rather than curing disease led to much emphasis on dietetics (e.g., *Su.*:i.46), and the texts contain instructions on how one should adapt oneself to the climatic changes of the Indian year. The relation of health and morals is not lost sight of. This is particularly stressed by Vāgbhaṭa, who devotes much of an important chapter to the subject. Besides pointing to diet and physical exercise (*A.H.*:i.2.9–10) as promoting health and longevity, he advocates the development of a mental attitude of unselfish affection as a potent health-giver: one should consider even worms and ants as equal to oneself, and one should be ready to help even an enemy intent on harm (*A.H.*:i.2.23–24). These moving ethical precepts, the more striking as they occur in the context of a medical manual, are no doubt inspired by Buddhism, for the introductory verse of the text shows that the author was a Buddhist.

THE *VAIDYA*

While the Vedic word *bhiṣaj* was still used in classical Sanskrit (*Su.*: i.25,31–32), the physician became increasingly known as *vaidya*. The term is derived by a common process of Sanskrit word formation from *vidyā*, "knowledge." Since the word *Veda* is also related, the term has religious overtones which *bhiṣaj* lacks. It is noteworthy that the corresponding Arabic word *hakīm* is similarly related to *ḥikmat*, also meaning "knowledge." The English "doctor" is semantically analogous, though here the emphasis is rather on the physician's giving instruction than on his acquiring it.

The term *vaidya* originally meant a learned man of any description. When the epic *Mahābhārata* states that among brahmans *vaidyas* are the best, it can only be using this word in the sense of those possessing Vedic knowledge (Dutt 1965:65–66; Kane 1946:581). By the time of Caraka, however, its special meaning was fully established. The *vaidyas* formed a recognized craft group, not yet a caste, but often following the profession of their fathers and forefathers. Vāgbhaṭa in one of his works states that his father and grandfather were both physicians (Vogel, 1965:7).

The medical profession was one which promised rich rewards, both material and spiritual. It fitted the prevailing ethical doctrine of the three aims of life: *dharma*, religious merit; *artha*, material gain; and *kāma*, personal satisfaction. By striving to relieve suffering, the *vaidya* follows *dharma*; by building up a rich practice, he achieves *artha*; and by acquiring renown for his cures, and by the satisfaction which he obtains from curing those whom he loves and respects, he serves the third end of pleasure (*Caraka*:i.30.29). The study of medicine was not the preserve of a special class, but it might be taken up by members of the three higher orders of Indian society—by the brahmans to give satisfaction (*anugraha*) to all beings; by the *kṣatriyas* (the ruling class) as part of their duty to protect their subjects; and by the *vaiśyas* (the middle class) as a means of earning a living (*Caraka*: i.30.29).

Buddhism, which encouraged the virtue of compassion and was less bound than Hinduism by considerations of ritual purity, seems to have been particularly conducive to the study of medicine. If we are to believe the tradition, the Buddha himself was interested in medicine and laid down many rules and regulations for the care and treatment of sick monks (*Vin.Mhv.*: viii.26). Indeed, it has even been suggested that the formula of the Four Noble Truths, the basic dogma of Buddhism, is based on medical precedent (Zimmer 1948:32–35). The early Theravāda school of Buddhism attempted to confine the monks to giving medical attention only to their own brethren, but this rule was not regularly observed and, with the Mahāyāna, medicine became one of the five secular sciences that the monk might study, and Indian medical knowledge was taken by Buddhist monks wherever they went (Demiéville 1937:226–227,240ff.).

Interesting in this context is the reference in Strabo (xv.60), based on Megasthenes (c. 300 B.C.). We are told that the highest of the seven classes of India, that of the philosophers, is divided into two sections, the *Brachmanes* and the *Garmanes* (Majumdar 1960:273–275). The identity of the first section is obvious. The latter is clearly an error for *Sarmanes*, equivalent to Sanskrit *śramaṇa*, and implying ascetics, especially unorthodox ascetics. The Garmanes are divided into several subgroups, the most honored of which are the *Hylobii*, who are forest hermits. Next in repute after these are physicians. These are frugal in their habits, and do not live in the open. They subsist by alms and begging. They are skilled in rites to produce offspring and they cure diseases, mostly by dietary methods. They have effective ointments and poultices, but their other remedies have much in them that is bad. They practice forms of penance, such as remaining in the same posture for long periods. The passage has been taken as applying to medical men generally (Dutt, 1931:292–293; Chattopadhyay 1968a:26), but it cannot refer to professional physicians, who were in no sense ascetics and certainly did not go begging for their food. It probably implies that even in Mauryan times Buddhist monks were obtaining a reputation for their medical and magical lore.

Later, Strabo (xv.70; Majumdar 1960:281) refers to the *Pramnae*, also different from the Brachmanes. This word seems also to be another corruption of the Sanskrit *śramaṇa*, since one group of Pramnae habitually go naked. As well as these Naked Pramnae, there are also Mountain Pramnae and City Pramnae. The last wear linen garments and live in the towns. The Mountain Pramnae wear deerskins and carry about with them bags of roots and drugs, with which they pretend to cure the sick, also making use of sorcery, spells, and amulets for the same purpose. These skin-clad wanderers can hardly be *vaidyas*, far less yellow-robed Buddhist monks. Can this refer to a class of non-Aryan hillmen who made a living as itinerant quacks among the more civilized plainsfolk?

The instructions of the textbooks can only be taken as normative, and not as having been universally applied. There is sufficient evidence to show that the many untrained quacks and charlatans, such as exist today in India, had their ancient counterparts in large numbers. Nevertheless, the norms established by the texts are so strict that one cannot believe that they had no effect on the standards of medical practice.

The training of the *vaidya* was analogous to that of the brahman religious student. He lived in the home of his teacher (*guru*) as a junior member of the family, and an intimate personal relationship was established, "a kind of magical union through which the master and pupil become one" (Zimmer 1948:76).

The student might be a member of any of the three higher orders of society (*Su*:i.2.3). Thus *vaidyas* did not form a caste. Some manuscripts of Suśruta would also admit members of the lowest of the four classes, the *śūdras*, who might be taught informally, without the solemn initiation ceremony undergone by students of the higher classes (Acharya 1945:7,fn.3), but the *vaidya* was normally a man of respectable parentage.

The initiation ceremony, performed on the student's embarking on his course of training, was a most solemn one. It was called *upanayana*, the same word as was used for the initation rite of a brahman religious student, and it involved the *guru* leading his student three times around the sacred fire, reminiscent of the similar rite in the Hindu marriage ceremony. Thus the young medical student was linked with his teacher by a supernatural and eternal bond. After this ceremony the student was thrice-born (*trija*), and this distinguished him from the ordinary man of respectable class, who was only twice-born (*dvija*) (*Caraka*:i.4.52–53).

The most impressive part of the initiation ceremony is the solemn address given by the *guru* to his student at its close. This seems more appropriate to the student's graduating than to the commencement of his studies, since it contains precepts of medical ethics reminiscent of the oath of Hippocrates. According to Caraka, the *guru* first directs the student to live a life of chastity, honesty, and vegetarianism during his studentship. He must not carry weapons, and he must be wholly subordinate and obedient to his master, unless instructed to commit major sins. He should pray every morning and night for the welfare of all beings. When he becomes a practicing *vaidya* he should strive with all his being for the health of the sick. He should not betray his patients for his own advantage. He should not have intercourse with other men's wives. He should dress modestly and avoid strong drink. He should be collected and self-controlled, measured in speech at all times.

He should constantly strive to improve his knowledge and technical skill. He should refuse to treat the king's enemies, evil-doers, loose women, and those who are obviously moribund. In the home of a patient he should be courteous and modest and should direct all his attention to the patient's welfare. He should not divulge any knowledge he may acquire concerning the patient or his family. If he knows that the patient is incurable, he should keep this fact to himself if it would cause any harm to the patient or others (*Caraka*: iii.8).

A similar address to the initiate is given by Suśruta. Here the student is told that he must always wear an ochre (*kaśāya*) robe, thus approximating him to the member of a religious order. This text adds an oath to be taken by the teacher: "If you behave well and I fail to care for you, may I participate in (the fruits of) sin and may my learning be to no avail" (*Su.*: i.2.6–7).

The training given by the *guru* was largely based on the treatise of the school to which he belonged. As with the study of the Veda, the pupil would repeat after the master passages from the text over and over again, until he had learned the whole work by heart. No outsiders were allowed to listen, lest the lore fall on unworthy ears—similar secrecy was observed in the imparting of Vedic learning (*Su.*: i.3.54). It was recognized that rote learning was not enough, however. The teacher would explain and elucidate the text as he taught it, and would introduce material from other texts from time to time, for "one *śāstra* cannot supersede all others" (*Su.*: i.4.5–6). The student was also given practical training in the use of surgical instruments, by practicing on gourds and similar objects (*Su.*: iii.9.3–6). He was tested throughout his course by oral examinations, and was given a final *viva voce* at the end of it (*Caraka*: iii.8.80–82).

The normal length of the *vaidya*'s training is not stated in the texts, but Jīvaka, a physician famous in Buddhist legend, is said to have studied for seven years under a famous medical teacher, Ātreya, of the city of Taxila in the remote northwest, and then only to have been allowed to leave reluctantly. Though we may not believe it as historical fact, the final test said to have been given by Ātreya to Jivaka is interesting for the light it throws on ancient Indian attitudes. Jīvaka was told by Ātreya to search for a *yojana* (about eight miles) on all sides of the city, and bring him specimens of any plants he could find which were of no use whatever in medicine. After some days, Jīvaka returned to his master's home with nothing in his hands. He was then allowed to go (*Vin.Mhv.*: viii.1.5–7; Keswani 1970:341).

The *vaidya*'s training did not end when he left his master. Caraka recognizes three sources of medical knowledge: instruction from an authoritative teacher (*āptopadeśa*), direct observation (*pratyakṣa*), and inference (*anumāna*). With a basis of authoritative instruction, the *vaidya* should continue to improve his knowledge by the study of his patients (*Caraka*: vi.4.5). Indian medical texts do not contain case histories of individual patients, or records of remarkable cures, but no doubt these were the subjects of discussions at the medical colloquia referred to by Caraka as among the most valuable means of widening the *vaidya*'s knowledge. As with philosophers and theologians, such gatherings (*sambhāṣā*) appear to have been regular features of the *vaidya*'s life. They were means of exchanging knowledge, and moreover in the heat of debate a *vaidya* might inadvertently disclose medical secrets not to be found in the textbooks, which he had learned orally from his teacher (*Caraka*:iii.8.15–18; cf. ii.32.72–85). Some texts advise the *vaidya* to gain knowledge of unusual herbal remedies from hillmen, herdsmen, and forest-dwelling hermits (*Su.*:i.36.10; *Dhanv.*:i.6–7).

A NOTE ON SURGERY AND DISSECTION

Sources of pre-Christian date, such as the *Rāmāyaṇa*, mention remarkable feats of surgery as having taken place in the legendary past. Thus we have reference to the transplantation of an eyeball (*Rām.*: ii.12.5); on another occasion the god Indra, rendered impotent by a curse, was cured by the transplantation of a ram's testes (*Rām.*:i.48.6–10). The semi-legendary Jīvaka, the famous physician of Buddha's day, is also reported to have performed remarkable cures involving deep surgery (*Vin.Mhv.*:viii,4–5). The best the Indian surgeons could do in internal surgery was the removal of calculi from the bladder; the replacement of bowels exposed as a result of a wound, stitching the stomach wall; and Caesarean section in the case of mothers who died before giving birth. They were brilliant, however, at external operations, and their achievements in plastic surgery were unrivaled anywhere in the world until the eighteenth century, when the Indian art of rhinoplasty was studied by European surgeons (Kutumbiah 1962:167–170; Müller 1958:42–49).

Yet the earliest Indian medical text, that of Caraka, does not mention surgical operations at all. Evidently, from the point of view of the compiler, surgery was an aspect of medicine beneath the notice of the *vaidya*, to be performed by low-caste persons such as barbers. The *Suśruta Saṃhitā*, however, devotes much space to the subject. From the point of view of the medical texts, the *vaidya* might incur what for other men of good caste would be grave ritual pollution. He might be compelled in his professional capacity to enter the homes of men of much lower caste than he, to touch the excreta of such people, and even to sip a few drops of their urine for diagnostic purposes. The texts do not apparently envisage purificatory ceremonies to expunge such impurity, and evidently the *vaidyas* generally took religious taboos quite lightly. As part of the student's training, it was not considered improper for him to practice dentistry by extracting the teeth of dead animals, or to gain command of the scalpel by trying to make an incision in an animal's inflated bladder without cutting through it and releasing the air (*Su.*:i.9).

The taboo on contact with human corpses was so strong, however, that even the emancipated *vaidya* dared not infringe it. The practice of dissection of corpses "had to fight against all the rules of archaic hygiene" (Zimmer 1948:175), and, against a taboo based essentially on many generations of practical experience, it could not win. Suśruta did the best he could to train his apprentices, by placing a new corpse in a basket in a running river for a week. Thus, if we are to believe the textbook, the flesh disintegrates so that it may be removed by scrubbing with a long, stiff brush to expose the intestines, which may thus be studied without physical contact (*Su*:iii.5.49). This method may have been followed in practice, because the texts show more accurate knowledge of the lower viscera than of the brain and lungs, which are covered by bones and would not be rendered visible by such treatment.

This is as far as the *vaidya* dared to go in the study of anatomy. No doubt he supplemented his knowledge by examining the bodies of those accidentally or judicially killed, as well as corpses on the battlefield. It would have been theoretically possible for him to hire the untouchables who served as executioners and cremation attendants to dissect corpses for him, but we have no record of this being done. Nevertheless there are accounts, all from texts of the earlier period, which show that the dissection of a corpse was not wholly unknown.

The *Arthaśāstra* ascribed to Kauṭilya, in its section on the detection and punishment of serious crime, recommends that the bodies of those dying in suspicious circumstances should be preserved in oil for examination as to the cause of death, and refers to the examination of the contents of the stomach for traces of poison (*Arth.*:iv.7.1.13; Mukhopadhyaya 1926:ii.363).

A remarkable story concerning the emperor Aśoka, occurs in a collection of Buddhist legends which exists in both Sanskrit and Chinese versions. We are told that Aśoka in his later years took a young wife, Tiṣyarakṣitā, who made amorous advances to the crown prince Kuṇāla, who indignantly rejected her, though he did not report his stepmother's evil conduct to his father. Soon after this, Aśoka was taken seriously ill with a rare disease involving the most unpleasant symptoms. Tiṣyarakṣitā feared that if he died Kuṇāla would come to the throne and punish her for her immoral behavior, and so she decided to restore Aśoka to health at all costs. She told him that if he would grant her whatever boon she desired she would cure him, and he put himself entirely in her hands. She ordered a search to be made for a sick man with exactly the same symptoms as the king. When one was found he was brought to her in her private apartments, and she killed him on the spot. She cut open his stomach and found that it contained an enormous worm. She treated the worm with strong and pungent substances such as pepper and ginger, but it was unaffected. At last she tried onions, and these killed it. So she fed Aśoka with large quantities of onions, which for obvious reasons are not normally eaten by high-caste people. He eliminated the dead worm, and was cured (*Divy.*:408–409; Przyluski 1923:285). This story, incredible though it may be, surely indicates that in some circles at least the idea of dissection for medical purposes was not wholly unknown.

Moreover, the drastic means used by the wicked queen to discover the cause and cure of the king's illness indicates that ideas prefiguring modern scientific methods of investigation and experiment were at work.

Nevertheless, the ineluctable taboo on contact with the dead prevented the development of anatomical knowledge, and it was not until 1835 that a *vaidya* strongly influenced by western ideas, Paṇḍit Madhusūdan Gupta, had the temerity to dissect a corpse (Keswani 1970:357). The complete ignorance and uncertainty of even the best-educated Indians of earlier times about the nature and functions of the various organs of the body is hard to realize nowadays. The interior of the body was almost as mysterious as the center of the earth, which was the realm of wonderful snake-spirits, *nāgas*, who dwelled in cavernous realms lighted by precious stones of unimaginable radiance. The body too contained a mysterious serpent power, *kuṇḍalinī*, which could be raised by yoga from its seat at the base of the spine to pass through the vein *suṣumṇa* in the spinal cord, progressing through the six centers of force (*cakra*) to the topmost *sahasrāra*, when the adept achieved highest bliss and immeasurable supernatural power.

The fantastic doctrines of later yoga were questioned in the latter part of the nineteenth century by a young ascetic, Dayānand Sarasvatī, who once on his wanderings came upon a corpse floating on a river, and decided to cut it open to examine the *cakras*. He found that they did not exist (Farquhar 1915:106); and as a result of this and other practical experiments he founded a reformed Hindu sect, the Ārya Samāj. Nevertheless, the practitioners of *haṭha yoga*, in India and elsewhere, still teach the reality of *kuṇḍalinī*, *suṣumṇa*, the *cakras*, and *sahasrāra*, though the more sophisticated claim that they are psychic entities, not made of solid matter.

THE *VAIDYA* IN PRACTICE

The qualified medical practitioner, as depicted by Suśruta, must have been an impressive sight as he went on his rounds in the ancient Indian city. Attended by an assistant, who no doubt carried his bag of surgical instruments for him (Jain 1947:179), and followed by a servant bearing a parasol; clad in white raiment, shod in sandals, a staff in his hand, "with a calm mind, speaking pleasantly, . . . the friend of all beings," he went from house to house on his rounds (*Su.*:i.10.3). In the homes of his patients he would be treated very courteously, and invited to a hot bath after his work was done (Jain 1947:179). The ideal *vaidya* was able to instill such confidence in his patients that they trusted him as fully as they trusted their parents and kinsfolk, and he cared for them as he would care for his own sons (*Su.*:i.25. 43–44).

Like the modern general practitioner, he would also see his patients in his own home (Jain 1947:179), where he had a storeroom filled with drugs and medical equipment (*Su.*:i.36.17). With the aid of his assistant he compounded his own drugs from herbs and other ingredients which he often collected himself. These were likely to be more efficacious than those obtained indirectly, for he could be sure that they were unadulterated and were collected at auspicious times, with the utterance of the correct *mantras*, and in a state of ritual purity (Zimmer 1948:105–106).

The pharmacopoeia of the *vaidya* was a very large one. Suśruta alone mentions over 700 medicinal herbs (Jolly 1901:25), and the number increased as time went on, with the introduction of drugs from western and central Asia. Particularly noted for medicinal herbs were the Himalayas, the home of the god Śiva, the lord of *vaidyas*, and of Soma, the king of plants, from which the narcotic beverage drunk by the brahmans at sacrifices was produced. Though not mentioned directly, there must have been a considerable trade in drugs from the mountains to the plains, and also from the humid tropical hills of the peninsula, where many herbs grew which would not thrive in the drier north, with its cool winters. In his prescriptions the *vaidya* was not bound by the usual taboos of upper-class Indians. He used animal products freely in compounding his drugs, and might recommend a meat diet in certain cases. Moreover, he was ready to prescribe alcoholic drinks, though he disapproved of intoxication (*Su.*:i.45.170–216).

The *vaidya* was not forbidden to advertise his skill. Jīvaka, the great physician of Buddhist legend, came to the city of Sāketa and walked through the streets saying "Who is ill here? Whom shall I cure?" He healed a rich merchant's wife who seemed to have an incurable malady, and he became a rich man overnight (*Vin.Mhv.*:viii.1.8–13). It appears from Caraka that fashionably dressed quacks would walk the streets in the hope of finding patients. "Immediately on hearing that someone is ill, they swoop down on him from all quarters and in his hearing speak loudly of their medical attainments. If a doctor is already in attendance ... they make mention of his failings. ... When they realize that the patient is at death's door, they make themselves scarce and seek another neighborhood" (*Caraka*:i.29.9). References to such charlatans occur in other contexts, and they were probably numerous (*Caraka*:i.1.128–132, i.9.16–17; *Su.*:i.25.31–32).

An interesting satirical passage on the *vaidya* is to be found in Kṣemendra's *Narmamālā* (ii.68–81, Kaul (ed.) 1924:20–21), a humorous poem from eleventh-century Kashmir. Here a *vaidya* is called in at short notice to attend to the wife of a petty official, who is feigning illness in order to escape her husband's attentions, which have become distasteful to her since she took a lover. He comes to the home of the official "after having quickly gone the rounds of a hundred houses," perspiring and panting. He wears a shabby ill-fitting garment, stained by his medicines.[1] He sits beside his patient,

---

1 Paṇḍit Madhusūdan Kaul, who edited the text, paraphrases the line "*vahann auṣadhasaṅketanām asaṃyogacīrikām*" as "he carries a bundle of prescriptions" (Kaul 1924:17). The passage is obscure, but we think "wearing an ill-fitting (ragged) cloth (*cīrikā*), indicative of (his medicinal) herbs," is more probable.

touches her breasts, and quickly gives his diagnosis and instructions: "She can't stand either fasting or overeating, ... but in my opinion she may eat everything. ... Her mind is dulled and her constitution is out of order. Give her first of all some smooth curd with sugar."[2] The *vaidya* then quickly goes away.

Kṣemendra's description of the *vaidya* portrays a dangerous quack, interested only in making money out of his patients. On occasions such as city festivals, pilgrimages, and weddings he is very happy, because he anticipates large profits from patients with stomach complaints due to overeating. He makes a habit of touching those parts of the bodies of his women patients which are normally kept covered. Numerous other uncomplimentary remarks are leveled at the *vaidya*, but none are very specific. He is compared to a beast of prey and a vampire. He is like a fierce wind, destroying the life of man. With the touch of his hand he wipes away all that is pure.[3] The description is qualified, however, in a verse which sums up the poet's thoughts on the subject: "*Vaidyas* devoid of learning, *kāyasthas* (clerks and minor government officials) ambitions for power, and *gurus* (religious preceptors) with corrupt morals cause the ruin of the people." The text is satirical and need not be taken too seriously.

Many passages in our sources indicate that the *vaidya* expected adequate rewards for his services, though the fabulously large fees said to have been received by Jīvaka are hardly typical. The *vaidya* might treat learned brahmans, ascetics, the poor and orphans free (*Su*:i.2.8; cf. iv.11.12–13), but we read of Jain monks being treated by a doctor who demanded a large fee which they could only raise with great difficulty (Jain 1947: 199).

The *vaidya* was assisted by trained nurses, normally referred to in the masculine (*paricāraka*). Nursing appears to have been a definite profession or trade and not merely a task performed by any domestic servant. Suśruta describes the ideal qualities of the nurse; who should be devoted and friendly, untiringly watchful, not inclined to disgust, and knowledgeable enough to fulfil the orders of the doctor (*Su*.:i.34.24; Zimmer 1948:93).

THE *VAIDYA* AND THE KING

The highest ambition of the more enterprising *vaidyas* must have been to enter the king's service. There may have been many physcians at the larger courts, attending on the enormous royal family with its innumerable courtiers and palace servants. These would form a hierarchy under the king's personal *vaidya*, who is placed by Suśruta almost on a par with the king's family priest

2 This translation differs somewhat from Kaul's (1924:18), which is an expanded paraphrase. The phrases "placed on a spit" (*hitaṃ śūle*), agreeing with "overeating" and "with me" (*mayā saha*), after "eat everything" do not make good sense, and we suspect that the text is corrupt.

3 We amend Kaul's text, *trimalakṣālaka*, to *vimalakṣālaka*, since the former, "wiping away the three impurities," is not in keeping with the tenor of the verse. Kaul (1924:17) finds a reference here to feeling the pulse, but this is unjustified.

(*purohita*), who was a very eminent personage indeed. The *purohita* and the *vaidya* would accompany the king on all his travels, and stand by him in all circumstances, for they were equally responsible for his protection—one guarding his soul and the other his body. As *āyurveda* is subsidiary to the four original Vedas, so the *vaidya* should yield to the *purohita* in matters where there were differences of opinion, but he obviously stood very high in the palace hierarchy (*Su.*:i.37.7–8).

The royal physician was not called in only when the king felt sick, but was constantly in attendance to promote his health, longevity, and virility. One of his main functions was the supervision of the royal kitchen. In this he had two ends in view—to ensure that the king had a health-giving diet, and to detect and prevent attempts at poisoning him (*Su.*:v.1.8–24). Such attempts appear to have been very common (*Arth.*:i.21). It is noteworthy that Cakradatta, the author of an important medical text of the twelfth century, the *Cikitsāsārasaṃgraha*, was the son of the kitchen superintendent of an eastern Indian king (Jolly 1901:6).

There were thus risks in the profession of the royal physician, even though the food of the king might be tasted by lesser royal servants under his supervision. Unexpected illnesses in the royal entourage would bring him under suspicion, and failure to effect cures might be fatal to the doctor himself. A Jain story tells of a physician who did not give a sick queen the proper treatment, and who was promptly put to death by the king (Jain 1947:179).

Another Jain account tells of a palace physician who became addicted to gambling and neglected his profession. His textbooks were lost and his surgical instruments became rusty, and his master at last dismissed him (Jain 1947:179). He represents another aspect of the palace life of the times, the easy-going parasitical minor courtier, who made a good living by doing nothing.

In war the *vaidya*'s services were much in demand. The king's personal physician accompanied him everywhere on campaign, and there was work for many lesser doctors with the army. There is no evidence that every ancient Indian kingdom organized an efficient army medical service, but the texts at least recommend this. The early *Arthaśāstra*, probably referring to conditions in the Mauryan period (third century B.C.), advises the king to organize a corps of healers (the word used, *cikitsaka*, may possibly connote a somewhat less qualified practitioner than *vaidya* or *bhiṣaj*), who should be in attendance in the rear of the army, equipped with surgical instruments, medicines, ointments, and bandages (*Arth.*:x.3.47). Physicians attached to the army are mentioned in the epic (*Rām.*:ii.77.14), and Suśruta recognizes the army doctor, whose quarters on campaign should be marked with a special flag, so that the wounded could easily find him (*Su.*:i.34.12–14).

MEDICINE AS A PUBLIC SERVICE

A phrase of uncertain meaning in Suśruta, stating that the *vaidya* should be "sanctioned by the king" (*rājānujñāta*), suggests that a system of licensing was known in early India (*Su.*:i.10.3). This at least is the explanation of the twelfth-century commentator Dalhana, who interprets it as a measure to prevent quackery (Jolly 1901:21). Further evidence that Suśruta envisaged some form of government control of the medical profession is contained in a statement that the quack doctor (*kuvaidya*) kills people out of greed, "because of the fault of the king" (*nṛpadoṣataḥ*), suggesting that the government has been negligent or corrupt in licensing poorly qualified practitioners (*Su.*:i.3.52). Other sources, however, say nothing about such licenses, and they may have been a special feature of the Gupta period (c. A.D. 320–550), during which the *Suśruta Saṃhitā* was probably compiled. The same text suggests that positively draconian measures were taken against the incompetent doctor, who was liable to be put to death by the king (*vadham carcchati rājataḥ*) (*Su.*:i.3.49).

This stern punishment is not advocated by legal texts, a few references in which show that the court took cognizance of the incompetent physician, but treated him more leniently. The *Arthaśāstra* prescribes a fine if a patient dies while receiving medical attention and the authorities are not informed, and a heavier one if his death is brought about by neglect or inadequate medical knowledge on the part of the doctor. A lesser fine is prescribed for permanent injury caused by bad treatment (*Arth.*:iv.1). The lawbook of Yājñavalkya, approximately contemporary with Suśruta, declares that a qualified and competent doctor incurs no guilt if his patient dies, but a quack in such cases should be punished (Kane 1946:19).

The *Arthaśāstra*, permeated with a spirit of centralized totalitarian bureaucracy very different from that of later Indian statecraft, declares that the physician should report to the local authorities all patients with suspicious wounds or apparently behaving strangely; otherwise, if such patients are convicted of crime, the physician should be treated as an accessory and should be liable to the same punishment as his patient (*Arth.*:ii.36). This prescription is not consistent with the lofty ethics of the medical texts, and it is perhaps from considerations such as these that the *guru* in Caraka advises his students not to treat patients "who hate the king or are hated by him" (*Caraka*:iii.8.13).

The government's interest in the health of the people was encouraged by the political ethic of Hinduism, according to which the main function of the king was the "protection" of his subjects. This function was not taken as the mere protection of life and property from internal and external enemies, but was interpreted in a positive sense. Indeed, Caraka declares that medicine should be studied and promoted by princes "for the purpose of protection" (*ārakṣārtham*) (*Caraka*:i.30.29). It is clear from a comparable passage in the Kāśyapa Saṃhitā, a later text owing much to Caraka, that the king is here advised to protect his subjects, not himself (Mehta et al. 1949:i.136). In fact we find considerable evidence of medical care provided free for the poorer people as a service or act of charity by kings and wealthy people.

HOSPITALS

It seems an article of faith among many scholars that ancient India was liberally endowed with free hospitals. Certainly a few sources do refer to institutions to which the sick went for treatment and where they apparently remained until they were cured, but the medical texts themselves are silent about them.

Many of the passages confidently taken to prove the existence of numerous hospitals are ambiguous and probably mean nothing of the kind. The *Artha-śāstra*, for instance, recommends that the king plan his capital city so that the *bhaiṣajya-gṛhas* are in the northwestern quarter (*Arth.*: ii.4). The term *bhaiṣajya* may mean "medical treatment" but it may also simply mean "a drug," and *gṛha* (house) does not suggest a very large building. In Suśruta, a similar term, *bheṣajāgāra* (*Su.*: i.36.17), clearly means the storeroom for herbs and drugs in the home of the *vaidya*, and the establishments referred to in the *Arthaśāstra* may have been only apothecaries' shops or dispensaries.

In the second pillar edict of Aśoka, the emperor states that he has provided *cikisā* for men and animals. Relying on references in later sources and on the Jain animal hospitals of western India much commented on by later European travelers, Bühler interpreted this as meaning that Aśoka established hospitals widely throughout his empire (Bühler 1883: 101), and later scholars have generally accepted this interpretation. The word *cikisā* (Sanskrit *cikitsā*) can only mean "healing," "cure," and is no evidence that in Aśoka's reign there was a fully developed hospital service. Nevertheless, this benevolent emperor may have done much to promote the health of his people, for in the same edict he claims not only to have brought healing to man and beast, but also to have caused medicinal herbs to be cultivated where they were not grown before.

The Jain scriptures contain several references to *tigicchaya-sālās*, and these may be interpreted as hospitals. *Sālā* suggests a larger building than *gṛha*, and we read of one such establishment with a hundred pillars and employing a number of doctors (Jain 1947: 179). *Tigicchaya-sālā* is the Prākrit equivalent of Sanskrit *cikitsakaśālā* ("hall of healers"), and more likely indicates a hospital in the real sense of the term than does the *bhaiṣajyagṛha* of the *Artha-śāstra*. The same is true of the *ārogyaśālās* ("halls of health") mentioned by the twelfth-century jurist Hemādri as worthy means of gaining merit by donating funds for their endowment (Bühler 1883: 101). The same word was used for the Khmer hospitals, which we mention below. But we must remember that in the India of recent times what is advertised as a "medical hall" is usually no more than a small chemist's shop.

A hospital in the true sense of the term is clearly described by Fa-hsien, the Chinese traveler who visited India at the very beginning of the fifth century A.D., when the Gupta empire was at its zenith. At Pāṭaliputra, the modern Patna, the pilgrim saw hospitals staffed by physicians, where the poor and sick received free treatment and were housed, fed, and cared for until they recovered. He specifically states that these establishments were endowed not by the state, but by wealthy private benefactors (Beal 1957:35). The fact that he mentions such hospitals only at Pāṭaliputra, and makes no reference to similar institutions in the numerous other cities which he visited, suggests that at that time they were rare.

The most famous of the Chinese travelers, Hsüan Tsang, does not mention hospitals. He does mention, however, the erection by king Harṣavardhana of rest houses along the highways, where food and drink were given to travelers and where there were stationed "physicians with medicines for travelers lers and poor persons round about, to be given without any stint" (Beal 1957:239).[4] We must be prepared for exaggerations in Hsüan Tsang's statements. The same passage speaks of Harṣa's 60,000 war elephants (an impossible number) and his forbidding the slaughter of animals and sale of meat "on pain of death without pardon," which seems intrinsically very unlikely. But we may be sure from this that the great emperor made some provision of medical aid to the poor and to travelers.

Numerous South Indian inscriptions refer to the endowment of medical establishments, usually attached to the larger temples (Sastri 1955:450,513, 623; Reddy 1941:passim). At at least one of these, in A.D. 1121, there was founded a school of medicine where students learned the works of Caraka and Vāgbhaṭa (Sastri 1955:632). Earlier, in the North, medicine was taught at the great Buddhist monastic university of Nālandā, and at other monasteries also (Beal 1911:112). But it was apparently in South India, especially under the benevolent Cola dynasty (ninth–twelfth centuries), that early Indian kings made the most sustained efforts at bringing medical care to their subjects.

Another impressive example of royal solicitude for the health of the populace is found in the *Ceylon Chronicle*, in its account of the benevolent fourth-century king Buddhadāsa. This king, a very pious Buddhist, had been trained in medicine and was himself the author of a medical digest. Wherever he went he carried surgical instruments and other equipment with him, and whenever he saw a sick or injured subject he treated him on the spot. Being a Buddhist, he cared little for the rules of ritual purity, and was not too proud to treat even untouchables and animals. He established a *vejjasālā* (Sanskrit *vaidyaśālā*, "hall of physicians," possibly a hospital), and appointed resident physicians for every ten villages, assigning lands for their upkeep. He also maintained horse and elephant doctors, and opened asylums (*sālā*) for the crippled and blind (*Cūlav.*:xxxvii.105–148; Zimmer 1948:87). No later kings of Ceylon are referred to as having done so much for the health of their subjects, but we cannot believe that his example was not sometimes followed.

4 In a footnote the translator points to a textual ambiguity which may mean either "doctors' medicines" or "physicians and medicines." The latter interpretation seems intrinsically more likely.

Our sources give us no clear indication of the organization of these medical establishments, whether hospitals or dispensaries, but the evidence is sufficient to show that the better rulers of early India, together with private bene-factors, did what they could to promote the health of the people. The provision of public medicine probably deteriorated in later times. Fryer, a seventeenth-century English traveler, notices the animal hospitals of western India, but little else in the way of public health services. "They have hospitals here for cows," he writes, "and are charitable to dogs, . . . being more merciful to beasts than [to] men" (Askari 1957:21).

The Indianized kingdoms of Southeast Asia, much under the influence of Mahāyāna Buddhism, may have outstripped most parts of India in the provision of medical aid. We are fortunate in having an inscription of the Khmer kingdom, now Cambodia, which gives us several details of the organi-zation of a hospital founded in 1186. There were at that time more than a hundred such establishments in the kingdom, under the guardianship of the heavenly Buddha Bhaiṣajyaguru ("Master of Healing"), who was looked on in the Mahāyāna as the special patron of medicine.

The hospital in question, at Sày-fòng on the Mekong river, had two doctors, each assisted by three nurses of both sexes, and 32 employees who lived on the premises, while 66 more lived elsewhere. The hospital was open to members of all classes, who were cared for and fed without charge, and even given clothing and other necessities three times a year. It seems, from their charitable character, and from the long periods which many of their inmates appear to have spent in them, that these establishments were homes for the aged and crippled poor as well as hospitals in the modern sense, but their very name, *ārogyaśālā*, meaning "hall of health," is evidence enough that the care of the sick was their main purpose. According to another inscription the hospi-tals established by the Khmer state used 11,192 tons of rice per year and a large quantity of drugs and medical supplies, including 3,402 nutmegs and 1,960 boxes of ointment for hemorrhoids! We are told that the great king Jayavarman VII, who developed this remarkable medical system, "felt the afflictions of his subjects more than his own, because the suffering of the people constitutes the suffering of the king, more than his own suffering" (Demiéville 1937:247; Coedès 1963:103–104).[5]

THE SOCIAL STATUS OF THE *VAIDYA*

It is clear from the medical texts that the *vaidyas* of early India were not a caste, but rather a fraternity of men drawn from various classes and castes who looked on themselves, in theory at least, as united by a common training and discipline for the high purpose of promoting human health and welfare.

5 For further details concerning the remarkable Khmer medical service see L. Finot, "L'ins-cription sanskrite de Say Fong," *Bulletin de l'école française d'extrême Orient* 3:18ff., and G. Coedès, "Les hôpitaux de Jayavarman VII," *ibid.* 40:344ff.

The *vaidya*, once he had completed his training, was not bound by a vow of celibacy, and he was encouraged to build up a rich practice. Nevertheless, his ideals had something in common with those of a religious order, and religious overtones are traceable throughout the medical texts. Like the *sannyāsī*, the religious ascetic, moreover, the *vaidya* did not adhere rigidly to the stringent rules of ritual purity which regulated the lives of the ordinary members of the higher classes. He would handle things which would normally incur pollution and even drink human urine in the course of his professional duties, apparently drawing the line only at touching and dissecting corpses. As far as the texts go, he made no attempt at defending such actions, no doubt considering that the end justified the means. In his own eyes, at least, the trained *vaidya* was ritually pure and of high status.

In the eyes of others, however, his status may not have been so clear. The texts on *dharma*, laying down the norms of conduct for Hindus of good caste, are very ambivalent in their attitude toward the *vaidya*. The lawbook of Manu, one of the oldest and most influential of its type, refers to a caste group called *ambastha* believed to be descended from brahman fathers and *vaiśya* mothers, who were specially equipped by nature for the art of healing (Manu:x.8,47). A later text, that of Parāśara, states that the function of the *ambastha* is to treat brahmans only (Dutt 1965:71). This would divide the ordinary *vaidya* from the *ambastha*, a clean caste, definitely below the brahman, but certainly well within the twice-born group. The term *ambastha* is still sometimes used in the sense of *vaidya*, but it appears that in earlier times it represented a small section of *vaidyas* who were specially favored by the orthodox brahmans.

Other *smrti* passages show that the average *vaidya* was looked down on by the brahmans, whose efforts at establishing a norm of conduct and a hierarchy of classes were increasingly successful with time. Manu, though he respects the *ambastha*, thinks ill of the *vaidya*. The latter must be avoided at mealtimes, for his very presence defiles the food (*Manu*:iii.152). The brahman should never accept food from the *vaidya* for he is just as impure as a hunter, an *ugra* ("fearsome," probably a tough bully in the service of a king or chief as a kind of irregular policeman), or a menstruating woman (*Manu*: iv.212; Jolly 1901:21). Here the motive is obvious: the *vaidya* is looked on as unclean because in the course of his duties he comes in contact with blood. A somewhat later *smrti*, that of Viṣṇu (*Viṣṇu*, 1.1.10), prescribes the penance for one who accepts food from a physician as living only on milk for seven days (Dutt 1965:67)—a very appropriate antidote, so to speak, for the blood which no ablutions can wash from the *vaidya's* hands.

Baudhāyana (ii.1.2), an earlier text, declares that the brahman who practices medicine is no better than one who becomes a professional actor or a teacher of dancing; his expiation is to live as an outcaste for two years (Dutt 1931:209; cf. Dutt 1965:66–67). A strange verse in the *Mahābhārata* mentions the *vaidya* as a caste different from the *ambastha*, being born of the hypogamous union of *śūdra* men and *vaiśya* women (Dutt 1965:70). Such miscegenation would produce offspring theoretically lower than either parent. The passage makes no reference to the profession of the *vaidya*; but there is little doubt that the brahman who inserted it in the text clearly distinguished between the *ambastha* and the *vaidya*, and thought little of the latter.

The same ambivalence in the social status of the *vaidya* has prevailed down to recent times. In Bengal, physicians have emerged as a very respectable caste with a history of several centuries during which it has gained in prestige. Technically they are pure members of the *śūdra* order, but from the mid-eighteenth century onward they have been claiming higher status, and some of them even declare that they are brahmans (Dutt 1965:72–75). Over the period from 1911 to 1931, about 50 percent of the Bengal *vaidyas* were employed in the higher professions and 54 percent were literate, while only 18 percent followed the caste's traditional occupation (Bose 1959:197).

Outside Bengal the term *vaidya* (appearing in modern languages in various forms such as *baid, bed, baijjo, vaithian*), has varying social connotations, and rarely implies a definite caste. The Nambūdiri brahmans of Kerala have six subdivisions, one of which is the *vaidiyan*, a class of physicians divided into eight clans. They are looked down on by the other Nambūdiris because they pay little attention to the study of the Vedas, but they hold a comparatively high rank in the social hierarchy (Iyer 1912:ii.175). Certain brahman groups in the region of Sagar (Madhya Pradesh) are also called *baid* (Russell 1916:i.344). In the Tamil country, where even a thousand years ago nearly every village had its *vaithiyan* who held land in service tenure (Sastri 1955:576), there is a subdivision of the low *Paraiyan* (Pariah) caste known by this title, though in fact āyurvedic physicians are often of higher caste (Thurston 1909:vii.267–270). Also in the Tamil country, there is a barber caste known as *Ambathan* (= Sanskrit *ambastha*) whose touch is polluting to brahmans. Some of them practice medicine and are more highly esteemed than the others, but all adopt the title *vaidya* (Thurston 1909:iv.449; Béteille 1965:89). In Orissa, a village *baidyo*, who claims to be a member of the warrior class, is a small landowner who effects cures as a sideline (Bailey 1957:113–114).

In the village India of recent times, the simpler aspects of medicine do not involve highly trained professionals. Bailey refers to a village headman in Orissa possessing a manuscript written by his grandfather and enlarged by his father, dealing with the local herbal medicines and their preparation (Bailey 1957:113). In South India, fractures are set by the *Kusavan*, the village potter (Thurston 1909:iv.195). In the Telugu country a low caste known as *Mandula* specializes in selling drugs, while the women practice midwifery (Thurston 1909:447). Everywhere minor operations such as extracting teeth and lancing boils are performed by the village barber (Blunt 1931:242; Thurston 1909:iv.195). Meanwhile the utter degeneration of the noble term used by Caraka and Suśruta is illustrated in Crooke's description of the *Mahāwat*, an itinerant medicine-man of western Uttar Pradesh, who attends to minor ills such as carious teeth and abscesses: "He wanders about the village calling *'Baid! Baid!* Who wants a doctor?' He is altogether rather a loathsome vagrant" (Crooke 1896:71–72).

NOTES ON ISLAMIC MEDICINE IN INDIA

Though the Muslim world learned much from India, its medical system was founded on that of Galen. Avicenna's (A.D. 980–1037) magnum opus, the *Kitāb al–Shifā'*, played a role of great importance in the development of Muslim medicine, and it was largely through the study of this great compendium of philosophy that the Muslim physician (*ṭabīb*) became known generally as a *ḥakīm* ("a learned man"). Since his system looks back to classical Europe, the Muslim *ḥakīm* in India practices *Yūnānī* (often spelled *Ūnānī*)—i.e., Greek medicine, as distinct from *āyurveda*, or a hybrid Muslim–Hindu system known as *Tibb* (Keswani 1970:354). A minor work of Albīrūnī (*Kitāb us-Sardāna*) emphasizes the differences between the two systems: "There is no people inclined so much to the sciences as the Indians. But this branch (medicine) particularly is based by them on principles which are opposite to the western rules to which we are accustomed. Moreover, the contrast between them and ourselves concerning religion, manners, and customs, and their excessive care concerning purity and uniformity, prevents intercourse and cuts short scientific discussions" (Askari 1957:10).

Albīrūnī's judgment, however, seems a little pessimistic in the light of history. Even before Islam, Indian medicine came to be known in western Asia; for Burzūya, court physician to the Persian emperor Khusrau Anūsharvān (*c.* A.D. 531), visited India, and brought back Indian medical texts and physicians who practiced at the great Persian medical school of Gundī Shāpur, which remained in existence after the Muslim conquest (Browne 1962:21). Later, at least fifteen Indian medical texts were translated into Arabic (Siddiqī 1959:40–41), and an Indian physician, Maṅka, who served in the famous hospital of the Barmecides in Baghdad, is said to have treated the Caliph Hārūn ar-Rashīd himself (Siddiqī 1959:36). The great thirteenth-century Persian doctor Rashīd ud–Dīn Faḍlu'llāh is said to have traveled at least as far as the Indus Valley, and to have brought back texts and drugs from India. At his medical school at Tabriz, doctors from India and China were employed as teachers, each having ten students (Browne 1962:103–109).

In Islam, medicine was part of the body of learning studied by the educated, and medical knowledge was widespread (Rashid 1969:165). Putting aside basic differences of theory, Islamic practice laid great stress on the study of individual cases, and Arabic medical texts contain many case histories, which are quite absent from the texts of *āyurveda*. Whether or not the Hindus had a fully developed system of hospitals, these are not mentioned in Hindu medical texts. On the other hand, they were essential aspects of the Muslim medical system, and the *tabīb* is advised to visit hospitals regularly (Browne 1962:55). Hospitals were established by both rulers and noblemen from the beginning of Muslim rule, but their endowment was looked on rather as a matter of philanthropy than as part of a ruler's administrative duties. The development of hospitals was encouraged in India by large numbers of Iranian doctors who migrated there in the reign of Akbar, and through them the number of hospitals increased in this and succeeding reigns (Askari 1957:15).

If their chroniclers can be believed, the Muslim rulers of India did more to develop medicine than their Hindu predecessors. Some of them, notably Muhammad Tughluq and Fīrūz Tughluq, were *hakīms* themselves, and many founded hospitals (Siddiqī 1959:xxvii–xxix). It is nowhere stated that unbelievers were excluded from these hospitals, but it is unlikely that Hindus of good caste would think of even entering such buildings. It is perhaps partly for this reason that we read of Hindu *vaidyas* being employed beside *hakīms* in these *bīmāristāns* (Siddiqī 1959:xxxvi; Askari 1957:19); they may have been required for the treatment of upper-caste Hindu patients who would be polluted by contact with meat-eating unbelievers. There was a full recognition on the part of the *hakīms* of the merits of the other system. The most important Muslim medical text produced in India, Miyān Bhowā's *Maʿdanu'l shifā'-Sikandarshāhī* (*The Mine of Medicine of King Sikandar*), completed in A.D. 1512 and dedicated to the Sultan of Delhi, Sikandar Lodī, fully recognized that the Yūnānī system in its pure form did not suit local conditions, because the climate was different, and many Yūnānī drugs were hardly obtainable in India. On the other hand, Indian medicine knew of many drugs equally efficacious, but not recognized in the Yūnānī system (Siddiqī 1959:99–101). The practitioners of the two systems seem to have collaborated, because each had much to learn from the other and, whatever the 'ulamā and the brahmans might say, we have no record of animosity between Hindu and Muslim in the field of medicine.

Literature Cited

Āchārya, N. R., and S. Pandurang, eds.
   1945 *Suśruta Saṃhitā*. Bombay: Nirnaya Sagar Press.
A. H.
   1965 *Vāgbhaṭas Aṣṭāngahṛdaya Saṃhitā*. See Vogel.
Arth.
   1960 *The Kauṭilīya Arthaśāstra*. R. P. Kangle, ed. Part 1, Text. Bombay: University of Bombay.
   1963 *Ibidem*. Part 2, Translation.
Askari, S. H.
   1957 "Medicines and Hospitals in Muslim India." *J. Bihar Research Society* 43:7–21. Patna.

A. V.
  1905 *Atharva Veda*. William Dwight Whitney, trans.; C. R. Lanman, ed. Cambridge: Harvard University Press.
Bailey, F. G.
  1957 *Caste and the Economic Frontier*. Manchester, Engl: Manchester University Press.
Baudhāyana
  1882 *The Sacred Laws of the Āryas as taught in the Schools of Āpastamba, Gautama, Vāsishtha and Baudhāyana*. Part 2, *Vāsishtha and Baudhāyana*. G. Bühler, trans. *Sacred Books of the East*, vol. 14. Oxford: Clarendon Press.
Beal, S., trans.
  1911 *The Life of Hiuen Tsiang by the Shaman Hwui Li*, 2nd ed. London: Kegan Paul, Trench, Trübner.
  1957 *Chinese Accounts of India*, 4 vols. Calcutta: Susil Gupta. (Indian reprint of *Si-yu-ki: Buddhist Records of the Western World*, 2 vols. London: Kegan Paul, Trench, Trübner, 1883.)
Béteille, A.
  1965 *Caste, Class, and Power*. Berkeley and Los Angeles: University of California Press.
Blunt, E. A. H.
  1931 *The Caste System of Northern India*. London: Oxford University Press.
Bose, N. K.
  1959 "Some Aspects of Caste in Bengal," in Milton Singer, ed., *Traditional India: Structure and Change*. Philadelphia: American Folklore Society.
Browne, E. G.
  1962 *Arabian Medicine*, 2nd ed. (Ist ed., 1921.) Cambridge: Cambridge University Press.
Bühler, J. G.
  1883 "Beiträge zur Erklärung der Aśoka Inschriften." *Zeitschrift der Deutschen morgenländischen Gesellschaft* 37:87–108.
Caraka
  1949 *Caraka Samhitā, with English, Gujarati, and Hindi translations*, 6 vols. See Mehta et al.
Chattopadhyay, Aparna
  1967 "Some Rules for Public Health in Kautilya." *Nagarjun* 11:158–161. Calcutta.
  1968a "Some Greek Impressions About Indian Medical System."
         J. Research in Indian Medicine 2:256–263. Banaras.
  1968b "Hygienic Principles in the Regulations of Food Habits in the Dharma Sūtras." *Nagarjun* 11:294–299. Calcutta.
  1969 "A Note on Some Hygienic Principles in the Manu Smṛti."
         Nagarjun 12:29–31. Calcutta.
Coedès, George
  1940 "Les hôpitaux de Jayavarman VII." *Bulletin de l'école française d'extrême Orient* 40:344ff.
  1963 *Angkor, an Introduction*. Hong Kong: Oxford University Press. (Original version: *Pour mieux comprendre Angkor*, 2nd ed. Paris, 1947.)
Crooke, W.
  1896 *Tribes and Castes of the North-Western Provinces and Oudh*, vol. 4. Calcutta: Government Printing Office.
Cūlav.
  1925 The *Cūlavamsa*. W. Geiger, ed. London: Oxford University Press.
Demiéville, Paul, ed.
  1937 "Hôbôgirin." *Dictionnaire Encyclopedique du Bouddhisme*, article Byo, fascicule 3:224–265. Paris.

Dhanv.
   1925 *Dhanvantarīya Nighaṇṭu.* V. G. Apte, ed. Ānandāśrama series no. 33. Poona.
Divy.
   1970 *The Divyâvadâna.* E. B. Cowell and R. A. Neil, eds. Amsterdam: Oriental
      Press. (Reprint of Cambridge University Press edition, 1886.)
Dutt, N. K.
   1931 *Origin and Growth of Caste in India,* vol. 1. London: Kegan Paul, Trench,
      Trübner.
   1965 *Ibid.,* vol. 2. Calcutta: K. L. Mukhopadhyay.
Farquhar, J. N.
   1915 *Modern Religious Movements in India.* New York: Macmillan. (Reprint, Delhi,
      1967.)
Filliozat, Jean
   1964 *The Classical Doctrine of Indian Medicine.* Delhi: Munshiram Manoharlal.
      (Original edition: *La doctrine classique de la médicine indienne.* Paris, 1949.)
Finot, L.
   1903 "L'inscription sanskrite de Say Fong," *Bulletin de l'école française d'extrême
      Orient* 3:18ff.
Iyer, L. K. A.
   1912 *Cochin Tribes and Castes.* Madras: Higginbotham & Co.
Jain, J. C.
   1947 *Life in Ancient India as Depicated in Jain Canons.* Bombay: New Book Co.
Jolly, J.
   1901 "Medizin." *Grundriss der indo-arischen Philologie und Altertumskunde* 3(10).
      Strassburg.
Kane, P. V.
   1946 *History of Dharmaśāstra,* vol. 3. Poona: Bhandarkar Oriental Research Institute.
Kaul, Madhusūdan
   1924 *The Deśopadeśa and Narmamālā of Kshemendra.* Kashmir series of texts and
      studies, no. 40. Poona.
Keswani, Nandkumar H.
   1970 "Medical Education in India Since Ancient Times," in C. D. O'Malley, ed.,
      The History of Medical Education. Berkeley and Los Angeles: University of
      California Press.
Kutumbiah, P.
   1962 *Ancient Indian Medicine.* Madras: Orient Longmans.
Majumdar, R. C.
   1960 *The Classical Accounts of India.* Calcutta: K. L. Mukhopadhyay.
Manu
   1886 *The Laws of Manu.* B. Bühler, trans, *Sacred Books of the East,* vol. 25. Oxford:
      Clarendon Press.
Mehta, P. M., et al.
   1949 Introduction and Notes to *Caraka Saṃhitā,* 6 vols. Jamnagar: Gulabkunverba
      Āyurvedic Society.
Mukhopadhyaya, Girindranath
   1926 *History of Indian Medicine,* 2 vols. Calcutta: University of Calcutta Press.
Müller, Reinhold F. G.
   1951 *Grundsätze altindischer Medizin. Acta historica scientiarum naturalium at medi-
      cinalium,* vol. 8. Copenhagen: Munksgaard.
   1958 "Eigenwertungen in altindischer Medizin." *Nova Acta Leopoldina* 20(138).
      Leipzig.
Narmamālā
   1924 *The Deśopadeśa and Narmamālā of Kshemendra.* See Kaul.

Przyluski, J.
  1923 *La légende de l'empereur Açoka* Paris. P. Geuthner.
Rām.
  1959 *The Vālmīki Rāmāyaṇa.* G. H. Bhatt et al., eds. Baroda: Oriental Institute.
Rashid, A.
  1969 *Society and Culture in Medieval India.* Calcutta: K. L. Mukhopadhyay.
Reddy, D. V. S.
  1941 "Medical Relief in South India: Centres of Medical Aid and Types of Medical Institutions." *Bull. of the History of Medicine* 9:385–400.
Russell, R. V.
  1916 *Tribes and Castes of the Central Provinces*, vol. 1. London: Macmillan.
R. V.
  1891 *The Ṛg Veda.* F. Max Müller, ed. *Sacred Books of the East*, vol. 32. Oxford: Clarendon Press.
  1897 *Ibid.*, vol. 46.
Sastri, K. A. Nilakanta
  1955 *The Colas*, 2nd ed. Madras: University of Madras.
Siddiqī, Muḥammad Zubayr
  1959 *Studies in Arabic and Persian Medical Literature.* Calcutta: University of Calcutta Press.
Su.
  1945 *Suśruta Saṃhitā.* See Āchārya and Pandurang.
Thurston, E.
  1909 *Castes and Tribes of Southern India*, 7 vols. Madras: Government Press.
Vin. Mhv.
  1881 *Vinaya Piṭaka, Mahāvagga.* H. Oldenberg and T. W. Rhys Davids, trans. *Sacred Books of the East*, vol. 13. Oxford: Clarendon Press.
  1882 *Ibid.*, vol. 17.
Viṣṇu.
  1880 *The Institute of Viṣṇu*, J. Jolly, translator. *Sacred Books of the East*, vol. 7. Oxford: Clarendon Press.
Vogel, Claus
  1965 "Introduction and Notes." *Vāgbhaṭas Aṣṭāngahṛdaya Saṃhita. Abhandlungen für die Kunde des Morgenlandes*, vol. 38, no. 2. Wiesbaden.
Zimmer, H. R.
  1948 *Hindu Medicine.* Baltimore: Johns Hopkins University Press.

Secular and Religious Features
of Medieval Arabic Medicine

J. CHRISTOPH BÜRGEL

My subject is an Asiaticized rather than an Asian medical system, and I will deal almost exclusively with the past. Like most other specialists on Arabic or Islamic medicine, I have concentrated on the period from about 750 to 1500 A.D. Indeed, little is known to survive of the scientific medicine of the Islamic Middle Ages. With the exception of India and Pakistan, no serious efforts are being made toward reviving the old system. In fact, my impression is that it is mainly in the wake of the revival of Āyurvedic medicine in India that similar pains have been taken toward a scientific renaissance of Arabic medicine. This Arabic medicine is called *Unani* by the Hindu- and Urdu-speaking people (to mention only the two leading language groups of Indo-Islamic culture). The name indicates the origin of this medical system. Unani is the English spelling of Yūnānī, which is derived from the Arabic language and means "Greek" (Ionian).

Ayurveda is an intrinsic part of the Indian culture, but this cannot be said of the Unani system with regard to Islamic culture. It is Greek medicine taken over during the early Islamic period and superimposed on a culture of different origin where, consequently, it met with reserve or even rejection by conservative and narrow-minded religious people. It even aroused a competitive movement based on indigenous Arabic medical traditions. These traditions were sanctified by attributing them to the Holy Prophet— who may, of course, have given medical advice occasionally. Thus Bedouin medical lore was transformed into an intrinsic part of the holy legacy of the Prophet.

The coexistence of different medical traditions during the early Islamic period shows some parallels to the situation in some Asian and other developing countries today. On the following pages I shall describe this medical dualism. To begin with, let us briefly consider the sources.

SOURCES

The great majority of the medical treatises of the classical period up to about 1000 A.D. were written in Arabic. During the first three or four centuries

44

after the *Hijra*, Arabic was the scientific language all over the Islamic world. After 1000 A.D. we also find medical books written in Persian; and some centuries later, medicine was treated in all the leading languages of Islam. For the most part, however, the later sources are of little value, their contents being translations or adaptations of Arabic sources. Thus, most of the material presented in this essay is gleaned from Arabic sources.[1]

These Arabic sources may be divided into various kinds. First, there are the translations from Greek and Syriac, on which the later medical writing of the Islamic world was essentially based—in literary form as well as content. Thus the great medical encyclopedia in which authors as far-famed as Ibn Sina excelled was inspired by the Greek prototypes created by Oribasios and Paulos of Aegina. And generally speaking this was also the case with monographs on special topics such as anatomy, physiology, fevers, pulse, etc.

Another classical form of recording medical knowledge was the commentary. The favorite form with practitioners was the epitome. It was the classic medical text relieved of every dispensable burden of speculative reasoning, polemics, etc. Many a work, especially of Galen's, fell victim to considerable abbreviation by this standard. Finally, there were the writings on the physician's ethical code and the history of medicine, but they played only a marginal role in medical literature.

All these literary forms and medical topics had been cultivated by the Greeks and were taken over by the Arabs, who "inherited" them by translating hundreds of Greek sources into Arabic. This work was done by a relatively small number of scholars, mainly during the ninth century. It cannot be overestimated as one of the great cultural achievements in the history of the human spirit.

The Arabs took over the Galenic system in its totality and clung to it until the European impact in the nineteenth century. Their own contributions, e.g., Razi's famous description of smallpox and measles, were based on this very system.

An unshaken confidence in the validity of the Galenic system characterizes even the few known instances of explicit criticism of Galen. Not the least idea of rebelling against the total system, or the slightest doubt about its principal soundness, can be perceived in these criticisms or corrections. On the contrary, the numinous weight, as it were, of the authority of Galen is felt in these observations perhaps more than elsewhere. For example, ʿAbd al-Latif al-Baghdadi discovered that the lower jawbone of the human body was not, as Galen had taught, composed of two parts, but that it was a

1 To a large extent I am drawing here on material I have gathered in a volume of essays, "Studien zum ärztlichen Leben and Denken im arabischen Mittelalter" (Studies in medical life and thought during the Arabic Middle Ages), which was accepted by the University of Göttingen in 1968 and will be published in an "ars medica" series by the Medical Historical Institute of the Free University, West Berlin.

single sutureless bone. This famous Egyptian scholar made his discovery in the course of osteological studies in an ancient cemetery in the northwest of Cairo—but not until he had investigated more than two thousand skulls did he realize that he had come across an error in Galen's teaching. In his account of this experience he expressed the conviction—which, self-evident as it may seem to us, was a bold statement in those times—that the evidence of the perception of our senses deserved more confidence than the teachings of Galen; though having said so, he added, typically enough that there might be found an interpretation of the words in question which would free Galen from the charge of error.

A similar attitude is nearly always met with when a daring physician voiced a doubt regarding a particular tenet of Galen's. But this is not the place to dwell upon the history of criticism of ancient authorities in medieval Islam. The point I want to emphasize is that the Arab physicians took over the Greek medical system in its totality.

Some treatises of Indian medicine were translated into Arabic. In his handbook entitled *The Paradise of Wisdom*, Rabban b.ʿAli at-Tabari, a famous author of the ninth century, gave a summary of the Indian medical system based on the chief sources: Caraka, Susruta, Vagbhata (Astangahrdaya) and Madhavakara (Nidana). However, he did not consult these sources in the original language; and, apart from a few drugs that were taken over by the Arabs, no discernible influence was exercised by Indian medicine on Arabic medicine (Ullmann 1970:103–107; Sezgin 1970:187–202).

Orthodox Muslims harbored a strong suspicion against the secular sciences taken over from the heathen Greeks. In regard to medicine this repugnance was intense, since Greek medicine claimed to care not only for the bodies but also for the souls of men. The Muslim opposition was not supported by the whole of the Muslim community, but was confined, at least in the beginning, to a comparatively small number of orthodox zealots. However, they did not content themselves with passive resistance but created a competitive medicine, the so-called medicine of the Prophet (Arabic: *tibb an-nabi*, or *at-tibb an-nabavi*). In its origin, it was based on the *hadiths*, or sayings and manners of behavior, attributed to the Prophet Muhammad, which were handed down, collected, and classified by the *muhaddithun*, the scholars of the Holy Tradition. Some of these sayings were authentic, while others were forged. On the whole, the authenticity of a given tradition may be established with some degree of probability if it is in line with the customs and beliefs of the people of Mekka and Medina at the beginning of the seventh century, and it must be held to be forged if it shows a clear influence of later developments. But modern scientific views on this question matter little or nothing for the role a *hadith* played, and sometimes even continues to play, in Muslim society. If a *hadith* is considered authentic by the Muslim community, which developed its own method of *hadith* criticism, it passes as sacrosanct.

As to the medical traditions, they may be described as a fragmentary extract of Bedouin medical practice.[2]

The totally different traditions of Galenic and of Prophetic medicine provide the subject for the following pages.

THE GALENIC SYSTEM

The essence of the Galenic system was the so-called humoral pathology which, having originated in the Hippocratic school of Kos, came to be modified by Aristotle and by medical schools such as the Pneumaticians. It was molded by Galen into a comprehensive and well-thought-out theory, the main point of which was that food, after having got into the body, was transformed ("boiled") by natural warmth in the stomach into different substances. Part of these substances was useful for the body, and after a second "boiling" in the liver was transported by the blood to the different organs and members of the body, while the rest was excreted. The main products of this process were the four cardinal humors: blood, mucus, yellow bile, and black bile. These humors combined with the four primary qualities: warmth (or heat), cold, moisture (or dampness), and dryness. According to this coordination, the blood was damp and hot, the mucus damp and cold, the yellow bile dry and hot, and the black bile damp and cold.

If the four humors and the qualities combined with them were in a state of mutual equilibrium (Greek: *eukrasia*, literally "the state of being well mixed" or "well tempered"), man was healthy. If one of the humors and, therewith, one of the qualities became so dominant that the balance was considerably disturbed, *eukrasia* was displaced by *dyskrasia* (state of being ill mixed, or "ill tempered"), which meant that a man was sick. While the Hippocratic school had believed in the existence of an ideal equilibrium of the four humors, Galen modified the theory by teaching that, in fact, no such ideal state existed. The influence of exterior factors such as climate, age, profession, customs, etc., caused a dominance of one of the four humors to be observed in every human body. This gave a man his individual habit and complexion, his "temperament," which may be sanguine, phlegmatic, choleric, or melancholic.

The Galenic system of therapy rested on the principle of *contraria contrariis*. In other words, the Galenic system was an allopathy par excellence, and so it seems strange that in India modern medicine is distinguished from the traditional Ayurvedic and the Yunani medicine by being labeled "allopathy." "Hot" diseases were cured by "cold" remedies, "moist" by "dry," and vice versa. Hearing these terms, a modern listener not familiar with Galenic medicine might think of cold and hot drinks, of baths and other hydropathic treatments; but these were only a small part of what Galen and his disciples meant when they talked of hot, moist, etc. These qualities were ascribed to

2 Cf. the exposition of this and other Arabic criticisms of Galen in my study "Averroes contra Galenum" (Bürgel 1968a:276–290).

every part of nature: musk was hot and dry, cucumber was cold and damp in the second degree, costus was hot and dry in the second degree, and so on. No drug taken from one of the three realms of nature could escape being categorized after this scheme.

The magic word of this system was *eukrasia* or, more comprehensively, *symmetria* (Arabic: *i'tidal*). It was by conserving symmetry in the different spheres of his life that a man protected his health, and it was by teaching his patients how to conserve or restore it that a physician made himself indispensable to them. Thus a strong ethical element was implicit in the Galenic system. The Galenic physician was meant to be a simple practitioner busy with curing bodily diseases, but he should be an ethical instructor as well.

Another characteristic feature of the Galenic system was the Aristotelian relation between the general (*to kat'holou*) and the particular (*to kat'hekastou*). What the medical textbooks contained were only the general facts of anatomy, pathology, therapeutics, etc. From these general rules—from this canon, as Ibn Sina's famous classic is called—physicians had to derive the appropriate individual treatment for a given case by means of logical procedure, especially by the so-called analogical conclusion (*analogismos*). This was why no one could be a good physician without having thoroughly learned the rules of logic.

The practical organization of medicine in medieval Islam was famous for its high standards. But how did it come into being? It was to a large extent erected on the pattern of a famous pre-Islamic institution: the medico-philosphical academy of Gondeshapur, a place near Susa, the ancient capital of Elam. This academy was probably founded in the first half of the sixth century after the closure of the Athenic Academy in 529. It was run by a number of Nestorian scholars and physicians, among them the famous family of Bukhtishuᶜ, who were to play an important role in the foundation and propagation of scientific medicine in the empire of the caliphs.

When al-Mansur, the founder of the Abbasid Caliphate, was troubled with a stomach disease, and the court physicians were at their wit's end, the chief physician of Gondeshapur, who belonged to the Bukhtishuᶜ clan, was called to Baghdad, where he successfully healed the monarch. He was followed for several generations by other members of this family, most of whom reached the highest rank possible at the court. They enjoyed—though not without various vicissitudes and interruptions—the most intimate confidences of their patrons. By their influence, presence, and teaching they were instrumental in modeling Arabic medicine after the theories of Galen and the practice of Gondeshapur.

Students of the medical arts were for the most part instructed in private circles, which were held in the homes of distinguished teaching physicians. Hospitals used to be equipped with teaching rooms, and students were encouraged or even obliged to attend hospitals for practical bedside training. The backbone of theoretical instruction was the so-called *Alexandrian Canon*, also labeled "the summaries of the Alexandrians." This was a selection of sixteen out of the hundreds of medical books written by Galen. These books, or summaries, were explained to students by a teacher, and after this instruction students were expected to possess sufficient knowledge for reading and understanding further texts on their own. In later times, the Alexandrian Canon gradually lost its central importance and was superseded by the works of Arabic authors, chiefly the encyclopedias compiled by physicians such as Razi, Ali ibn Abbas al-Majusi, Ibn Sina, and others.

We gain precious information from a work on medical education (*Adab at-tabīb*) written by an otherwise unknown physician named Ishaq ibn Ali of Edessa. This author said that each student should choose a branch of medicine for special study, and that nobody should be accepted for an examination if he pretended to posses the knowledge of the whole art. This very pretension would be proof of ignorance, because no one could master such vast knowledge![3] The special disciplines of medicine mentioned in this and other Arabic sources were: physiologist (*tabā'i^cī*, literally specialist of the "natures," which means the humors), oculist, orthopedist (*mujabbir*, literally bone-setter), surgeon, phlebotomist, and cupper. The last two specialists played only a subordinate role, being usually mere underlings to the theoretically trained physicians.

The list of specialists engaged by Adud ad-Daula for his hospital in Baghdad comprised physiologists, oculists, surgeons, and orthopedists. This hospital, founded in 981; that of Nur ad-Din in Damascus, founded in 1154; and that of the Mamluk al-Mansur Kala'un in Cairo, founded in 1284, were equipped with special rooms or halls which corresponded more or less with the aforementioned specializations. The only remarkable additions were rooms for cholerics or melancholics (*mamrur*, literally somebody suffering from a disease in the *mirra*, the bile).[4] We are also told that maniacs were treated in these rooms, but this should not be confounded with the modern standard treatment of mental diseases, as is sometimes done. Recourse to chains and whipping in the treatment of the insane was a normal proceeding of the time.

After a certain period of instruction, the future physician could finish his studies by an examination. Much source material exists about this examination. For example, we have collections of questions and answers; and we may, I think, be sure that teaching physicians used to examine their pupils and to give some sort of certificate to the successful ones. But we know very

3 The "Adab at-tabib" ("Education of the Physician") which is extant in a unique manuscript (Edirne, Selimiye Kütüphanesi Nr. 1658), has been translated into English (Levy 1967). This translation is full of mistakes (cf. Bürgel 1968b). I am preparing a German translation of the text and have discussed its importance in two papers (Bürgel 1966, 1967).

4 All three hospitals had such halls, as is proved by anecdotes set in the "hall of the maniacs" (*qa^cat al-mamrūrīn*) in the hospitals of Baghdad and Damascus (Müller 1884: vol. 1, p. 254, line 23 and vol. 2, p. 242, line 1 from bottom) and the description of the hospital of Mansur in the Khitat al-Maqrizi (vol 4, p. 260)—where, however, the word *mabrūd* has to be changed into *mamrur*. The same correction is, accordingly to be made in Issa's translation of this description (Issa 1929:121).

little about the role played by the state or the government in these examinations, or about the official control of the healing art as a whole. Of course, one has to mention the *Hisba*, an office known to have existed as early as the third century of the *Hijra*. Its purpose was to be a kind of industrial and moral inspection board in the towns. The *muhtasib*, the holder of this office, was bound to control public morals. He had to look to it that the merchants were upright and used honest weights and measures—and, according to an influential handbook for *muhtasibs*, he had to control and, if necessary, examine physicians.[5] But how could he do that without some medical training? The mentioned handbook told him what to ask the examinee. But if the knowledge indicated by those questions was deemed sufficient for an official license, then the acknowledged level of medical practice must have been deplorably low. This would indeed be in line with the growing decline of the time. The author died in 1329.

Serious physicians carried on a constant struggle against quackery. Even during the most prosperous period of Arabic medicine, critical voices painted a gloomy picture of the alleged decay in contemporary medicine, and called for severe control by the government and strict adherence to the ancient authorities. These measures were considered the only protection against the otherwise irremediable decline of the Hippocratic art. It is difficult to decide how much these Cassandra-cries were mere repetition of a topic already in the writings of Galen and even of Hippocrates, and how much was realistic. That quackery existed, and that it was increasing, is beyond all doubt. But since I will describe Prophetic medicine later in this essay as quackery piously disguised, let me now proceed to the practice of the ethical Galenic physician.

The physician—if he was not one of the court physicians to whom most of our biographical source material refers, and as long as he did not work in a hospital—would receive his patients either in his home or in a special shop in the town called *hanut*. He had apprentices who helped him in the preparation of drugs. According to an admonishment in *Adab at-tabib*, drugs should always be prepared by the physician himself or in his presence. Errors in this respect were said to have fatal outcomes. If treatments requiring special knowledge or skill were necessary, the physician should consult a specialist.

The physicians were bound to follow ethical rules based mainly on the Hippocratic oath. They were forbidden to kill or help to kill somebody by poisonous drugs, a temptation to which a court physician might be exposed more than once during his life. They were also forbidden to perform abortions, and they were not to reveal secrets confided to them by their patients. The proscription not to accept patients whose cases appeared to be hopeless was to avoid the risk of an almost certain failure which would be harmful to the renown of the medical art. The ideal of treating poor patients without fees

---

5 Cf. the chapters referring to the different types of practitioners and physicians in *Ibn al-Ukhuwa's Handbook on the Rules of Hisba* (Levy 1938).

was important, but it could only be realized on the basis of sufficient wealth or a self-denying way of life. In *The Fountains of Information* by Ibn abi Usaibiᶜa, a collection of about 450 biographies of famous physicians up to the thirteenth century, only a few are expressly reported to have treated patients without fee, and in most of these cases we are incidentally informed of extraordinary riches in the possession of those benefactors. This does not mean that there were no true idealists among the Arab physicians. Although Ibn abi Usailiᶜa's collection is an excellent source, it is oriented toward success and glory, and this may be why we know so little about the idealists.

Some rules of demeanor handed down from Greek to Arabic sources took account of the psychological relationship between a physician and his patient. The practitioner should wear white, well-scented clothes, have his hair and his nails cut so that they are not too long or too short (this in accordance with the ideal of symmetry). Likewise, he should proceed to the bed of the patient at a moderate speed[6], and when talking to him put no unnecessary questions.[7] This behavior to win the patient's confidence was regarded as one of the chief factors in the process of healing. Such ideas bring to our mind the considerable role that Greek and Arabic medicine assigned to psychological factors in general. Among the elements such as climate, rest, and motion, or sleeping and waking, which had to be kept in a moderate and well-balanced state, were the so-called psychological accidents (*al-aᶜrād an-nafsānīya*). Physicians warned people of the consequences of unbalanced emotions: excessive joy promoted obesity, boundless mourning made a man meager, fright set the humors in motion. These and other psychosomatic interrelations might also be used in therapies. A high-ranking person who suffered from obesity and was unable or unwilling to follow the diet prescribed to him was finally cured when his physician foretold his imminent death and left him in this fear until the necessary degree of emaciation had been reached (Müller 1884:1, 150–151).

The great Razi healed an emir of Raiy (the Rhagae of ancient Persia), struck by a chronic paralysis of his legs, by a combined therapy: after a long hot bath and a drink which was "to ripen the humors," he suddenly threatened the prince with a knife as if he intended to kill him, whereupon the prince sprang to his feet. Razi fled on a horse kept in readiness, and after reaching a safe place wrote a letter to the *emir* in which he explained his "psychological therapy" (*ᶜilādj-e nafsānī*). This, however, was only the most spectacular in a series of similar cures (Browne 1921:82).

To the heritage of Greek medicine belonged the famous treatise on melancholy by Rufus of Ephesus. Its Arabic translation was worked on and considerably supplemented by Ishaq ibn Imran, a court physician in the Kairouan of the beginning of the tenth century. His monograph was to become the base

---

6 These rules are to be found in the spurious "Testament of Hippocrates" which was translated into Arabic.

7 This rule was given by the author of the *Adab at-tabīb*, who was very concerned about how to keep the high standard of the healing art.

of the *melancholia* of Constantine the African, a most influential book in the history of medieval Latin medicine. Melancholy was treated by drugs as well as by psychiatric measures, with music playing an important part in this connection.

One of the most remarkable achievements of ancient psychiatry is till to be mentioned: the healing of maniacs, i.e., of persons possessed by fixed ideas. Rufus cured a person who was suffering from the delusion of having no head—in another Greek source this man is said to have been a bloody tyrant—by ordering him to wear a helmet of lead (Flashar 1966:99). The same treatment for the same ailment was successfully administered by the just-mentioned Imran ibn Ishaq of Kairouan (Matran:fol.48r.). Galen cured a person haunted by the fancy of having swallowed a snake by having the patient describe the imagined snake. He procured such a snake, blindfolded the patient, gave him an emetic, and when he began vomiting Galen smuggled the snake into his vomit and removed the band from his eyes. Beholding the snake, the patient was said to be convinced he had gotten rid of his evil.[8]

The principle of these cures was to take the fixed idea seriously, and it was perfectly grasped and imitated by great Arab and Persian physicians. Several cases of the kind were reported in Ibn abi Usaibiᶜa's *Fountains of Information* and in other sources. We need not argue whether manias may in fact be cured by so simple a measure. What I want to point out is the acute awareness on the part of those physicians of the influence a man's belief has on the state of his body and on the success or failure of therapeutic measures. It was therefore logical for them to admit, or at least not to deny the possibility of a healing effect of remedies outside the Galenic framework, provided the sick persons believed in their effectiveness. We shall return to this point in discussing Prophetic medicine.

On the whole, and with only a few exceptions, the contributions of the Arabs and of the Islamic Middle Ages to the development of medicine do not reside in sensational discoveries. One of the rare exceptions is a rather correct description of the pulmonary circulation by Ibn an-Nafis about four centuries before the European discovery of it by William Harvey. Progress was also made in the diagnosis and description of certain diseases. The main achievements of medieval Arabic medicine must, however, be looked for in five fields: systematization, hospitals, pharmacology, surgery, and ophthalmology.

The development of Arabic medical literature may to a considerable degree be described as a constant process of reshaping and rearranging the Greek heritage by shortening, broadening, commenting on, and systematizing the ancient source material. "Ibn Sina concentrated the legacy of Greek medical knowledge with the addition of the Arab's contribution in his gigantic *Canon of Medicine* (*al-qanun fi t-tibb*), which is the culmination and masterpiece of Arab systematization" (Meyerhof 1931:329).

I have already discussed the importance of hospitals during the golden

8 This case is related by the author of the *Adab aṭ-ṭabīb*. I do not know its Greek origin.

age of Islamic culture. The base of pharmacology was the *Materia Medica* of Dioscorides, but it was enlarged by many excellent Arabic authors who added about 500 names of simple and compound drugs to the ancient stock (Dubler 1959).

As for surgery, it flourished mainly in Andalusia. In the East it was usually looked upon as a lowly craft. The outstanding figure in this field was Abu l-Qasim az-Zahrawi, who died in 1013. He was a court physician of Cordova, known to the Latin West as Abulcasis. His name is associated with a great medical *Vademecum* (*at-tasrif*) in thirty sections, the last of which deals with surgery. Based largely on the sixth book of Paul of Aegina, it is enlarged with numerous additions and contains illustrations of instruments. It influenced other Arabic authors and especially helped to lay the foundation of surgery in Europe (Meyerhof 1931:330–331).

Finally, ophthalmology flourished in Egypt and Mesopotamia, where diseases of the eyes abounded. Meyerhof wrote:

The Christian oculist Ali ibn Isa of Baghdad, known to the Latins as Jesu Haly, and the Muslim Ammar of Mosul, known as Canamusali, left two excellent treatises, increasing the Greek canon of ophthalmology with numerous additions, operations, and personal observations. Both were translated into Latin. They were the best text-books on eye diseases until the first half of the eighteenth century, when the renaissance of ophthalmology set in in France. (1931:332)

THE DECLINE OF GALENIC MEDICINE

After a golden age from about the tenth to the twelfth century, Arabic medicine came to a standstill, which gradually changed into a slow decline leading to the most deplorable decay imaginable. Some reasons for this are very clear. One of them was the lack of an evolutionary conception of science. Ibn Sina, no doubt one of the most prominent figures in the phalanx of those universally learned scholars who typify the golden age of Islamic culture, tells us in his autobiography that at the age of eighteen he had already finished the courses in all the sciences and did not learn anything new afterward (Arberry 1959:9–24). To him, and to most of his colleagues, science seems to have been the detailed knowledge of a complete set of facts which did not call for any essential supplement but only needed to be brought into a clearly arranged system.

There were a few representatives of the opposite outlook. Among them Razi and Averroes were well aware of the gaps in human knowledge, and dreamed of a future completion of science by the storing up of knowledge from generation to generation. But they could not pass beyond the limits set to scientific progress by the technology of those times. There was no microscope, the most important instrument for piercing through the veils of nature and thereby breaking the fetters of the Galenic system. And the dissection of human bodies, which might have improved anatomical and physiological knowledge without a microscope, was strictly prohibited by religion. Our sources do not contain the slightest indication of anybody having dared to trespass against this custom. Yuhanna ibn Masawaih, a great physician of the earliest period (died 857) who was a Christian in name and a free-thinking rationalist by demeanor, dissected apes. I know no parallel to this exception, and he is reported to have said that he would kill his insane son and dissect his body if he did not fear the sultan's punishment (Müller 1884:1, 180).

These reasons for the lack of progress do not sufficiently explain the steadily increasing decline. Other reasons must be at the bottom of this, and some of them we do know. The Mongols played their part, destroying hundreds of libraries and, probably, dozens of hospitals. They started by destroying the Adudi hospital in Baghdad, which had prospered for more than two and a half centuries. But a society incapable of resisting nomadic invaders must have been largely rotten, at least in its leading circles, and the Mongols cannot be charged with having destroyed Islamic civilization or even science. On the contrary, after having won power they encouraged and revitalized science and culture on a large scale.

If we want to know which spiritual forces were most potent in paralyzing the scientific impetus of the golden age, we have to ask what the essentials of science are. I think that one essential is immanent to science, its very soul and lifeblood, and this is rational argumentation propelled by an insatiable curiosity. The other thing essential for science belongs to the history of economy as well as to the history of science, and it is the interest in, the demand for, and the consumption of scientific products.

What forces were harmful to these essentials? As for the economic element, a strong and ever-increasing influence was exercised by Islamic mysticism, which turned people to the inner instead of the outer world so that they restricted their natural demands to a minimum. As to curiosity, I have noted the prevailing concept of science as a constant stock of knowledge. Rational thought had several renowned enemies, some of whom could trace their origins to antiquity. I refer to astrology, alchemy, magic—and, finally, of Islamic origin, the so-called Prophetic medicine. These four were looked upon as sciences by the great majority, and even by most of the scholars. Nevertheless, they were hothouses of irrationalism, the rational disguise making them only the more harmful.

PROPHETIC MEDICINE

The classical collections of the sayings of the Prophet Muhammad comprise many chapters on the spheres of daily life, among them illness, health, and healing. In the most famous of these collections, the *Sahih* by al-Bukhari (died 870), eighty paragraphs, or about 2.3 percent of the whole collection, are more or less directly concerned with medical questions. The author has grouped these paragraphs into two chapters, one "on the sick" and the other "on healing." To form an idea of this material, we shall use the following division: theological problems, ethical and social concerns, popular health rules, drugs and other remedies, and magical healing and apotropeic measures.

Theological Problems

Pious people were confronted with two basic questions when they were ill: What was the religious meaning of disease? Were rational remedies and secular therapies compatible with pious striving and trust in God's omnipotence? The latter question was especially urgent where predestination or determinism was a religious or philosophical tenet. Thus it is easy to understand why the problem was discussed by orthodox Muslims sometimes along the same lines that had been followed by Greek stoics.

Muhammad's answer to the first question was rather distinct: "A believer will suffer no sickness nor even a thorn to pierce his skin without expiating one of his sins" (Bukhari 1376: mardā, bāb 2). The positive sense assigned to suffering in this saying, as in similar ones, was stressed even more by two other traditions in which people suffering from epilepsy or blindness were promised paradise because of their patience (Bukhari 1376: mardā, bāb 5 + 6). From here it was only a small step to the conviction of many pious Muslims that suffering was a religious virtue and disease a sign of holiness. The Prophet was reported to have said: "He who dies on a sickbed, dies the death of a martyr and is secure against the inquisition of the tomb" (cf. the article "*Shahīd*" in the Shorter Encyclopaedia of Islam 1953). This conviction was incompatible with the resort to medical cure.

The religious meaning of illness was linked with the question of secular therapy, toward which the attitude of the *Hadith* was less clear. The glorification of suffering and of doing without medical help depended on belief in predestination, one of the speculative consequences of which was to deny the so-called secondary causes (*causae secundae*). The argument was that no such thing as natural causality existed. The apparent relation between cause and effect was a delusion of the senses, and all actions and phenomena were immediately caused by the prime cause, which was God. This attitude was called *tawakkul*, meaning a boundless and totally passive reliance on the Almighty, and it involved abstention from—among other things—any medical treatment (*tark at-tadāvī*) (Reinert 1968:207–213). Although this attitude claimed the example of the Prophet, it was not a true imitation of Muhammad. The affirmative view on medical cure expressed in the larger part of the medical sayings was more typical of the active and pragmatic character of the Prophet than the life-denying *tawakkul* of the later pietists and mystics.

The defenders of medicine drew upon holy traditions to provide the lawfulness of their standpoint. One saying was usually quoted in the introductions of medical books, "God did not send down any disease without also sending down a medicine (or cure)" (Bukhari 1376:tibb, bāb 1). An amplification of this tradition clearly made the point that the pietistic interpretation of tawakkul was not in line with the Prophet's view on medicine:

A companion of the Prophet fell ill during the battle of Uhud. The Prophet, thereupon, called for two practitioners from Medina and asked them to cure him. They said: "O Apostle of God! In the *Djahiliya* ["time of ignorance," meaning the pre-Islamic period] we used to treat our patients by diverse measures. But since Islam has appeared, there doesn't exist anything save *tawakkul*!" He said: "Treat him! God who sends down disease sends down the remedy and then puts into it the [power of] healing." (Levy 1938:165–166).

This later amplification is a good example of the way that *Hadith* developed by being used (and forged!) as a weapon in struggles between different parties and movements.

Another sentence must be mentioned because it is frequently met with in the sources. It usually passes for a saying of the Prophet, though it did not figure in the early collections, and Suyuti, well-known scholar of the fifteenth century, expressly ascribed it to ash-Shafi i, the founder of the Shafi͑ite rite. The sentence is: "Science is twofold: the science of bodies and the science of religions (al-͑ilmu ͑ilman ͑ilmu l-abdan wa ͑ilmu l-adyān)." This saying is still quoted by Muslims who want to prove the favorable views of Islam of learning and science.[9]

An affirmative attitude toward the use of medical treatment must not, however, be confounded with a favorable view on rational scientific medicine. On the contrary, Prophetic medicine was meant to be the religious counterpart of the suspected Galenic medicine.

Ethical and Social Concerns

The *Sahih* chapter "On the Sick" contained instructions for the correct behavior toward ill people, especially at the bedside. Visiting the sick was a religious duty. Women were allowed to visit and nurse sick men. The Prophet even visited a heathen member of his family, on which occasion he invited him—and, of course, not in vain—to embrace Islam. In a number of cases the Prophet was reported to have performed the ritual washing at the bedside and afterwards to have let the patient drink the water he had used. This was apparently a magic healing in religious disguise.

9 A typical example occurred recently in Istanbul: The leading Turkish magazine *Hayat* (*Life*) showed colored photographs on prenatal life, at the same time publishing opinions of the Mufti and another spiritual authority in Istanbul. The Mufti not only thought the possibility of such photographs improbable, but declared the photographing of a pregnant woman, married or single, as *haram*, a sin. Whereas the other man welcomed the event as a marvelous confirmation of the description in the Koran of the evolution of an embryo. There should be no objection to these pictures, he said, for Islam never opposed science, especially not medicine, but rather promoted it (!), the words proving it: "al-͑ilmu ͑ilmān ͑ilmu l-abdān wa͑ilmu l-adyan." Eventually, this authority regrets that this progress was achieved in another religion instead of Islam, a sign that one ought to turn to science even more intensively than hitherto.

Popular Health Rules

The chapter "On healing" contained a number of rules for protecting one's health, most of which originated in Bedouin folklore. "Travel! It keeps you healthy!" is one of these rules (Ibn ʿAbd Rabbih 1948:6271). Another instruction that did not figure in Bukhari's *Sahih*, but very frequently appeared in later sources of Prophetic medicine, is the rhyme: "*al-miʿdatu baitu d-dāʾ, al-himyatu raʾsu d-dawāʾ*," which translates, "The stomach is the house (or tent) of disease. Caution (diet) is the head (i.e., the best method of) healing" (Spies 1968: fol. 6 r.,7).

The basic theory of Bedouin pathology was evidently that all diseases were ultimately caused by a disorder in the stomach, by wrong nutrition or indigestion. Reasonable nutrition was therefore the chief prophylactic against falling ill, and diet the best remedy for sickness. However, the leading role this saying came to play in medical literature might be based on the fact that it was closely related to the central Greek idea of symmetry. The same relation could have helped a verse of the Koran to a similar importance. It was, "Eat and drink, but do not yield to excess!" (surah 7, 31). A typical anecdote in later Prophetic medical literature related how a certain physician of the "People of the Scripture" (Jews and Christians), on being confronted with the saying attributed to the Prophet and the verse of the Koran, felt that the hundred medical books he had written were superseded. He embraced Islam, exclaiming, "Verily your Book and your Prophet have left nothing for Galen [no gap to be filled by his teaching]!"[10]

Drugs and Other Remedies

If on the whole the rules for protecting health were rather reasonable, the dangers of Prophetic medicine come to light in many therapeutic prescriptions. The range of remedies in the medical chapters of the early Hadith collections is very narrow. According to one of the traditions, Muhammad knew, or acknowledged, only three treatments, one of which he disliked. "Healing resides in three things: a draught of honey, a cut by the cupping-glass (scarification), and a branding by fire (cauterization). But as for branding I forbid it my people" (Bukhari 1376:tibb, bāb 3). Besides bleeding, cupping, and branding, which represented the surgery of Prophetic medicine, apparently the only other outward therapy in the early traditions was to treat fever by water pourings. Reasonable in appearance, this therapy was based on superstition: "Fever is vapor of hell; extinguish it with water!" (Bukhari 1376:tibb, bāb 28).

Even more dubious were the drugs recommended by Muhammad. Sometimes their enigmatic character seemed to be intended: "Use this black

---

10 I know two versions of this anecdote, both from Arabic manuscripts, dealing with the so-called Prophetic medicine. The one is contained in as-Surramarri's Shifāʾ al-lām (fol. 1 v.-2 v.), the other in a work written for the Osmanic Sultan Beyazit (reigned 1389–1402 A.D.) by one ʿUmar ibn Khidr Sufi, Istanbul Nuruosmaniye 3546 (first folio).

grain, it heals everything except death!" (Bukhari 1376: tibb, bāb 7). Commentators later explained that the black grain meant the black cumin—but the original meaning, if there was one at all, is unknown. Another drug was the Indian costus, which effected seven cures (Bukhari 1376: tibb, bāb 10). And another tradition maintained that on the advice of the Prophet, two men successfully cured a disorder in their stomachs by the milk and the urine of camels (Bukhari 1376: tibb, bāb 5 + 6).

With such drugs and treatments, Prophetic medicine had no chance of winning the battle against its scientific competitor. The representatives of Prophetic medicine were not physicians but scholars of the Koran and the Tradition. From about the ninth century they started mixing scientific with Prophetic medicine. This would not have been a bad enterprise, if it had had no other consequence than to give prophetic medicine a more critical approach to medical theory and practice. Thus, for example, Suyuti regarded the tradition of the universal healing qualities of black grain to be apocryphal, and added that even to maintain that it healed most diseases would be an exaggeration (Elgood 1962:*passim*). But the enterprise of mixing Galenic with Prophetic medicine did not increase critical thinking; it introduced magic and religious superstitions into the rational system of the ancients.

Magical Healing and Apotropeic Measures

Though the Prophet, in the sayings assigned to him, showed reserve toward magical things, he nevertheless regarded them as real. The world-view reflected in the holy tradition of Islam was essentially the same as that of the Koran with its *djinns* and its witches. While black magic (*sihr*) was strictly forbidden, other forms of magic were implicitly permitted. *Ruqan* was allowed as a remedy against the evil eye, and it consisted in reciting the last two *surahs* of the Koran and in magic gestures such as blowing in the four directions or stroking one's face and other parts of the body (Bukhari 1376: tibb, bāb 32–42).

Later, with support from the orthodox and the authors of Prophetic medicine, magical healing developed into gross forms of religious sorcery. Amulets were worn not only against the evil eye but also against all kinds of evil spirits. They were used, for example, by pregnant women as a means of guarding against the difficulties of childbirth. An especially widespread practice was to write words of the Koran or the Prophet on a washable material; the script was rinsed out, and the rinsings administered to the sick as medicine. This practice was approved by Ahmad ibn Hanbal, the founder of the most rigid of the four schools of Islamic rites (Elgood 1962: 155).

The boundary between empirical medicine and magic in Hadith literature was not clear. Unexplainable phenomena were regarded as magical, and this magicizing of natural phenomena, together with his reserve about magic, induced Muhammad to make an assertion which later puzzled scholars trying to harmonize Prophetic with scientific medicine. One tradition of the

Prophet denied the existence of contagion, together with oracle birds and an obscure disease of the stomach with a magic etiology (Bukhari 1376:tibb, bāb 43–45). But, as in the case of cauterization and the admissibility of medical help, the Hadith material was inconsistent. It also contained the advice to flee from a leper and not to enter a land where a plague or a pestilence was raging.

For this and other problems of consistency, later commentators found a solution in recourse to the negation of the secondary causes: if there was any such phenomenon as contagion—which could hardly be denied in countries frequently visited by the plague—this did not mean that the disease was caused by contact, unless God as the only cause of everything should make the contact the vehicle of a man's falling ill (De Somogyi 1957:66). The same viewpoint was advanced with regard to the use of any therapeutic treatment, whether it be medical or magical. Both were admissible on the condition that the sick did not rely on the remedy, but put their confidence in God alone. Religiously sound as this rule may seem, it abolished the difference between medicine and magic by putting them both on the same level. This was expressly stated in Suyuti's monograph on Prophetic medicine: "The recitation of charms and the wearing of amulets are a form of taking refuge with God for the purpose of securing health, just as is done in the case of medicine" (Elgood 1962:154).

THE ASCENDANCE OF PROPHETIC MEDICINE

The most important principle of Prophetic medicine was the shift of authority from the ancients to the Prophet and from reason to religious belief. It was no longer a matter of discretion and reasoning whether a certain medicine should be administered or not, but primarily one of knowing whether the Prophet had approved it. A typical report in a fourteenth-century monograph on Prophetic medicine claimed that a certain scholar doubted the authenticity of a tradition in which the Prophet said that he who is scarified on a Saturday will fall ill with leprosy. In order to prove that he was right about this, the scholar had himself cupped on a Saturday. As soon as he did he was struck by leprosy, and only after repenting and confessing his contrition to the Prophet, who appeared to him in a dream, did he recover from his illness (Bachmann 1968:33).

"The relation of Prophetic medicine," says Surrammarri, one of its most fanatic defenders, "to the Galenic system is correspondent to the relation of the latter to quackery." (Dietrich 1966:117). And he frankly stated that the purpose of his book was to prove the data of scientific medicine by the statements of the Prophet.[11] This was the Islamic dethronement of Galen, which took place long before his supersession by the progress of European science.

11 "I have adopted the method of the Jurists (*fuqaha'*)—i.e., putting forward proofs according to the texts of the Koran and the Hadith—for each question I treated. Thus, I name a drug and quote what the practitioners had said about it, then I give proofs in accordance with sayings and actions of the Prophet. Likewise, I name a disease and begin with mentioning what was said about its treatment by the practitioners, therefore what occurs about it in the Hadith" (fol. 13r.).

It was a dethronement in favor of Bedouin quackery and superstition sanctified by religion.

This judgment would sound too severe if it had not already been made by a Muslim scholar in the Middle Ages. No doubt many physicians of the rational party were well aware of the dangers of Prophetic medicine. But we seldom come across an open criticism, for physicians, especially if they were non-Muslims or notorious rationalists, feared the orthodox reaction if they were to put forward too candid a criticism of this part of the holy tradition. We may be sure, however, that much of the indirect criticism referring to shameful intruders who had stolen into the art and pretended to have knowledge of things in reality they knew nothing about, was directed against those who espoused Prophetic medicine.

Ibn Butlan, a famous Christian physician of the eleventh century, made fun of people who resort to faith healing instead of using some well-tested medical remedy (Zalzal 1901:19). But it is by two famous Muslim scholars that an open criticism of Prophetic medicine was finally advanced. The renowned Ibn Khaldun (died 1406) repudiated the authority of the Prophet in medical concerns. Proceeding from the antagonism between nomads (Bedouins) and inhabitants of towns, which was the central idea of his social theory, he stated that diseases came into being as a consequence of the refinements of advanced civilization and were almost nonexistent among nomads. Therefore, nomads had no science of medicine and no physicians, but only a rudimentary knowledge and a primitive practice. The so-called medicine of the Prophet was of this kind, since it was not part of the Prophet's mission to teach medicine. These words were clear enough, but even Ibn Khaldun did not dare to go further. He closed this heretical passage by the placable remark that the dubious remedies would not do any harm to those who used them piously (Browne 1921:13–14).

The second critical voice was that of the Andalusian poet, politician, and bel esprit Ibn al-Khatib, whose fame is scarcely inferior to that of Ibn Khaldun. In a treatise on the plague he repudiated, or at least restricted, the validity of traditions that were incompatible with the evidence of the senses (Ullmann 1970:246).

These voices came too late, and even if advanced at an earlier time they would scarcely have been influential enough to rescue the scientific spirit from the steadily growing religious reaction. Scientific medicine survived, but it survived like a senile old man who had lost all the vital energy of his youth.

The Islamic world has for over a century entered upon a new period of acculturation. From its very beginning, Islam has revealed a peculiar skill in accommodating and amalgamating foreign cultural influences without losing its own identity. It is just now proving that it has lost nothing of this marvelous faculty. But if there is no chance for the Galenic system as a whole to be revived in our day, one may think of reviving particular achievements—

for example, certain well-tried therapies and old drugs—which are in fact now being scientifically tried out and reproduced on a large scale by Unani pharmaceutical companies and state pharmacies in Pakistan, India, and Sri Lanka.

Finally, one thing that should certainly be revived, or kept alive if it is still surviving, is the spirit of humanity which prevailed in the golden age of Greek as well as Arabic medicine, and which manifested itself in the deep understanding of psychosomatic interdependence as one of the basic facts of human ease and disease.

Literature Cited

Ibn ʿAbd Rabbih,
  1948 *Al-ʿIqd al-farīd*, edd. A. Amīn et al. Kairo.
Arberry, A. J.
  1959 *Avicenna on Theology*. London.
Bachmann, P.
  1968 "Zum Medizin-Kapitel des Buches 'al-Baraka' von al-Habaši." In *Medizinhistorisches Journal*, Vol. 3, pp. 28–39.
Browne, E. G.
  1921 *Arabian Medicine*. Cambridge: University Press (reprint 1962).
Bürgel, J. C.
  1966 "Die Bildung des Arztes. Eine arabische Schrift zum ärztlichen Leben aus dem 9. Jahrhundert." In *Sudhoffs Archiv*, Vo. 50, pp. 337–360.
  1967 "Adab und iʿtidāl in ar-Ruhāwīs Adab aṭ-ṭabīb. Studie zur Bedeutungsgeschichte zweier Begriffe." In *Zeitschrift der Deutschen Morgenländischen Gesellschaft*, Vol. 117, pp. 90–102.
  1968a *Averroes 'contra Galenum'. Das Kapitel von der Atmung im Colliget des Averroes als ein Zeugnis mittelalterlich-islamischer Kritik an Galen* eingeleitet, arabisch hrsg. u. übersetzt von J. C. B. In *Nachrichten der Akademie der Wissenschaften in Göttingen* I. Philologisch-historische Klasse. Jahrgang 1967, Nr. 9. Göttingen: Vandenhoeck & Ruprecht.
  1968 "Martin Levey: Medical Ethics of Medieval Islam..." (review). In Göttingische Gelehrte Anzeigen, Vol. 220, pp. 215–227.
ʿal-Bukhārī, Abu ʿAbdallāh
  1376h *Saḥīḥ al-Bukhārī*, ed. M. A. Ibrahim. Kairo: Matbaʿat al-Fajāla al-jadīda.
Ibn Buṭlān
  1901 Daʿwat al-aṭibbā', ed. B. Zalzal. Alexandria.
De Somogyi, J.
  1957 "Medicine in Ad-Damîrî's Ḥayāt al-ḥayawān." In *Journal of Semitic Studies*, Vol. 2, pp. 62–91.
Dietrich, A.
  1966 *Medicinalia Arabica. Studien über arabische medizinische Handschriften in türkischen und syrischen Bibliotheken*. Abhandlungen der Akademie der Wissenschaften in Göttingen, Philologisch-historiche Klasse. Dritte Folge, Nr. 66. Göttingen: Vandenhoeck & Ruprecht.
Dubler, C.
  1959 "Die 'Materia Medica' unter den Muslimen des Mittelalters." In *Sudhoffs Archiv*, Vol. 43, pp. 329–350.

Elgood, C.
1962 "Tibb ul-nabi or Medicine of the Prophet." In *Osiris*, Vol. 14, pp. 33–192.
Flashar, H.
1966 *Melancholie und Melancholiker in den medizinischen Theorien der Antike*. Berlin: De Gruyter.
Issa Bey, A.
1929 "Histoire des Bimaristans (hôpitaux) à l'époque islamique." In *Comptes Rendues du Congrès International de Médecine et d'Hygiène-Tropique*, Vol. 2, pp. 81–209. Kairo.
Levey, M.
1967 *Medical Ethics of Medieval Islam with special reference to al-Ruhāwī's 'Practical Ethics of the Physician'*. Transactions of the American Philosophical Society, New Series, Vol. 57, part 3. Philadelphia.
Levy, R.
1938 See: Ibn al-Ukhūwa
Maqrizi
1324h *Al-Khiṭaṭ al-Maqrīzīya*. Kairo.
Ibn al-Maṭrān
13th century
"Bustān al-aṭibbā' (Orchard of the Physicians)." Unique manuscript in the Army Medical Library in Cleveland, Ohio.
Meyerhof, M.
1931 "Science and Medicine." In *The Legacy of Islam*. Ed. by T. Arnold and A. Guillaume, pp. 311–355 Oxford: University Press (many later reprints).
Müller, A.
1884 See: Ibn abi Uṣaibiᶜa
Reinert, B.
1968 *Die Lehre vom tawakkul in der klassischen Sufik*. Studien zur Sprache, Geschichte und Kultur des islamischen Orients, Neue Folge, Band 3. Berlin: De Gruyter.
Ṣāᶜid ibn al-Ḥasan
1968 *Das Buch At-Tashwīq aṭ-ṭibbī des Ṣāᶜid ibn al-Ḥasan. Ein arabisches Adab-Werk über die Bildung des Arztes* hrsg. und bearbeitet von O. Spies. Bonn: Selbstverlag des Orientalischen Seminars der Universität Bonn.
Sezgin, F.
1970 *Geschichte des arabischen Schrifttums*, Band 3—Medizin, Pharmazie, Zoologie, Tierheilkunde bis ca. 430 h. Leiden: Brill.
Shorter Encyclopaedia of Islam
1953 Ed. on Behalf of the Royal Netherlands Academy by H. A. R. Gibb and J. H. Kramers. Leiden: Brill; London: Luzac & Co. (many later reprints).
Spies, O.
1968 See: Ṣāᶜid ibn al-Ḥasan
Surramarrī, Jamāl ad-dīn
14th century
"Shifā' al-ālām fī ṭibb ahl al-islām. Manuscript Fatih 3584 in Istanbul.
Ibn al-Ukhūwa
1938 *Maᶜālim al-qurba fī aḥkām al-ḥisba*. Ed. with abstracts of contents, glossary and indices by R. Levy. Gibb Memorial Series, Nr. 12. London: Luzac & Co.
Ullmann, M.
1970 *Die Medizin im Islam*. Handbuch der Orientalistik. Erste Abteilung, Ergänzungsband VI, Erster Abschnitt. Leiden: Brill.
Ibn abiᶜUṣaibiᶜa
1884 ᶜUyūn al-anbā' fī ṭabaqāt al-aṭibbā'. Ed. A. Müller. Königsberg and Kairo.
Zalzal, B.
1901 See: Ibn Buṭlān

The Intellectual and Social Impulses Behind the Evolution of Traditional Chinese Medicine

MANFRED PORKERT

Whoever tries to appraise the status of indigenous Chinese medicine today is confronted by conflicting evidence. On the one hand, more than a century of contact with Western science has up to now failed to stimulate any significant effort at a theoretical reassessment of the heritage of traditional medicine in terms of universal modern medicine. On the other hand, the traditional methods continue to stand up remarkably well against the competition of Western medicine, not only in China but also in Formosa, Hong Kong, and Singapore. To resolve these apparent contradictions, it will be useful to consider the intellectual and social constants of Chinese medicine, operative throughout its history.

THE EPISTEMOLOGICAL PREMISES OF CHINESE MEDICINE

What is true of Chinese thought in general holds equally true for its practical applications in Chinese medicine: It is primarily interested in function as opposed to substratum.

The cognitive mode leading to the systematic perception of functions is called inductive and synthetic; the cognitive mode by which substratums are perceived rationally is called causal and analytic. The scientist who uses the inductive and synthetic mode of cognizance will observe first, and then speculate on his observations; the scientist who applies the causal and analytic mode will first speculate and act, and after that he will observe. The analytic and causal exploration of substratums requires that active effort precede receptive cognition. The synthetic and inductive perception of functions calls for no initial action, but requires the observer to consciously suspend any activity that would interfere with the functions to be observed.

My hypothesis is that, at the dawn of systematic speculation, philosophers of all civilizations first adopted the inductive and synthetic mode of cognition because of its directness and simplicity. Causal analytic thought apparently did not enter the scene before the 4th century B.C. In China it then only constituted a brief interlude in the works of the mohists and of Hsün-tzu;

in the West, the opus of Aristotle marked the beginning of a tradition that was to continue into our days. From the 13th century A.D., the analytic approach gradually became established as the leading mode of inquiry in the West. The synthetic argument was almost completely pushed out of science until the development of electrodynamics and nuclear physics necessitated its camouflaged reintroduction in the middle of the 19th century.

The analytic and the synthetic approach each have heuristic advantages and shortcomings that can be particularly well demonstrated in medical science. The phenomena with which medicine is concerned can be divided into those that may be reduced to efficient causes—e.g., the impressive advances in histological pathology, biochemistry, or bacteriology—and an equally large number of phenomena for which analysis only yields tautological results. The reasons will be apparent if we consider certain regular relationships between functions and substratums.

Every function is based upon a substratum. *Rule 1*: there is a direct relation between the temporal dimension of the function and the spatial dimension of the substratum. A prolonged or intensive function presupposes a large, dense, or heavy substratum; inversely, a light or small substratum may only produce a function of short duration or small intensity. *Rule 2*: there is an inverse relation between the apparent homogeneity of substratums and their dimension. In other words, the smaller the size of individual substratums, the greater appears to be their collective homogeneity. From these two rules I derive *Rule 3*: the apparent homogeneity of a substratum is in inverse relation to the temporal dimension of its corresponding function.

When a physicist enumerates the specific qualities of the iron molecule, his data have not been derived from the persistent examination of one individual molecule, but from the collective appraisal of millions of them. The fact that his data gleaned from the investigation of a limited number of iron molecules may, for all practical purposes, be generalized with a probability 1 to all iron molecules, is due to the great homogeneity of the substratum called iron. This homogeneity of inorganic matter decreases in direct proportion to the increase in complexity of substratums. When a level of complexity is reached that corresponds to the average between the most simple and the most complex substrative elements with which medical science deals, the method of drawing inferences from an analysis of the substratum ceases to furnish integrable data. In other words, the empirical data that analysis collects can no longer be related in an exact manner to other data. This is because the homogeneity of the substratum has diminished to such an extent that the probability of any inference is lowered to a 50/50 average.

At this juncture an outlook confined to the causal and analytic mode of observation considers that science ends and empirical techniques take over. However, by drawing out and applying the implications of Rule 3, what appeared to be an impenetrable methodological wall is revealed as the threshold to description of the world of dynamic phenomena. The decrease of substrative homogeneity is always paralleled by an increase of duration and apparent stability, and hence of the significance and ease of observation of functions. The conclusion is that to achieve a logically stringent and consistently systematized description of all positive phenomena, the inductive and synthetic method can and must step in at the point where the causal and analytic mode no longer furnishes integrable data.

Traditional Chinese medicine has consistently relied upon inductive and synthetic method; consequently it did not develop any anatomy worth speaking of, has known no histology or biochemistry, and instead has evolved organic energetics, a number of interrelated, highly consistent physiological subdisciplines such as orbisiconography (*tsang-hsiang*) and sinarteriology (*ching-luo*), pharmacodynamics (*pen-ts'ao*), and even a methodically imperfect yet fairly extensive climatology and immunology called phase energetics (*yün-ch'i*). These specifically Chinese disciplines are completed by the Chinese versions of all our clinical disciplines, with the exception of surgery of the organs, and implemented by diverse healing techniques.

THE THEORETICAL INSTRUMENTARIUM OF CHINESE MEDICINE

The crucial task of any inductive science is to determine and define the relationships between different functions. Since every relationship implies a direction, and since direction is equivalent to a quality, inductive science primarily aims at the qualitative definition of functions. To comply with the requirements of science in the narrow sense, such definitions must be given in unequivocal and universally significant terms. Consequently, the qualitative statements of traditional Chinese medicine are, as a rule, made with constant reference to conventional standards of value.

The principal and basic standards of value used in Chinese medicine and shared by all Chinese sciences are the polar combination *yin/yang* and the cycle of the Five Evolutive Phases (*wu-hsing*). The terms *yin* and *yang* originally designated topographical aspects—the shady and the sunny side of a mountain, or the southern and northern bank of a river, respectively. At the constitutive stage of Chinese science, during the second half of the first millenium B.C., they were adopted as designations for the polar aspects of interrelated phenomena. Hence, in modern terms, *yang* corresponds to all that is active, expansive, centrifugal, aggressive, competitive, negative, and *yin* implies all that is structive, substantive, contractive, centripetal, responsive, conservative, positive.

Classifying all phenomena by *yin* and *yang* furnishes a rough and ready picture as to which effects complete one another and which effects, on the contrary, are neutral toward one another. Effects neutral toward one another may coexist or simultaneously appear at a given effective position. Effects completing one another—complementary effects—are on the contrary diametrically opposed to one another; consequently they exclude one another and may not be perceived simultaneously at a given effective position.

For more subtle qualitative graduations, in medical literature the *yin* aspect may be graded into Shrinking Yin (*chüeh-yin*), Minor Yin (*shao-yin*), and Major Yin (*t'ai-yin*), and the *yang* aspect into Minor Yang (*shao-yang*), Resplendent Yang (*yang-ming*), and Major Yang (*t'ai-yang*), thus describing a six-partitional cycle of graduated polar opposites.

A still more perfect graduation is achieved by the complementary use of the cycle of the Five Evolutive Phases. Four of the Five Evolutive Phases mark four critical phases in any evolutive (i.e., biological, physiological, meteorological) cycle, *viz.* potential activity (*Wood*), actual activity (*Fire*), potential structivity[1] (*Metal*), actual structivity (*Water*). The fifth Evolutive Phase (*Earth*) stands for neutral indifferentiation, or for what empirically produces the same impression, the transitions between phases of specific quality. The cycle of the Five Evolutive Phases likewise had gained systematic significance throughout the Chinese sciences since their beginnings in the middle of the first millenium B.C.

In Chinese medicine, the utmost precision in the evaluation of functions is made possible by (a) systematic derivations and combinations of the basic quality standards just described—e.g., *yin* in *yin*, *yin* in *yang*, *yang* in *yin*; *yin* of the first Evolutive Phase, *yang* of the first Evolutive Phase, *yin* of the second Evolutive Phase, etc., and then first Evolutive Phase of the first Evolutive Phase, second Evolutive Phase of the first Evolutive Phase, etc.—and (b) establishing systems of technical correspondences in the terms of these basic quality standards. The most widely applied and best known of these technical correspondences are those of *orbisiconography*, describing the interaction of the functional orbs of the organism; of *sinarteriology*, dealing with the interdependence of physiological signs, pathological symptoms, and therapeutic measures perceptible at or applicable to the body surface; and of *phase energetics*, postulating criteria for determining the influence of cosmic (i.e., meteorological, immunological) functions on the functions of the organisms.

These technical correspondences in turn constitute the theoretical framework of all applied and clinical disciplines of Chinese medicine, of which we must at least mention *pharmacotherapy* (*pen-ts'ao*)—i.e., the administration of vegetable, animal, and mineral drugs—and *acu-moxi-therapy* (*chen-chiu*)—i.e., the application of needles or cauters to sensitive spots at the body surface. And, of course, all the specialties that Western medicine today shows, with the notable exception of surgery of the organs, also developed in China.

THE PRACTICAL EFFECTIVENESS OF CHINESE MEDICINE

Having reviewed the theoretical and methodological background of Chinese

---

1 "To struct," "structive," "structivity," superseding the epistemologically incorrect terms "to react," "reactive," "reactivity," are the terms used for the substantive, positive, concretive *yin* aspect.

medicine, it is possible to reflect on how it meets the practical demands of medicine as we define them today.

To apply specific remedies, to rationally diagnose disease, seems to be the absolute minimum definition for scientific medicine. Chinese medicine, there can be no doubt, is capable of furnishing detailed and rational[2] diagnoses. Western physicians may disparagingly compare the simple means by which Chinese doctors may arrive at a diagnosis to the elaborate tests by which they strive for a precise assessment of causes. But the Chinese physician is interested in the present functions and actual symptoms of his patient. His four diagnostic methods (*szu-chen*)—inspection, interrogation, auscultation/olfaction, and palpation—aim for a complete appraisal of the momentary functional situation of the patient. Since the data he looks for are directly open to the senses, the Chinese diagnostician's job consists in their rational appraisal by applying the inductive method and its qualitative standards. The fact apparently so difficult to grasp is that because of their epistemological complementarity, Chinese and Western medicines, without one being basically inferior to the other, cannot and do not produce results mutually identical.

The strengths of Chinese medicine are:

1. The diagnosis and treatment of diseases that are manifest essentially through symptoms—i.e., irregularities of function without as-yet concomitant alterations of the substratum. Against a vast number of disturbances Western medicine can only offer unspecific treatment, since no specific organic disorder can be diagnosed, while Chinese medicine, keyed to the observation of functions, has differentiated symptoms and a specific therapy.

2. The diagnosis and treatment of so-called chronodemic (*shih-ch'i*) diseases. A number of diseases which flare up simultaneously over vast territories are, according to Western medicine, probably caused by virus. But they are explained in Chinese theory as deficiencies or redundancies of energy in certain orbs, conditioned by the momentary immunological situation.

3. The early diagnosis and prevention of organic disease. There is general agreement that serious organic diseases such as cardiac failure, diabetes, or cancer are preceded by stages of growing functional disorders. If they are given a specific diagnosis and treatment, they can be prevented from entering the organic stage which, in the opinion of Chinese doctors, represents an advanced if not terminal stage of every disease.

By contradistinction, the strength of Western medicine resides in:

1. The diagnosis and treatment of accidental or sudden organic disease. Organic damage due to sudden accidents or organic disorders with imprecise symptoms in the eyes of traditional Chinese physicians—e.g., an advanced tubal pregnancy—may be completely corrected by modern surgery.

---

2 "Rational" here meaning, of course, that logical connections are established between the symptoms perceived and the factors that may have brought on these symptoms.

2. The causal diagnosis, prevention, and treatment of disease favored by the physical milieu. The hygiene based on the findings of bacteriology and virulogy today has, of course, also been accepted by Chinese doctors.

3. The diagnosis and treatment of serious organic disease. If, due to negligence of the patient or incompetence of the doctor, diseases like cancer have developed into manifest organic disease, the more radical therapeutic measures of Western medicine may give better results.

By reflecting upon what has been said on the intellectual impulses actuating the development of Chinese medicine, it is now easy to see the reasons why Chinese medicine to this day has not attained the status of a full-fledged science in the narrow sense of the term. The classical Chinese medical theories were put into written form at very nearly the same time that in Asia Minor the *Corpus hippocraticum* was constituted—that is, during the 3rd century B.C. But the ease of observation of the functional phenomena in which Chinese medicine was primarily interested led to a greater wealth of positive empirical data upon which a general medical theory could be founded. Western medicine did not reach a comparable stage of theoretical stringency and systematic cohesion until the second half of the 19th century, when complex technical instruments for analyzing the substratum became available. The core of Chinese theories was cast in exact terms and was susceptible to as little later "improvement" as the theorem of Pythagoras. Of course, they had to be completed in accessory details, and their practical application and interpretation have occupied the minds of Chinese doctors to our day.

The relative ease of observation of functions in Chinese medicine led to a sensibly better ratio between therapeutic efforts and curative effects than could ever be achieved by the causal Western medicine. Yet this immediate practical advantage engendered two drawbacks that were perhaps decisive in keeping Chinese medicine at the level of a very highly developed technique, but never letting it pass over the threshold of a science in its own right.

1. Before its confrontation with Western science, and even today, the relatively high efficiency of its measures lets Chinese medicine perceive much less keenly the basic limitations of its therapeutic scope.

2. The relatively greater simplicity and stringency of its theoretical framework meant that run-of-the-mill Chinese practitioners could achieve fair results with a much smaller investment of time and talent than their Western colleagues. These lower requirements, and the ensuing intellectual mediocrity of the average Chinese medical practitioner, were reflected in the correspondingly lower social status of Chinese doctors.

THE SOCIAL STATUS OF THE CHINESE HEALER

Throughout Chinese history, the social status and influence of the physician were essentially determined by the rank assigned him in the Confucian social pyramid, and by the degree of social and psychological independence he succeeded in attaining through affiliation to Taoist philosophy and methods.

During the first Han dynasty (2nd century B.C.) Confucianism had become established as the political orthodoxy of the Chinese state, and from then up to 1912 it never ceased to shape the political order of Chinese society and the policies of its government after the ideals of its founders. The central and very often the only concern of Confucian philosophy was social ethics, the relation of the individual to society. Every quality, skill, or activity that contributed to the cohesion and boon of society was considered morally good (*shan*), and the individual thus endowed deserved the estimation (*kuei*) of his fellowmen. The social hierarchy resulting from the application of this reasonable precept placed the official literatus and the tiller of the soil in the two highest ranks of society, and put the soldier and the merchant in the two bottom positions. Medical men were considered to be technicians (*shu-shih*), and consequently, together with artists, engineers, craftsmen, and skilled laborers of all sorts, were assigned to the middle ranks of society. This intermediate position gave medical men wide latitude for professional and social development. Depending upon their education, skill, and inherited means, they could mingle with all classes of society, practicing medicine only occasionally and as a sideline, or making it their profession.

In numerically few cases, especially since the T'ang and Sung (8th century) dynasties, physicians could rise to official rank in the central administration. There is no case on record of anyone gaining the confidence of the emperor or one of his ministers because of his medical skill, but men of learning who occupied high positions might take a truly scientific interest in medicine. The most prominent examples are the poet and statesman Su Tung-p'o and his contemporary Shen Kua, who compiled a critical collection of prescriptions (*liang-fang*). Yet proficiency in medicine hardly ever solely procured a man official honors, let alone historical celebrity. Men like Chang Chung-ching (c. 150–219), the author of the *Shang-han tsa-ping lun*, and Li Shih-chen (1518–1593), the author of the Great Pharmacopeia *Pen-ts'ao kang-mu*, are very rare exceptions to this rule.

The Confucian social philosophy never offered much encouragement to explorers of the individual psyche, or of surrounding nature. Taoism amply filled this gap. Taoism represented the complementary philosophy to Confucianism, taking care of the private needs of the Chinese mind, its desire for individual salvation and for control over the forces of nature. Taoism, and especially its more popular form, Didactic Taoism (*tao-chiao*) favored an attitude of inquiry into the causes, but of receptive observation of recondite agents of sensuous phenomena. The similarity of style and terminology between Taoist and medical texts is no accident, nor is the fact that many of the early compilers of medical classics were even better known as Taoist adepts—e.g., Huang-fu Mi, Ko Hung, T'ao Hung-ching, and Sun Szu-mo. The reputation of being a Master of the Tao (*tao-shih*), at least up to the T'ang (9th century) and perhaps well into the Sung era (10th to 13th centuries), carried with it a strong flavor of otherworldliness and a reminiscence of priestly or shamanistic functions. Consequently, a medical man who was a *tao-shih,* or at least succeeded in giving himself the air of a *tao-shih,* could transcend the barriers of the Confucian society. His absorption in studies that otherwise would have been considered trivial and of no consequence was condoned.

These conditions changed gradually, parallel to the consolidation of the Confucian administration. Up to the 6th century A.D. all traditions were transmitted from master to disciple, and the only way to become a doctor was to apprentice oneself to a practicing physician. Then under the T'ang, first attempts were made to set up a regular medical school at the capital. From the Sung period, the Great Medical Office (*t'ai-i-chü*) became a permanent institution, receiving some 300 medical students; and the academy-trained physicians inherited some of the prestige, but not the social independence, of the Taoist practitioners. It is still hard to gauge the effect of these institutions on the situation throughout the country. Very probably it improved only slightly. Most of the graduates of the Medical Office stayed on at the capital, to be delegated only temporarily to the provinces.

For to the transmission and continuous evolution of Chinese medical science, its institutionalization and integration into the Confucian administration was a doubtful benefit. For a while the concentration at the capital of hitherto dispersed medical traditions led to a critical reappraisal of their accumulated data, and gave powerful impulse to systematic clarification of their theories. But in the long run the wealth of neatly ordered knowledge, together with the disparaging attitude of the Confucianists toward the observation of nature, paralyzed further empirical research in the medical disciplines. The qualitative decline of Chinese medical science, and with it the social downgrading of its practitioners, began under the Yüan in the 14th century. It continued under the Ming, and became rife by the middle of the Ch'ing era—i.e., since the end of the 18th century. And to all evidence traditional Chinese medicine, despite strong efforts during the past three decades to revive its procedures, has to this day not recovered from the methodological sterilization it suffered as a consequence of its marriage with Confucianism.

HISTORICAL DEVELOPMENT

It is to be supposed that an oral medical tradition had existed in China from at least the second millenium B.C. Only thus can the high degree of sophistication of the first record of medical theory, the *Huang-ti nei-ching* (Inner Classic of the Yellow Sovereign), be explained. It is safe to assume that many parts of today's version of this text were compiled not later than the 3rd century B.C. In them we find the essence of the orbisiconographic and sinarteriological theories valid to this day, as well as developments on the therapy by means of needles, moxas, and drugs. The rational sobriety of this book is underscored by the fact that it contains nothing that can be construed as an allusion to religious or magical procedures.

The documents of the Han dynasty—which extended roughly from 200 B.C. to 200 A.D.—reflect an increased awareness of problems of public welfare and hygiene, as is evidenced by decrees on sweeping public streets, on prophylactic examinations, and on the building of public nursing homes and of public toilets in some cities. Historians of Chinese medicine formerly quoted the *Chou-li* (*Rites of the Chou Dynasty*), one of the Confucian classics, as the first evidence of public awareness of problems of hygiene and sanitation. Yet today there is general agreement among scholars that this text does not reproduce the historical organization at the Chou court, but was written as the theoretical blueprint for ideal organization of a Confucian administration. And indeed, not a few of the organizational reforms of Chinese rulers were prompted by the desire to reenact the ideas of the *Chou-li*.

The outstanding medical figure of the Han period was Chang Chung-ching, who lived from about 150 to 219. His *Shang-han tsa-ping lun* (*Treatises on Cold Noisome and Other Diseases*) may be called the first clinical manual in Chinese medical literature. In it he made extensive use of the terminology introduced by the *Huang-ti nei-ching su-wen*, yet sometimes assigned different values to its standards of quality. This fact became a source of embarrassment to Sung- and Ming-period commentators, who believed it was their duty to gloss over apparent differences between two equally classical texts. From this we may deduce that during his lifetime the tradition of the *Su-wen* had not yet become established in every detail. However that may be, Chang Chung-ching furnished 397 rules bearing on diagnosis and therapy, and 379 drug prescriptions. Among the practical items was the use of emetics and enemas against poisonings, and instructions on how to apply artificial respiration to drowned persons. The *Shang-han tsa-ping lun* became the classic text on clinical medicine throughout the sphere of Chinese culture.

Of the physicians at the end of the second Han era, we should also mention Hua T'uo, who was probably a contemporary of Galen. If one relies on the accounts of his life in official sources, he may have been the first and only Chinese doctor to attempt and succeed at surgical cures of acute organic disorders. A treatise on therapeutic gymnastics was also attributed to him; but the *Chung-tsang-ching* (*Treasure-House* Classic) today bearing his name is certainly of later date. Although his surgical feats, embellished in the popular *San-kuo yen-i*, were to evoke the wonderment of all later generations, he would have preferred to be considered a literary man. He was put to death, according to the official sources, because of his reluctance to serve the Lord protector Ts'ao T'ao. According to the popular version, he was executed because his proposal to trepanate Ts'ao T'ao's skull was construed as an attempt to assassinate the usurper.

At this juncture two classical texts by anonymous authors must be discussed, the *Nan-ching* and the *Shen-nung pen-ts'ao-ching*. The Chinese term *nan* means "difficulty, difficult issue, objection." Hence the *Nan-ching* purports to contain the replies given to 81 difficult problems raised by the yellow Sovereign of hoary antiquity and not solved in the *Nei-ching*. The terminology and some rather analytical developments in today's text of this book suggest that it was, at the earliest, compiled during the second Han era, and may have been written as late as the 4th century A.D. The *Shen-nung pen-ts'ao-ching* (*Classic Pharmacopeia of the Divine Husbandman*), attributed to the legendary patron of agriculture, was probably written in the same period. It was a systematic inventory, according to the criteria set forth in the *Nei-ching*, of 347 drugs, including mercury compounds. These drugs were given with information on the degree of their toxicity, their occurrence, preparation, indications, and contraindications.

The political chaos following the collapse of the Han empire had no adverse repercussions on the evolution of medicine. Consequently, the 3rd century saw a number of fundamental texts appear. The historian and medical author Huang-fu Mi (215–282) compiled the *Chen-chiu chia-i ching* (*Systematic Classic on Acu-Moxi-Therapy*), a book which essentially consists of the critical reproduction of all passages of the *Huang-ti nei-ching* dealing with sinarteriology, acupuncture, and moxibustion. Because of its consistency, terminological precision, and systematic transparence, this text for centuries superseded and displaced the original *Ling-shu ching* from which it had first been culled. Wang Shu-ho (c. 265–316) re-edited the text of the *Shang-han tsa-ping lun* and also became famous for his lucid and detailed book on pulse diagnosis, the *Mo-ching* (*Classic of the Pulse*). This first monograph on the subject became the point of reference for all later investigations of this theme and, in the course of the 10th century, even influenced Arabic medicine.

For clarity's sake we must renounce discussing all of the treatises and booklets that in many details enhanced the tradition of Chinese medicine between the 4th and 8th centuries. But we have to mention the *Chu-ping yüan-hou lun* (*Origins and Symptoms of All Diseases*), an elaborate pathognostic compendium giving the differential diagnoses and therapeutic prospects for 1,720 diseases. This work by Ch'ao Yüan-fang, a professor at the Imperial Medical Academy, was completed in 610. It gave very circumstantial descriptions of smallpox, bubonic plague, measles, dysentery, and phthisis. The earliest corollary version of the *Nei-ching*, entitled *Huang-ti nei-ching t'ai-su*, also dates from this period. A significant fragment of this text has come down to us through a manuscript conserved in Japan.

At the beginning of the T'ang era, the time had come for a first inventory of therapeutic techniques and prescriptions. This was produced by Sun Szu-mo, born in 581, who was equally famous as a Taoist adept, alchemist, and physician. The two collections today transmitted under his name, the *Ch'ien-chin yao-fang* and the *Ch'ien-chin i-fang* (*Essential Prescriptions Worth a Thousand* [*Pieces of Gold*] and *Accessory Prescriptions Worth a Thousand*), com-

prise a number of drugs that had quite recently been introduced as a consequence of the intensive commercial exchange with India, Persia, and the
Arab countries. With more than 10,000 items, these texts did not neglect
any practical aspect of medicine. Acupuncture and obstetrics, respiratory
gymnastics and dietetics, the preparation of drugs, medical ethics, and
many other subjects were recorded. Another manual for practicing physicians,
entitled *Wai-t'ai pi-yao* (*Hermetic Essentials from the Outer Terrace*) was completed
in 750 by Wang T'ao. Taking up again the differential descriptions and the
terminology set forth in the *Chu-ping yüan-hou lun*, it furnished prescriptions
and therapeutic advice for the treatment of 1,104 diseases or syndromes.

The definitive edition of the *Nei-ching su-wen* (*Candid Questions on the Inner
Classic of the Yellow Sovereign*)—i.e., henceforth the first part of the *Nei-ching*—
was produced in 762 by Wang Ping. In the course of the full millenium
that had elapsed since its compilation, the text of the *Huang-ti nei-ching*
had become obscure and contradictory in many places. Wang Ping—
according to most sources an official of medium rank at the Court of Imperial
Carriages, a Taoist adept and uncommon connoisseur of Taoist and medical
literature—presented an exceptionally complete version of the *Nei-ching
su-wen*. After the example of the Confucian classics, he added a running
commentary on the entire text. Since then, but definitely since its revision
and special approval by the Bureau for Editing Medical Treatises set up
in 1057, this text of the *Su-wen* completely displaced all other versions of
the first part of the *Nei-ching*.

Wang Ping's work is of interest for two reasons: (1) By adding an authoritative commentary to the *Nei-ching su-wen*, he not only revived interest in
this basic and venerable text, but also established a self-conscious classical
tradition. None of the medical texts before his time, and very few additional
ones in the future, were distinguished by a commentary. (2) Wang Ping,
in the preface to his edition, says that he was prompted in his work by being
confided with an exceptionally clear and readable secret copy of the *Su-wen*
by his Taoist teacher. A comparison between his edition of the text and
inventories and fragments of former editions reveals that Wang Ping, un-
wittingly or intentionally, incorporated the whole development on phase
energetics (*yün-ch'i*), thus increasing the text by at least one third of its previous volume, and adding an entirely new discipline to the curriculum of
Chinese medical theory.

In the histories of the Sui and T'ang dynasties, repeated mention was
made of an institution called *T'ai-i-shu*—Great Medical Bureau under the
T'ang—which had teaching facilities and a garden for raising medicinal
plants. However, the small staff of this Bureau and its temporary neglect
under some rulers suggests that this institution was solely intended to supply
the needs of the Court. This limitation must not have existed for the Great
Medical Office (*T'ai-i-chü*) established in 1078 under the Sung dynasty.
The greatly enlarged staff; separate departments for the compilation,

collation, editing, and publication of medical texts; and permanent training facilities for some 300 students, with annual examinations and grading of students and staff, indicate that an institutionalization and standardization of medical science throughout the empire was intended. The disciplines taught there are separately enumerated as: (1) general inner medicine (*lit.*, prescriptions and treatments for adults); (2) exogenous fever diseases (*feng-k'o*); (3) general pediatrics (*lit.*, prescriptions and treatments for infants; (4) ophthalmology; (5) ulcers and swellings; (6) obstetrics; (7) oto-odonto-laryngology; (8) acupuncture and moxibustion; (9) surgery and hermetic theories. As has been explained, this more intensive promotion of medical studies by the state at first brought on an effervescence of theoretical invention and a corresponding boom in publications.

In 980, official compilers had completed the *T'ai-p'ing sheng-hui fang* (*Prescriptions of Exemplary Indulgence of the T'ai-p'ing Era*), the first of a whole line of similar collections of prescriptions and cases to be published under the auspices of this and the following dynasties. Among the books of general theory, the contribution of Ch'en Yen, *San-yin chi i ping-cheng fang-lun* (*Practical Discussions on How the Three Kinds of Pathological Agents Lead to Every Disease*), perhaps published in 1161, must be mentioned. Ch'en, developing the theories of Chang Chung-ching of the Han era, held that any disease may be traced to one of three inductive relationships: external, internal, and neutral. His work has influenced medical thinking in China up to our day. In 1085, Ch'ien I completed *Hsiao-erh yao-cheng chih-chüeh* (*Secret Precepts Set Forth on the Prescriptions and Symptoms Applying to Infants*), which became the standard textbook of pediatrics, and in which effective remedies against measles were described.

Sinarteriological theory was checked against experience, and new aids to teaching acupuncture were produced, when in 1026 Wang Wei-i completed life-size bronze models for practicing the detection of the sensitive points. He then set forth their topology in the *T'ung-jen shu-hsüeh chen-chiu t'u-ching* (*Illustrated Classic on Acu-Moxi-Therapy Based on the* Foramina inductoria *of the Bronze Figure*). A comprehensive book on all aspects of gynecology, the *Fu-jen ta-ch'üan liang-fang* (*The Woman's Compendium with Wholesome Prescriptions*) was compiled from ancient sources in 1237 by Ch'en Tzu-ming.

A particularly brilliant accomplishment of the official medical compilers were the pharmacopeias of the Sung era, the first of which appeared in 973. In 1108 the first edition, and in 1116 the revised edition of the *Ching-shih cheng-lei pei-chi* [resp. *pei-yung*] *pen-ts'ao* (*Practical and Critically Systematized Pharmacopeia* [*Incorporating Material from the*] *Classical and Historical Texts*) was published. This compilation brought together all pharmacological data that had been transmitted in the traditional pharmacological and medical texts, as well as by Confucion, Taoist, and Buddhist authors and in the histories. The beautifully printed text is illustrated with woodcuts considered to be among the finest examples of Sung printing art. Also among the remarkable medical works of the Sung era, the *Hsi-yüan lu* (*Catalogue for Rectifying Injustices*) by Sung Tz'u was published in 1247. For many centuries it was the standard reference book of forensic medicine.

During the 13th and 14th centuries, four distinctive medical doctrines crystalized within the hitherto fairly uniform tradition. This splitting up had no doubt been favored by the extension of medical training and by the rapid dissemination of medical texts through printing, and perhaps also by the fact that speculation had started to outbalance empirical data. Each of these doctrines was based upon the teachings of a physician famous in his time. The first, Liu Wan-su (c. 1120–1200), held the opinion that any energetic configuration is prone to "ignite"—i.e., to produce fever spontaneously or by the wrong application of remedies. Thus he recommended the frequent administration of refreshing and cooling drugs, and his followers became known as the *Han-liang-p'ai* (*School of Cold and Cool* [*Prescriptions*]). Secondly, Chang Tzu-ho (1156–1228), a disciple of Liu Wan-su, expatiated on the advantages and methods of purging. He became the patron of the *Kung-hsia-p'ai* (Purgatory School).

The third doctrine was founded by Li Tung-yüan (1180–1251), one of the few medical figures who succeeded in captivating popular imagination with the airs of a Taoist adept. He considered the roboration of the central orbs (i.e., of the *orbes lienalis et stomachi*) basic to any curative measure. Later advocates of this idea came to be known as the *Pu-t'u-p'ai* (School Strengthening the Evolutive Phase Earth; "Evolutive Phase Earth" stands for the conventional quality of the *orbes lienalis et stomachi*). The fourth doctrine advocated by the *Tzu-yin–p'ai* (School of Bolstering Up the Yin) traced its origin back to Chu Tan-hsi, who was also a Taoist adept. Chu Tan-hsi (1281–1358) came from South China, and recommended to the agile Southern Chinese that they must not spend too freely the energy potential received at birth.

During the following centuries under the Ming and Ch'ing dynasties, the administration of Chinese medicine continued in the ruts fixed under the Sung and Yüan dynasties, with the slow but continuous deterioration of empirical verification of the venerable theories. This qualitative decline did not prevent outstanding achievements such as the work of Li Shih-chen (1518–1593) on pharmacology and on the iconography of the pulse. Li Shih-chen had been trained by his father, a practicing physician. After several unsuccessful tries at an official career, he made his living from modest sinecures and from practicing medicine. His scientific leanings led him to check and revise the traditional pulse lore. He wrote *Pin-hu mo-hsüeh* (*Pulse Studies of* [*Master*] *Pin-hu*), *Chi-ching pa-mo k'ao* (*Investigations of the Eight Pulses* [*Corresponding to the*] *Paracardinales*), and *Mo-chüeh k'ao-cheng* (*Critical Investigations of Some Traditional Pulse Theories*). But his everlasting fame rests upon his *Pen-ts'ao kang-mu* (*Standard Inventory of Pharmacology*), a monumental collection bringing together the complete pharmacological knowledge of

Chinese medicine, and containing the detailed characteristics of 1,892 drugs and more than 10,000 prescriptions. This book was completed in 1578, after twenty-six years of research and compilation in which three of his sons and one of his disciples also took part. Because of its exceptionally high standards of scholarship, this work is to our day indispensable for research into the pharmacological traditions of China.

CHINESE MEDICINE TODAY

What follows is recent history. Some physicians of the Ch'ing era attained fame by their practice, but they did not leave any lasting impression upon the inner structure of Chinese medicine. And of course they could not halt its general decline. It is to be hoped that such will not be the verdict of future historians on the evolution of traditional Chinese medicine during the 20th century. As a consequence of the drive initiated by the Chinese government during the 1950s to collect and reassess the medical heritage of China, conditions of research into the tradition have dramatically improved. Besides new critical editions of all classical texts, a number of ancient collections unavailable for centuries have been reprinted. Moreover, before and after the All-China Congress on Teaching Materials of Traditional Chinese Medicine held in 1963, quite good modern textbooks have been compiled in which all the essentials of theory and practice are set forth with clarity.

This will not discharge us or the Chinese from serious efforts to reinterpret the message of the ancient theories in modern terms. Such reinterpretation cannot consist in the primitive attempt to stick new Western analytical terms on the ancient synthetic terms of Chinese medicine—by translating *ch'i* "air," or "breath"—but must instead start from an integral comprehension of the Chinese theories within their original logical and historical setting.[3] Only in this way may a seamless transition between Chinese and Western medicine be achieved, confirming the positive results of each system, yet ameliorating once and for all the intellectual antagonism that today still opposes them.

3 A number of examples of how this can be done are given in my book, *The Theoretical Foundations of Chinese Medicine* (Massachusetts Institute of Technology Press, 1974).

PART II

The Structure and Character of Cosmopolitan Medicine

D ESPITE the example of a few scholars who have worked cross-culturally, medical historians and sociologists have been overwhelmingly concerned with European and American institutions. This pattern has resulted from the accessibility of data and research opportunities, but it has been reinforced by an ethnocentric view of science.

Western scholars often assume that the only significant ideas and events for the history of science occurred in Europe. In the introduction to a collection of essays by anthropologists and philosophers on the nature of rationality, we read, "Only in advanced western societies is the detached and systematic approach to social (and perhaps also to natural) phenomena at all commonly adopted—or adoptable. It is in this society that the dilemma of how to understand the world arises as an intellectual problem . . ." (Wilson 1971: xiii). The author is a sociologist, but he might have been a philosopher or historian of science. Like bureaucrats who write the specifications for a new job so that a cousin will be the only qualified applicant, they define science so that only the Greek tradition will qualify.

Joseph Needham once gathered a number of ethnocentric statements by fellow historians, among them A. C. Crombie's assertion that the "technical achievements" of Chinese and Indian societies lacked "the essential elements of science," for "it was the Greeks who invented natural science as we know it" (Needham 1963:140). On the contrary, Needham argued, Chinese traditions in some fields of knowledge were more advanced than those of Greece, and although modern science originated in Europe, it utilized Hindu–Arabic notation, trigonometry, and other knowledge borrowed from Asia. To describe the relationship of modern science to the traditional civilizations, Needham paraphrased the revolutionary Cuban slogan, "Western science, no, . . . modern universal science, yes." As we improve our knowledge of the Asian medical systems, we will learn to recognize the ethnocentric attitude toward Western science in previous studies of cosmopolitan medicine.

The essays in this section illustrate current approaches to the social structure and research traditions of cosmopolitan medicine. The diagrams and tables that accompany Mark Field's essay help us to think about differentiated bureaucratic systems that serve enormous populations in modern nation-states—systems that compete with other bureaucratic structures for capital, manpower, and other "inputs." Field's categories indicate the parameters for comparing the scale, organization, cost, and performance of these systems, and his data are suggestive: the lack of autonomous professional associations in Russia, the large proportion of women physicians, the ratio of doctors to population, the use of feldshers in rural areas, and the delivery of medical care as a public service to all segments of the population contrast sharply to the American system.

I want to draw attention to one aspect of the differences between the Soviet and the American medical systems that Field touches on when, for example, he mentions how an Indian bureaucrat once compared the utility of these systems as models for health planning in India. The ways that different medical systems serve as models for policy-makers are important phenomena for research on cosmopolitan medical institutions. The primary model for India has been the English system, and contacts with English and American medicine have in the past been more influential than contacts with Soviet medicine; yet cosmopolitan medicine in India is distinctly Indian, for it has evolved in a social system and among cultural traditions different from those of other countries. New research should show us how this happens, so that we can compare the evolution of cosmopolitan medicine in India with that of other countries.

In another section of this volume Dr. Yasuo Otsuka writes that the German system served as a model for Japan in the late nineteenth century (at the same time, incidentally, that the Johns Hopkins University medical school led reforms in the United States by following the German model). This use of models indicates a way that scientific progress and structural innovation in one cosmopolitan medical system affects other systems. The real significance of Chinese propaganda in recent years about acupuncture and barefoot doctors is not that other societies will greatly benefit by borrowing therapeutic practices from traditional Chinese medicine, but that the massive utilization of briefly-trained personnel and of indigenous therapies provides a new model for Asian and African countries that seek with limited resources to modernize their medical systems.

The social power of cosmopolitan medicine is justified by the ability of its practitioners to use knowledge created by new research, Renée Fox describes the value orientation of research in cosmopolitan medicine, and contrasts the ethos of this work with the world-view of "traditional Bantu African medical thought." The scientific ethos that she describes is one of the shores of light toward which liberal thinkers hope the human spirit strives. When she refers to experiments on human subjects by Nazi physicians, however, I think involuntarily of secret medical research on chemical and biological warfare during the period that she calls a golden age of research in the United States. And, going on to recall accounts of research that uses prisoners and other institutionalized subjects in the United States, I imagine how Nazi doctors might have described their work as secular, rational, universalistic, probabilistic, and so on, using the very categories Fox enumerates for work of a different character.

Because Renée Fox analyzes the ethic of medical research, her essay provokes questions about the whole relationship between the organization of professional work and humane values. What are we to make of the fact that excellent scientists, engineers, and physicians have performed with alacrity in fascist, communist, and liberal democratic states, not only to save lives or improve material well-being, but to invent and produce agents of biological warfare, bombs, and guided missiles? Is the professionalization of scientific research a mode of moral progress, or is it merely a consequence of technological advances and of changes in the scale and organization of society? The poise with which Fox writes shows that she is not a stranger to the dark thoughts these questions generate. Her poise illustrates the attitude of mind that she calls "detached concern," and her essay reminds us that cosmopolitan medicine is a force in modern history not only because it is technologically effective, but also because its scientific institutions and practitioners exemplify ideals of the moral order.

Charles Leslie

Literature Cited

Needham, Joseph
    1963 "Poverties and Triumphs of the Chinese Scientific Tradition," in A. C. Combie, ed., *Scientific Change*. New York: Basic Books.
Wilson, Bryan R.
    1971 *Rationality*. New York: Harper and Row, Harper Torchbooks.

The Modern Medical System:
the Soviet Variant

MARK G. FIELD

THE MEDICAL SYSTEM[1]

For any professional to provide his services to clients, certain elements of social organization must be present. There can be no doctor–patient relationship, in the sense of a fully differentiated medical system, unless the following structural features are present:

1. There must be a person identified as a physician who is available, motivated, and ready to provide services to patients.

2. The physician must have knowledge and techniques that the patient does not have (Freidson 1970). This specialized skill is acquired either through a special educational program or through experience, or both.

3. The physician's activities must be formally defined and sanctioned by the society, and particularly by its values. What the physician does must be recognized as consistent with social values and beliefs, and thus proper, legitimate, and desirable.

4. Terms must be arranged to exchange the time and services of the physician for payment, either by the patient, an insurance fund, or a governmental or other agency. At the same time, economic resources must also be invested in hospitals, clinics, and other facilities.

The aggregate of persons and resources concerned primarily with medical care constitutes the medical system of a society in its static state. The performance of personnel in that system constitutes its dynamic aspect, and becomes a part of the total functional contribution of medicine to society. A society may, and often does, have more than one medical system, and they may well overlap each other, but it may be argued that the totality of such systems constitutes *the* medical system of that society, in contrast with other (non-medical) systems. The point I want to make now is that the medical system of modern society is characterized by a complex division of labor in which, for example, physicians constitute only a small minority of health personnel.

1 I have described the basic features of the medical system of modern society at length in two other essays (Field 1971a, 1973). The present section is an abbreviated version of that conceptual scheme.

Similarly, types of medical facilities have proliferated with the increased sophistication and complexity of medical instruments and techniques (Field 1970, 1971a).

The medical system is thus a specialized and differentiated subsystem of society. It is bounded and can be conceptually identified in the same way that one identifies the family and the economic, educational, or political systems (Miller 1965). The borders of the medical system may sometimes be fuzzy. For example, is the mother who nurses a sick child a member of that system? Is the American pharmacist who sells cosmetics as well as prescription drugs a health specialist? Nevertheless, the overall identity of the medical system vis-à-vis other systems in the society is not problematic. The problems it deals with have been called the five D's: death, disease, disability, discomfort, and dissatisfaction (White 1968).

Medical personnel cope with these health problems by performing six types of services, which I call the basic modalities of the medical system (Figure 1).

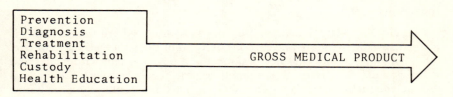

FIGURE 1. Modalities of the medical system.

The transactions that constitute the services of the medical system to cope with health problems are the manifest functions of the system. I call the aggregate of these services the Gross Medical Product. However, two other formal components are integral structural parts of the medical system: education and research.

The educational component is the totality of manpower, facilities, and resources invested in training medical personnel of all types (I exclude the elementary or secondary schools that provide a general education prior to professional or vocational medical training).

The research component is the aggregate of manpower, facilities, and resources invested in creating new knowledge and techniques relevant to health. The research component is primarily an elaboration and application, in the medical system, of generally available scientific knowledge and technology—e.g., the use of laser beams for eye surgery, or the application of computers for diagnostic and record-keeping purposes. Scientific knowledge is universally available and applicable, but the fact that it may originate in a society of one type may create problems of acceptability and compatibility for a society of another type. This is particularly important to cultural anthropologists, and I will return to this later.

Putting these elements together, I conceive a medical system as composed of educational and research components that train and equip, and a service component that produces a Gross Medical Product which addresses itself to society's health problems (Figure 2).

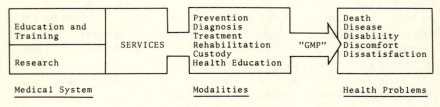

FIGURE 2. Components of the medical system.

The medical system is no more self-sufficient than the solo physician, and must be structurally supported in analogous ways, though I shall label them differently:

1. The medical system must not only be considered trustworthy, but is given a specific mandate and responsibility from the society. This mandate, often embodied in law and licenses, must also be congruent with values and belief systems. Society, so to speak, enters into a contract with the medical system and delivers it a charter. Such a charter is tantamount, in many instances, to a monopolistic license, and all that this implies, for the exclusion of other medical traditions and practitioners.

2. The medical system needs an input of knowledge and technology, an accumulated "state of the art." This state of the art, wherever a medical system is based on verifiable knowledge, excludes eternal truths or sacred revelations, since every aspect of it is open to challenge and change through research and experience. The scientific method has been shown to be a most effective way of dealing with health problems, and it claims universal validity —but it is primarily, though not exclusively, the product of Western culture, and it is identified with the West. These historical facts pose important problems for attempts to diffuse the scientific method to non-Western cultures, which have their own concepts, and traditional approaches to health problems grounded in their values.

It should be noted that scientific knowledge is the only input to the medical system that is intrinsically nonfinite. Knowledge once acquired, or technique once developed, are not diminished when they are used. Such knowledge, on the other hand, has wide implications regarding the use of finite resources such as manpower and funds.

3. The medical system depends on individuals who are specially motivated, screened, trained, tested, certified or licensed, and deployed within the occupational roles of the system. This is a scarce resource, since educated manpower in any society is finite, and other subsystems in the society compete

for it. Within limits, one society may import trained manpower from another society, but at any one time the supply of health manpower in the world is finite.

4. The medical system depends on economic resources to support health personnel, to purchase hospitals, clinics, medicines, and other equipment, and to pay running, maintenance, and capital costs. Society devotes a certain determinable percentage of its Gross National Product to medicine and health care, whether this allocation is a planned political administrative decision, as in the Soviet Union, or a more spontaneous mix of the use of tax monies and private expenditures affected by market mechanisms, as is the case in the United States. This allocation may be further analyzed by using two initial categories:

a. The percentage of the Gross National Product that goes to health, in comparison to other sectors of the society.
b. Within the health sector, the proportion of "allocated" economic resources that goes to different public and private services, and within these services to preventive, clinical, rehabilitative, and other purposes.

The same calculations can be used to describe the allocation of manpower. In both cases, the scarcity of resources increases competition for them by other, equally functionally significant, sectors. Using the schema already presented, I diagram the structural supports of the medical system as shown in Figure 3.

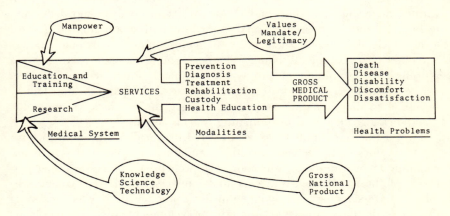

FIGURE 3. Structural supports of the medical system.

Thus my conceptual model yields a formal definition: *The medical system (or systems) of any society may be defined as a societal mechanism that transforms generalized inputs (manpower, mandate, knowledge, money) into specialized outputs in the form of medical services aimed at the health problems of society.*

The structure, the organization, the management, the internal integration of the health system play a critical role in the efficiency of transforming generalized resources into medical services. Since that organization is affected by the culture and the history of a society, medical systems vary the world over, and the transmissibility of the application of medical knowledge reflects fundamental differences of values, organizational and management forms, types of practitioners, and so on. For example, John Bryant points out that in Thailand, medical and nursing education follow the more advanced countries while the health ministry, quite separately, develops a system of medical care. The educational and medical care institutions function almost as separate subcultures, so that the product of one is often not well suited to serve the other. Bryant interprets this problem as a consequence of religious differences between Buddhist and Western traditions.

In the West, organizations have an administrative hierarchy with graded responsibilities and levels of supervision. There is a flow of policy or instructions from the top down, and a feedback of information on field experience from the bottom up. These principles, important to the effectiveness of a Western enterprise, may not work in a Buddhist society. The flow of information is almost exclusively from the patron to the client. There is a reluctance to criticize and confront another person. This harms the harmony of interpersonal relationships. Supervision is difficult, because it may involve confrontation and criticism. Thus essential elements of the organizational mechanism may be weak or missing, but this may be overlooked because on the surface the organization looks the same as its Western model. (Bryant 1969:79)

The medical system coexists with other subsystems of modern society, each with its own values, mandate, and legitimacy, its own body of knowledge and techniques and its own functional contribution to maintain the general level of societal functioning. Each subsystem must obtain a share of manpower and of the Gross National Product. Whether through deliberate planning or a pluralistic confrontation of supply and demand, every society allocates scarce resources to different subsystems in some kind of equilibrium. It may be useful to diagram these elements, to place the medical system in the macrosociological context of competing systems (Figure 4).

Two of the four inputs have been altered drastically in modern society: (a) the values of the society and the mandate of the medical system are changing to provide better and more comprehensive services to larger segments of the population, and eventually universal medical coverage; (b) science and technology are changing medical practices at an ever-increasing rate. The dramatic aspects of this latter development, such as open-heart surgery, are well known, but many other improvements cause great changes in medical practice, particularly in the large clinical centers.

As a result of these changes, the medical system seems to increase in size at a faster rate than most other sectors of modern society, with the possible exception of education. With increasing size and the growing scientific nature of medical practice, the system becomes more internally differentiated: specialization changes the roles of physicians and brings about a proliferation

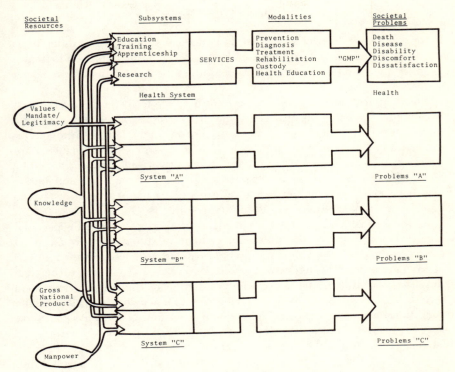

FIGURE 4. The medical system in the macrosociological context of competing systems.

in paramedical personnel (Magraw 1966; Rutstein 1967). As the health system becomes more scientific and differentiated, the care of the individual often becomes more impersonal and segmented (Field 1970, 1971a). This advanced division of medical labor, with its increasingly narrow and varied elements, potentially increases errors and communication failures within the system as well as adding to the alienation of the patient, who faces an often impersonal physician and a frightening bureaucratic system when his vulnerability and anxieties about illness are at their highest. The "medical" component seems to squeeze out the "pastoral" aspects of health care.

It is therefore not unlikely that a formal differentition between the specialist and the generalist may evolve among physicians, with the latter entrusted with the pastoral functions of medical care as well as the coordination and integration of specialized services (Field 1970). A similar phenomenon may be happening in developing societies, where the national or indigenous medical culture may claim to meet needs for pastoral care better than the foreign scientific import.

THE SOVIET MODEL

If we seek two industrial societies whose medical systems are as different as can be while remaining firmly grounded in the scientific approach to health problems, we can do no better than to contrast the American and the Soviet systems.

The American medical system was built by discrete accretions over almost two hundred years, with physicians and other professional curers operating mainly as private practitioners who evolved strong and relatively autonomous associations. Until recently, and still today to a large extent, medical care proceeds within a framework of private, voluntary arrangements. The public sector has traditionally been relegated to preventive medicine and public health, to people who either cannot afford private medical services or who deserve care on the basis of service to their country.

An ideological tenet of American medical practice is the essentially personal and private nature of the physician–patient relationship. Another tenet conceives the physician as an entrepreneur who nevertheless puts the interests of his patients above his own (Parsons 1951:428–479). These ideological simplifications did in fact reflect the orientation of the American medical system for a long time. Structural changes that would alter the working conditions, autonomy, status, and economic position of the physician have been vigorously opposed by the medical profession, particularly the American Medical Association. The primary arguments have been that such changes would destroy the privacy of the doctor–patient relationship, and would thus damage the scientific efficacy of medical practice. The success of the organized medical profession in maintaining and enhancing its social position gives it a practical monopoly in the formation of public policies regarding medicine.

It is instructive for Americans to look at Soviet medicine because it represents a radically different approach to health services for a large population. From an American perspective it also involves innovative devices for organizing, financing, and managing medical services. Furthermore, the Soviet health service may be more relevant to Asian medical systems than the American system. A former health minister for India told me once that American medicine was technologically well advanced but much too expensive for India, while the Soviet model was more germane.

When the Communist Party seized power in the fall of 1917, it inherited problems which threatened the country's stability for many years. Russia in 1917 was in the third year of a ruinous war; the Tsarist regime had left a heavy legacy of administrative ineptness and corruption; the economy was inefficient. In addition, the population had suffered a general decline in health, and epidemics were taking a frightful toll. Commenting on typhus, Lenin remarked tersely: "Comrades, either the lice destroy socialism or socialism destroys the lice" (Vinograd and Strashun 1947).

To create a health program, the Communist Party set out to radically alter the nature, status, and power of the medical profession. In spite of the auto-cratic nature of the Tsarist regime, the medical profession had evolved in Russia as it had in other European countries, and by the opening of the 20th century had achieved a relatively high degree of autonomy. The Society of Russian Physicians in Memory of N. I. Pirogov had looked forward to a change of regime as an opportunity to reshape the health system along more progressive lines, but it expected to remain, as a corporate body, in charge of these reforms. This conception of autonomy in professional matters was not consonant with the Communist *Weltanschauung*, and led to a confrontation soon after the seizure of power (Field 1960, 1972).

The Communist world-view claims to provide a comprehensive picture of society, and asserts that the medical profession is not and never can be "apolitical." It has always served the interests of the ruling class, and would help the exploited classes only so that workers could produce more for the benefit of capitalists. The task of the new (Soviet) regime was to make medicine serve the interests of the proletariat. It was to be "class medicine." In 1918 Khirin declared: "Workers and peasants must take into their hands the protection of health in the same way as they have seized all the political and economic power in the republic" (Gurevich 1947).

Although the regime had fairly well formulated ideas about what the medical profession must do in a socialist system, these ideas did not find a receptive audience among most physicians. The idea, for example, that physicians should give priority to the proletariat was held to contradict the ethical principle that a sick person deserves attention regardless of social status. The Bolsheviks replied that this was pure sham, since the physicians had always favored the upper classes. Another aspect that rankled the physicians was that they were to be demoted from authority over subordinate medical personnel. The physician was to be considered a "medical worker" on a par with or even ideologically inferior to the "medical proletariat," which it had formerly "exploited": nurses, feldshers, hospital orderlies, and so on.

The issue was joined over the alleged refusal of physicians to treat wounded revolutionaries, leading to the charge of "medical sabotage." The flavor of these accusations is contained in a book by Barsukov which gives examples of purported refusals to care for Bolsheviks, and using medical installations to hide "counter-revolutionaries." He quotes A. Okhapkina, who wrote about events in Moscow shortly after the Revolution:

They brought the wounded to the secondary school. ... In the school there were White wounded. I, myself, with difficulty, found the doctor in another room; he started to beat around the bush and to bare his teeth; knowing that we were Reds, he found a pretext to refuse to operate. I called some of our own people, ordered the doctor to go to the operation room, forced him to boil the instruments, asked the attendants to look after the wounded, put someone on duty, and then brought in the rest of the wounded. (Barsukov 1951:74)

The professional associations were dissolved, and the regime established its own medical trade unions that would do its bidding. The epitaph of the Pirogov Society conveys the irreconcilability of the two conceptions of medical practice:

Soviet public health historically was built and grew in the struggle against reactionary bourgeois medicine, among whom were the reactionary ideologists from the "Pirogovist" camp. . . . The ideologists of bourgeois medicine, emanating chiefly from the reactionary part of the Pirogovists, were hostile to the Soviet regime, not only rejected the term "Soviet medicine," but also rejected the very possibility of its existence.

The Pirogovists rejected the class character of medicine, endowing it with above-class (*nadklassnii*) elements. Standing on the idea of the solidity of the bourgeois order in society, not recognizing the dictatorship of the proletariat as a new world-historical type of proletarian democracy, Pirogovists opposed the idea that public health should be a state matter under the conditions of Soviet society. They felt that medicine should be autonomous, independent from the Soviet state, and that it must be turned in its entirety to the community, i.e., to the bourgeois Zemstvo self-government, with the leading role given to the medical corporation. (Barsukov 1951:27)

Abolition of the medical profession as a fairly autonomous social force was a *sine qua non* for the building of a new system of medical services, and a half-century of development permits us to draw some generalizations, as well as comparative data, on the nature and the performance of a national health service. Tables 1–7 at the end of this article provide some data on Soviet personnel and hospital resources and vital statistics compared with the American performance.

The Soviet health system represents a rational attempt to make medical care accessible to every citizen, despite scarce resources and the immensity of the task. From the regime's viewpoint the primary desideratum was functional, in that the medical system must address itself to the working and fighting capacity of its people—i.e., it must reduce the negative impact of morbidity and premature mortality, and the resultant devastatingly low life expectancy.

Furthermore, there was never any doubt about the monopoly enjoyed by the state to provide health services based on modern medical science. The Marxist doctrine required the medical system to conform to scientific principles by rooting out the "superstitions" of traditional medicine. Medical research was to be for the solution of immediate problems, rather than to achieve theoretical advances. Manpower inputs were to be centrally planned. Women were to serve as physicians, releasing men for the more technical occupations. At the present time about three-fourths of all practicing physicians are women, though the percentage is now declining (Field 1966, 1971b). The state was to finance the medical system with budgetary allocations made in full consideration of other needs. The fact that physicians were to be salaried meant that the state could determine with great accuracy what these costs would be.

The Soviet medical system is said to be governed by the following principles (Field 1967:42–48):

1. Public health and medical care are a responsibility of the state, and are provided as a public service.

2. All medical policies evolve within the framework of a single plan, integrated with the needs, commitments, policies, and programs of the regime.

3. Although the system is centralized and bureaucratized, in practice a fair amount of local administrative latitude is permitted. Health facilities are organized in tiers of increasing sophistication as one moves from local facilities to those that serve larger areas, up to those of national significance.

4. Personal medical services are available to the population at no direct cost at time of service. They are financed from taxation. The one major exception is drugs prescribed for outpatient use.

5. Preventive medicine stands in theory at the center of the Soviet system and is said to guide all activities of the health service.

6. The Marxist concept of the unity of theory and practice rejects the ideal of knowledge for its own sake. Medical research must be oriented toward the solution of practical problems such as the reduction of industrial absenteeism due to illness.

7. The efforts of medical personnel must be backstopped by voluntary and community efforts.

8. As long as medical services remain a scarce resource, those who perform the more important jobs must have priority over others.

Access to health services is provided through two networks of primary-care facilities: the territorial and the occupational network. In the first case, the individual is assigned to an outpatient facility on the basis of his residence. Four thousand persons (about 3,000 adults and 1,000 children) form a medical micro-district (*ushastok*). Primary care is given in an outpatient clinic that typically serves the population of ten micro-districts, called a medical district (*raion*). Two physicians and one pediatrician, plus one or two nurses, are usually directly and personally responsible for the population of one micro-district. They have office hours at the clinic, and also visit patients at home. Specialists are also available in the outpatient clinic, but they serve more than one micro-district. Several clinics are in turn affiliated with hospitals to which patients can be referred.

The occupational network operates on the same principle, except that individuals, who are usually industrial workers, are assigned to facilities maintained by their plant. In addition, a whole gamut of facilities are reserved for members of the Soviet political and cultural elite and their families. Access to these facilities is a perquisite of rank.

Private practice still exists, although frowned upon as the remnant of a bourgeois past. There are some polyclinics where, for a relatively modest fee a patient can have the services of a better consultant or specialist. As far as I know, there are no private medical (inpatient) facilities in the Soviet Union.

In this system the physician is trained at state expense, and works as a salaried state employee in state-owned facilities. Even the few who have a private practice must have at least one full-time job. Physicians are not an organized profession to be reckoned with, for example, in such questions as salaries or hours of work, or number of patients to be seen.

The one major conspicuous failure of the system has been its inability to deploy professional manpower to the countryside. Like their counterparts the world over, Soviet physicians prefer to remain in the cities. It is therefore instructive to note that even a centralized and politically monolithic system cannot freely dispose of its professional resources as it sees fit. The practice has been, until recently, to assign medical school graduates immediately upon completion of their studies (and without an internship year) to a post in the countryside for two to three years, an assignment that most graduates fear for a variety of reasons, and which they often manage to evade successfully. One loophole is the regulation that a woman cannot be assigned to a job that would separate her from her husband, and about three-quarters of the physicians are women. Other physicians are able to manipulate the bureaucratic structure of the ministry and remain in, or return to, the cities, where there is often a surplus.

It is in this respect that it is worth examining the role of the feldsher, for this semi-professional health worker may well be relevant to Asian countries as well as to the Soviet Union. Under Tsarism, physicians' assistants, or feldshers, played an important role in Russian medicine, particularly in the countryside, where they provided the bulk of medical care to the peasants. Western countries phased out practitioners similar to the feldsher toward the end of the nineteenth century. Liberal physicians in pre-revolutionary Russia considered "feldsherism" to be a second-class medical practice that should also be eliminated, and Soviet health authorities originally intended that every citizen should receive medical care from qualified physicians rather than from feldshers, who are considered "middle-level" personnel. But this plan has not been fully realized, for reasons adduced above; and as a result feldshers continue to provide many primary medical services in the rural areas (Field 1957:97–100; Mueller et al. 1972).

The use of the feldsher represents, in my opinion, a rational utilization of manpower and educational resources in a situation where the task is huge, population density is low, distances are great, transportation is poor, and medical resources are still scarce. The training of full-fledged physicians in all countries, and particularly in developing ones, is lengthy and expensive, and the insistence that only medical graduates be allowed to practice, particularly in the countryside, is tantamount to condemning large numbers of people to no medical care at all (Jensen 1967). The Soviet experience reveals that when feldshers are integrated into a well-designed medical structure, they amplify the work of physicians and are very useful (Sidel 1968). When feldshers work by themselves, the experience has not been uniformly favorable, because of the feldsher's tendency to misdiagnose, overtreat, and fail to refer patients to physicians in time. But in the aggregate, the feldsher provides a modicum of medical care where otherwise there might be none, or where the population might have to rely on unqualified personnel.

The Soviet medical system makes it possible for the Health Ministry to decide what kinds of medical personnel the country needs, and to train them without having to gain approval from a well-organized independent medical profession. The relative isolation in which Soviet medicine operates makes it easier than would otherwise be the case for the USSR to train the kinds of physicians it needs without having to worry about the equivalency of the training with other countries. Most developing nations, on the other hand, are under pressure to provide training equivalent to Western standards and thus to produce physicians poorly trained to meet the medical needs of their *own* country.

Another aspect of the Soviet medical system is the monopoly it gives modern scientific medicine, and its suppression of potential competition from traditional practitioners. The rise of professionalism throughout Western countries was associated with new scientific approaches to health problems, and gave almost exclusive legitimacy to physicians trained in the modern system. The apothecaries, midwives, bone-setters, blood-stoppers, baruchers, wart doctors, and practitioners with esoteric medical theories or secret remedies (Jones 1949) were displaced during the past century, and survive in Western countries as irregular or quack healers outside the medical system. These marginal practitioners most often cater to patients whose conditions are not amenable to scientific treatment, or they provide the pastoral element of medical care so often lacking in the scientific medicine available to lower- and middle-class patients. The point is that the Soviet system stresses scientific medicine exclusively, as do the systems of other Western countries.

Problems of a different nature occur in Asian nations with substantial medical traditions represented by large numbers of folk and learned practitioners. Importing from the West medical knowledge and practices that claim the universal applicability of modern science was bound to cut the ground from under indigenous specialists, to provoke critical attitudes toward indigenous culture, and to lead in medicine as well as in other fields to the reactive nationalism that is common whenever a people is challenged by an alien society and culture. This has led to pluralistic medical systems and the dual professionalization of traditional and modern medical institutions quite different from either the Soviet or the American medical systems (Croizier 1968; Leslie 1969).

Although the Soviet regime did not encourage medical practices from the past, the famous Russian priority campaign launched by Stalin after World War II did to some degree affect Soviet medicine. Historians were enjoined to establish the priority of Russian medicine over Western medicine, to look into the archives for often dubious "firsts," and to stop kowtowing to the West.

But it should be noted that the campaign was couched in scientific terms: in other words, Russian scientists using the canons of science and the inherent wisdom of the Great Russian people had discovered the scientific truth before their foreign colleagues, but the credit had been appropriated by a mendacious West. There was no appeal to obsolete humoral theories, or to the alchemy and astrology favored by medical revivalists in South Asia (Leslie 1971). After Stalin died, this campaign was relaxed, but traces of it may still be found here and there. For example, until recently Pavlov was virtually canonized in Soviet medicine.

There was also, it is true, some talk about folk medicine and folk remedies and the superiority of certain medicinal herbs used by the Russian peasants over pharmaceutical compounds (one may suspect because of the perennial shoratege of the latter). But even the injunction to reexamine the clinical merits of these remedies was usually coupled with the admonition to separate what was scientifically valid from what was useless. The development of two parallel systems was never encouraged. As might be expected, charlatans, quacks, faith healers, and native practitioners have not completely disappeared in such a vast country, where a sizable proportion of the population still lives under rural conditions (about half, at the present writing) They are stigmatized in official publications as the last remnants of superstition and ignorance to be rooted out by an enlightened and scientific approach, and not as the valuable heritage of a national culture.

In conclusion, I would submit that the Soviet national health service, with more than fifty years of experience behind it and attempting (with reasonable success) to provide health care to a large population spreading over two continents, deserves the attention of scholars interested in the comparative study of medical systems and the recurrent problems of improving medical care in modern society.

Literature Cited

Barsukov, M. I.
    1951 *Velikaia Oktiabrskaia Sotsialisticheskaia revolutsia i organizatisiia sovetskogo zdravookhraneniia (The Great October Socialist Revolution and the Organization of Soviet Health Protection—October 1917—July 1918)*, Moscow.
Bryant, John
    1969 *Health and the Developing World*. Ithaca: Cornell University Press.
Croizier, Ralph C.
    1968 *Traditional Medicine in Modern China*. Cambridge: Harvard University Press.
Field, Mark G.
    1957 *Doctor and Patient in Soviet Russia*. Cambridge: Harvard University Press.
    1960 "Medical Organization and the Medical Profession," Cyril C. Black, ed., *The Transformation of Russian Society Since 1861*, pp. 541–552. Cambridge: Harvard University Press.
    1966 "Health Personnel in the Soviet Union: Achievements and Problems," *Am. J. Public Health*, 56:1904–1920.

1967 *Soviet Socialized Medicine: An Introduction.* New York: Free Press.
1970 "The Medical System and Industrial Society: Structural Changes and Internal Differentiation in American Medicine," Alan Sheldon, Frank Baker, and Curtis P. McLaughlin, eds., *Systems and Medical Care*, pp. 143–181. Cambridge: MIT Press.
1971a "The Health Care System of Industrialized Society: The Disappearance of the General Practitioner and Some Implication," Everett I. Mendelsohn, Judith P. Swazey, and Irene Taviss, eds., *Human Aspects of Biological Innovation.* Cambridge: Harvard University Press.
1971b "Evolutions structurelles de la profession médicale aux USA et en URSS," *Cahiers de Démographie et Sociologie Médicales*, 11(2):104–119.
1972 "Taming a Profession: Early Phases of Soviet Socialized Medicine." *Bull. N. Y. Acad. of Medicine* 48(1):83–92.
1973 "The Concept of the 'Health System' at the Macrosociological Level," *Soc. Science and Medicine* 7:763–785.

Freidson, Eliot
1970 *Profession of Medicine.* New York: Dodd, Mead.
Gurevich, G. E.
1947 "Istoricheskii S'ezd (Historical Congress) *Sovetskoe Zdravookhranenie* VI:39." Statement by Khirin at the First Regional Congress, 1918.
Jensen, R. T.
1967 "The Primary Medical Care Worker in Developing Countries." *Medical Care* 5(6):382–400.
Jones, Louis C.
1949 "Practitioners of Folk Medicine." *Bull. History of Medicine* 23:480–493.
Leslie, Charles
1969 "Modern India's Ancient Medicine." *Trans-action*, June issue pp. 46–55.
1973 "The Professionalizing ideology of medical revivalism," Milton Singer, ed., *Entrepreneurship and Modernization of Occupational Cultures in South Asia.* Durham: Duke University Press.
MaGraw, Richard M.
1966 *Ferment in Medicine.* Philadelphia: Saunders.
Miller, James G.
1965 "Living Systems: Basic Concepts." *Behavioral Science* 10:193–237.
Mueller, James E., Faye G. Abdellah, F. T. Billings, Arthur E. Hess, Donald Petit, and Roger O. Egeberg
1972 "The Soviet Health System: Aspects of relevance for medicine in the United States." *New England J. Medicine* 286:693–702.
Parsons, Talcott
1951 *The Social System.* Glencoe, Ill.: Free Press
Rutstein, David D.
1967 *The Coming Revolution in Medicine.* Cambridge: MIT Press.
Sidel, Victor W.
1968 "Feldshers and 'feldsherism'," *New England J. Medicine* 278:934–992.
Vinogradov, N. A., and I. D. Strashun
1947 *Okhrana zdorovia trudiashikhsia v Sovetskom Soiuze (Health Protection of the Workers in the Soviet Union).* Moscow.
White, Kerr L.
1968 "Organization and Delivery of Personal Health Services: Public Policy Issues." *Milbank Memorial Fund Q.* 46(1):225–258.

TABLE 1
Total Labor Force and Health Workers, USA and USSR, 1930–1969
(in thousands and percentage of labor force)

		1930	1940	1950	1960	1969
	Total	48,686	51,742	62,208	69,628	77,347
USA	Health	900	1,090	1,440	2,040	3,515
	Percentage	1.8	2.1	2.3	2.9	4.5

		1932	1940	1950	1967	1969
	Total	24,200	33,926	40,400	62,032	87,922
USSR[a]	Health	399	1,512	2,051	3,461	4,927
	Percentage	1.6	4.5	5.1	5.6	5.6

SOURCES: USA: *Estimates and Projections of the Labor Force and Civilian Employment in the USSR: 1950–1975*, U.S. Dept. of Commerce, Bureau of the Census (Washington, D.C.: U.S. Government Printing Office, 1967), International Population Reports, Series P-91, No. 15, p. 26.
Health Manpower Perspective, 1967, U.S. Dept. of Health, Education, and Welfare, Public Health Service, Bureau of Health Manpower (Washington, D.C.: U.S. Government Printing Office, 1967), p. 5, table 1.
Health Manpower Source Book: Allied Health Manpower 1950–1980 (Washington, D.C.: Public Health Service Publication No. 263, 1970), p. 48, sec. 21.
USSR: *Narodnoe khoziaistvo SSSR v 1969 g.* (Moscow, 1970), pp. 529, 530, 531.
a. Excluding members of collective farms.

TABLE 3
Women in Medicine, USA and USSR, 1913–1970
(in percentage of all physicians)

	1913	1920	1930	1940	1950	1960	1970
USA	NA	NA	4.5[b]	5.0[b]	6.0	7.0	7.0

	1913	1920	1928	1940	1950	1960	1968
USSR[a]	10	—	45	62	77	76	72

SOURCES: USA: *World Sanitary Statistics Annual, 1966, Vol. III: Health Personnel and Hospital Establishments* (Geneva: World Health Organization, 1970), p. 36.
Datagrams, Association of American Medical Colleges, vol. 7, no. 8 (Feb. 1966), table 2
USSR: *Zdravookhranenie v SSSR: Statisticheskii Sbornik* (Moscow, 1960), p. 50.
Narodnoe khoziaistvo SSSR v 1959 g. (Moscow, 1960), p. 787.
Narodnoe khoziaistvo SSSR v 1961 g. (Moscow, 1962), pp. 743–744.
Narodnoe khoziaistvo SSSR v 1969 g. (Moscow, 1969), pp. 729–731).
a. Including stomatologists and dental doctors (*zubnie vrachi*).
b. Percentage of women completing their medical studies.

TABLE 2
Physicians, USA and USSR, 1913–1970
(in absolute numbers and in physicians per 10,000 of population)
(for the USSR, unless otherwise indicated, not counting stomatologists and dental physicians, (*zubnie vrachi*) and without the military)

		1913	1921	1931	1942	1950	1960	1969
USA	Physicians	NA	145,404	156,406	180,496	219,997	260,484[a]	340,000
	Physicians per 10,000	NA	13.4	14.1	13.4	14.3	13.2[b]	16.3

		1913	1920	1928	1940	1950	1960	1970
USSR[a]	Physicians	23,200	18–20,000[c]	63,900	134,900	236,900	385,000	577,249
	Physicians per 10,000	1.5	NA	4.0	7.2	13.6	20.0	22.4[c]

SOURCES: USA: *Statistical Abstract of the US, 1958*, p. 75, table 84 (Washington, D.C.: U.S. Government Printing Office). *Statistical Abstract of the US, 1967*, p. 66, table 80 (Washington, D.C.: U.S. Government Printing Office). *Statistical Abstract of the US, 1970* (Washington, D.C.: U.S. Government Printing Office).

USSR: *Zdravookhranenie v SSSR: Statisticheskii Sbornik* (Moscow, 1960), p. 50. *Narodnoe khoziaistvo SSSR v 1968 g.* (Moscow, 1969), pp. 729–731. "The Soviet Health System: Statistical Materials" in *Sovetskoe zdravookhranenie*, vol. 31 (1972), no. 2, pp. 91ff.

a. Without osteopaths and physicians in the Federal service.
b. Figure for 1967.
c. Estimate.

TABLE 4

Hospital Beds, USA and USSR, 1909–1970
(by total numbers of beds and beds per 1,000 of population)

	1909	1920	1930	1940	1950	1960	1970
USA Total number of Beds	421,065	817,020	955,869	1,226,245	1,455,825	1,657,970	1,649,663
Beds per 1,000	4.7	7.7	7.8	9.3	9.6	9.2	8.2

	1913	1917	1928	1940	1950	1960	1970
USSR Total number of Beds	207,300	149,300	246,500	790,900	1,010,700	1,739,200	2,567,300
Beds per 1,000	1.3	1.0	1.6	4.0	5.6	8.1	10.6

SOURCES: USA: US Bureau of the Census, *Statistical Abstract of the US, 1950* (71st edition), p. 83; also *1971* (92nd edition), p. 68.
USSR: Central Statistical Board of the USSR Council of Ministers, *40 Years of Soviet Power* (Moscow, 1958) p. 309.
Narodnoe khoziaistvo SSSR v 1969 g (Moscow, 1970) p. 732.

TABLE 5

Crude Birth Rate, Crude Death Rate, and Natural Increase of the Population, USA and USSR, 1910–1970
(per 1,000 of population)

		1910	1920	1930	1940	1950	1960	1970
USA	Birth Rate	30.1	27.7	21.3	19.4	24.1	23.7	18.2[a]
	Death Rate	14.7	13.0	11.3	10.8	9.6	9.5	9.4[a]
	Natural Increase	15.4	14.7	10.0	8.6	14.5	14.2	8.8[a]

		1913	1926	1937	1940	1950	1960	1969
USSR	Birth Rate	47.0	44.0	38.7	31.7	26.5	24.9	17.0
	Death Rate	30.2	20.3	18.9	18.3	9.6	7.1	8.1
	Natural Increase	16.8	23.7	19.8	13.4	16.9	17.8	8.9

SOURCES: USA: *Statistical Abstract of the US, 1968,* p. 55; *1971,* p. 48.
USSR: *Narodnoe khoziaistvo v 1969 g,* p. 31.
a. Provisional.

TABLE 6
Infant Mortality, USA and USSR, by Sex, 1913–1970
(expressed as number per 1,000 born alive and dying within one year of birth)

		1915	1920	1930	1940	1950	1960	1970
USA	Total	99.1	85.8	64.6	47.0	29.2	26.0	19.8
	Male	109.9	95.1	71.3	52.5	32.8	29.3	—
	Female	89.4	76.1	57.5	41.3	25.5	22.6	—

		1913	1920–22	1926–27	1940	1950	1959	1969
USSR	Total	269[a]	334	187[b]	182	81	40.6	26
	Male	—	—	201	—	—	44.2	—
	Female	—	—	172	—	—	36.7	—

SOURCES: USA: *Statistical Abstract of the US, 1950*, p. 77; *1971*, p. 55.
Vital Statistics Rates for the US, 1940–1960, Public Health Service Publication No. 1677, National Center for Health Statistics, p. 206.
USSR: *Narodnoe khoziaistvo v 1969*, p. 31.
World Health Statistics Report, vol. 24, no. 6 (1971).

a. For USSR within boundaries prior to September 17, 1939, the figure is 273.
b. European part of the USSR only.

100

TABLE 7

Average Life Expectancy at Birth, USA and USSR, by Sex, 1920–1969

		1920	1930	1940	1950	1960	1968
USA	Total	54.1	59.7	62.9	68.2	69.7	70.2
	Male	53.6	58.1	60.8	65.6	66.6	66.6
	Female	54.6	61.6	65.2	71.1	73.1	74.0

		1926–27	1930	1938–40	1950	1960	1968–69
USSR	Total	44[a]	—	48.4	68	70	70
	Male	42[a]	—	46.7	64	65	65
	Female	47[a]	—	50.2	71	73	74

SOURCES: USA: *Statistical Abstract of the US, 1971*, p. 53.
USSR: *Narodnoe khoziaistvo v 1956 g*, p. 271.
Narodnoe khoziaistvo v 1969 g, p. 588.

a. European part of the USSR only.

The Sociology of Modern Medical Research

RENÉE C. FOX

Medicine as an institution turns around the relationship between health and illness, and the physical and psychic capacity of individuals to perform in their social roles. Medicine is concerned with the ultimate conditions of man's existence and the problems of meaning associated with them.[1] It is linked with birth, life, pain, suffering, anxiety, mortality, and death. Medical research is a way of inquiring into and striving to control the body, mind, psyche, and environment as they bear upon health and illness.

Medical research occupies a strategic place in modern society. Like modern science, of which it is an important part, it is accorded strong and extensive value. It is a symbolic as well as concrete expression of the social structure and cultural tradition. And it epitomizes some archetypically modern forms of competence, achievement, and yearning.

This paper will consider medical research in a cross-cultural and evolutionary framework. Medical research has flourished more in modern than in pre-modern societies, and it is more firmly and centrally institutionalized in some Western societies than in others. I will not take these facts for granted, or consider them accidental. As the distinctive features of modern medical research are identified, I will suggest the implications that variations in them have for ongoing scientific inquiry. Finally, I will comment on nascent trends visible in the current historical phase of modern medical research.

COGNITIVE ASSUMPTIONS AND MODE OF THOUGHT

The mode of thought on which modern medical research is based is an emergent, eclectic product of the biological and behavioral sciences. In its ideal form, it applies logico-rational thought to phenomena that are related to health and illness. Through observation, interviewing, and experimental

---

1 "Ultimate conditions" is a phrase of Robert N. Bellah (1964:359). "Problems of meaning" is a concept of Max Weber that has been further developed by Talcott Parsons.

techniques, information is amassed and refined. Instruments that enhance observation and increase the control of data range in power and complexity from the stethoscope to the electron microscope. The data collected are ordered by conceptual schemes, the highly generalized and systematic sets of ideas that constitute the framework for scientific thought (Conant 1951:25 and *passim*). They provide investigators with insight-provoking ways of formulating questions and seeking answers about an otherwise intricate and confusing empirical reality.

At the same time, conceptual schemes bind the investigator to a particular way of conceiving reality, so that he tends to find what he looks for. Other characteristics of medical scientific thought help curtail this penchant. Great methodological and ethical value is attached to null hypothesis reasoning, the rigorous attempt to systematically disprove or rule out the premises on which a piece of research is founded. The medical researcher is expected to be a specialist in uncertainty who is engaged by the tentativeness and incompleteness of medical knowledge. He advances knowledge by laying bare these uncertainties, as well as by mitigating or dispelling them.

The highest prestige in modern medical research accrues to contributions that constitute a "breakthrough" in knowledge. This is a primary factor in the numerous disputes over priority that have occurred in the history of scientific research (Merton 1957). In medical research such breakthroughs have the added cogency of promising relief or cure to suffering patients. Clinical investigators in the dual role of caring for and conducting experiments upon patients with conditions outside of current medical competence nourish this hope in themselves and their patients.

The value system in which modern medical research is rooted is associated with transcendent assumptions about the nature of man and the universe. Nevertheless, the problems and questions with which it deals are sharply distinguished from religious concerns: it addresses itself to the mechanisms of health and illness, life and death, rather than to the meaning of their occurrence. Although it is ethically self-conscious, and respects the subjects it investigates, its outlook is disenchanted, in Max Weber's sense of the term. It does not consider the sacred to be located in any of the spheres it explores, or to constrain inquiry into them. Modern medical research also tries to detach itself from what it regards as the biasing effects that the ideas of specific religious traditions would impose on investigation. The relationship between modern medical science and a religious view of the world might best be characterized as a state of "creative tension," rather than one of reciprocal repudiation (Bellah 1965:194). On the other hand, modern medical thought is resolutely anti-magical in intent, if not always in fact.

A comparison of these cognitive traits of modern medical research with a different tradition throws into relief what is distinctive about them. Traditional Bantu African medical thought, like that of modern medical science, seeks an explanatory theory in a causal context and is concerned with classification and taxonomy.[2] But in contrast to modern medical science, it exhibits an "imperious, uncompromising demand ... for determinism" (Lévi-Strauss 1966:11). Health and illness are determined primarily by super-natural, psychic, and interpersonal forces within a closed system of thought and belief, whose logic is that of the "self-fulfilling prophecy" (Merton 1949). Explanations for illness are limited in range, and fixed. When evidence contrary to traditional interpretations is encountered, there is a tendency to develop "secondary elaborations" that excuse or explain it away (Evans-Pritchard 1937). No room exists for the concept of probability or the formal acknowledgement of uncertainty. Objective and subjective reality, ideas and empirical happenings are not dissociated from one another. Health signifies that one's life-force is intact, and that one is sufficiently in harmony with the social, physical, and supernatural environment to enjoy what is positively valued in life, and to ward off misfortunes and evils. Illness is the antithesis of health, prototypical of the most negative, tragic life experiences that beset man. It is also unnatural. It ought not and would not occur without the intervention of transhuman forces, mediated by human agents. With limited exceptions, illness is believed to be caused by the evil thoughts, feelings, or motives of other people, through the medium of sorcery or witchcraft.

Traditional Bantu medical thought is consonant with the concepts and beliefs of a primitive or archaic religious system (Bellah 1964). It forecloses the kind of systematic, sacred-free questioning that lies at the heart of modern medical research. At the same time, it provides answers to problems of meaning associated with health and illness that modern medical science circumvents and, in some ways, increases.

VALUE-ORIENTATIONS AND SOME VARIANTS

The cognitive assumptions and mode of thought of modern medical science are interrelated with the value-orientations on which it is premised.[3] The value of rationality provides the *raison d'être* for all forms of modern scientific inquiry, and a strongly-felt commitment to progress in rationally understanding health and illness is institutionalized in medical research. The pursuit of logical, orderly, generalized but open-ended knowledge is valued for its own sake, and as an expression of man's higher intellectual and moral faculties. But this pattern of rationality derives even more sustenance from the supposi-tion that it is the primary means through which diseases will be vanquished and adventitious death overcome. Thus, rationality intersects with a dynamic, melioristic value complex that Talcott Parsons has called "instrumental activism" (Parsons 1967:225–226).

2 My analysis of Bantu medical thought is based on field work in the Democratic Republic of the Congo (now renamed Zaïre) during the period 1962–1967, and on English, French, and Belgian anthropological monographs on other Bantu African societies.

3 My discussion of the value-orientations of modern medical science is based on Talcott Parsons (1951:326–383), Robert K. Merton (1949:295–316), and Bernard Barber (1952:60–83).

The role that affect is supposed to play in this rationality is shaped by a value conception of detached concern.[4] The medical investigator is supposed to be emotionally involved in the search he conducts, to care about the knowledge it may bring forth and the practical fruits of that knowledge. At the same time, he is to maintain a detachment that blends objectivity with organized doubting. The truth that he seeks is concepts, facts, and techniques that transcend those he would achieve if he were influenced by unexamined and unbridled sentiments.

This value-orientation shades into universalism. Judgments of the reliability, validity, and import of the findings of medical investigators, along with eligibility for the status of researcher, are supposed to be dissociated from particularistic considerations. Scientific competence and excellence are considered to be the only appropriate criteria for these judgments, and the scientist's personal qualities or the social attributes of sex, age, race, nationality, class, religion, and political persuasion are believed to be irrelevant.

Finally, modern medical research is poised between individualism and collectivity–orientation. The investigator is enjoined to follow the paths of knowledge that scientific inquiry opens up to him, no matter how lonely or heterodox they seem to be. But he is also expected to recognize that the knowledge he utilizes and that he helps to create does not belong to him. It is the property of a community that extends far beyond social groupings of which he is a member, and beyond his own historical time. The medical scientist is expected to be aware of the social consequences of his research, though the content and scope of these responsibilities are not clearly designated.

Rationality, instrumental activism, detached concern, universalism, individualism, and collectivism describe the ethos of science as it has developed in modern Western societies. They have not been perfectly realized in any society. Within the social systems that are both modern and Western, considerable variability exists in the form and in the degree to which they are institutionalized. For example, medical research in Belgium is conducted by institutions affiliated with the country's four major universities (Fox 1962, 1964). Each university represents a different combination of the social and cultural distinctions of Belgian life. Brussels is a Free Thought, preponderantly anticlerical, private university, with separate French and Flemish sections. Ghent is a state university, officially neither Catholic nor Free Thought, but with a sizable number of practicing Catholics in the student body and on the faculty. Since the early 1930s, all its teaching is done in Flemish. Liège is a state university, neither Catholic nor Free Thought, but with at least a plurality of its students and faculty non-practicing Catholics or non-Catholics. All classes at Liège are taught in French. Since 1969,

---

4 I formulated this concept in a paper that I co-authored with Miriam Massey Johnson in 1950–51, but it was not until 1963 that I used it in a publication (Fox 1963 : 12–35).

Louvain, Belgium's venerable, private, Catholic university has split into two separate universities, a French one and a Flemish one (Leuven).

Thus, to a significant degree, the Belgian university settings in which medical research is conducted are particularistic. A person's linguistic, ethnic, and religious-philosophical affiliations, along with his related social class membership and political persuasion, are as much determinants of his appointment to a faculty position in which he can do research as are his scientific talent, training, and achievement. Furthermore, each university tends to recruit its faculty from its alumni. All this reinforces the tendency of the universities to seal themselves off from each other. In the opinion of many Belgian medical researchers, the result is cloistered academic milieux that curtail the interchange of ideas between colleagues, the mobility of personnel, and a sharing of facilities that would enhance medical research. This entrenched and pervasive particularism is a pre-modern value-orientation and feature of the social structure. Although it is not totally incompatible with viable, modern medical research, it constrains its volume and originality.

SCIENTIFIC MAGIC

As a traditional element, particularism is analytically different from another pattern in modern medical research that is ostensibly pre-modern and incongruous with scientific rationality. I refer to various forms of what I have called "scientific magic" (Fox 1959). The particularistic retention exemplified in Belgian medicine impedes the full development of research, but scientific magic helps to further it.

Precisely because he approaches matters related to life and death in a scientific way, the modern medical investigator lives with the problems of uncertainty and the therapeutic limitations of medical science. He also confronts the unanswered why's of illness that fall outside the boundaries of science. These challenges help to trigger and shape the search for more adequate medical knowledge; but they are also a source of considerable strain. One of the coping mechanisms investigators develop is essentially magical, though it may be disguised to some extent in research procedures. Scientific magic tends to be more elaborate in groups of medical researchers with physicianly responsibilities to care for patients who are also their subjects. Scientific uncertainty, the limitation of therapy, and problems of meaning are compounded for these physicians, who make and use more scientific magic than their colleagues whose investigations are confined to the laboratory.

A pattern of scientific magic that characterizes all genres of modern medical researchers consists of investigators making levity-accompanied wagers with each other about what the results of particularly important and/or risky experiments will be. This ironic ritual symbolically comments on the apparent lack of order, predictability, and sense in the phenomena they are exploring. In it they express self-mocking chagrin over their inability to understand, know, predict, and control; and they protest against what seem to be existentially absurd processes or entities associated with illness, and with the efforts to comprehend it. Finally, this game of chance is an affirmative petition for success. The investigators who engage in it pit their own intelligent guesses against the unknown in ways that mimic the more speculative aspects of scientific research. They hope that their projections will have a positive relationship to the answers they seek.

Scientific magic seems to grow directly out of the limitations of rationality in modern medical research, and the strains that this imposes on investigators. Although scientific magic parodies the basic value premises of rationality and of instrumental activism, it is a latently institutionalized pattern in modern medical research. It ritualizes the optimism of medical investigators concerning the meaningfulness of their activities (Malinowski 1948:70). It appears to be a necessary condition, enabling investigators to further knowledge and technique according to the cognitive and moral canons of modern science.

SOCIAL STRUCTURE AND ORGANIZATION

A mural at the Institut Jules Bordet in Brussels honors the distinguished medical scientist after whom the institute is named.[5] Though perhaps not intended by the artist to do so, the mural romanticizes the pre-modern conditions under which medical research was conducted in Western universities in the nineteenth century. These are not the conditions most conducive to innovation and productivity in twentieth-century, modern medical research; yet they are perpetuated in many European societies to this day.

The mural depicts Bordet as an elderly man, white-haired and white-mustached, lean, erect, dignified, and elegant; clad in a dark suit, his vest properly buttoned over a white shirt and dark tie, white handkerchief neatly arranged in his jacket pocket, a small ribbon rosette of honor affixed to his buttonhole. He stands with hands in his trouser pockets, a solitary figure in the midst of the laboratory where so much of his work was done. The laboratory is a cluttered, but orderly and austere, white-tiled room, lit from overhead by three gas lamps. The tables, shelves, cupboards of the

5 The artist who painted the mural is P. Delvaux. Jules Bordet was awarded the Nobel Prize for medicine and physiology in 1919. His early studies showed that anti-microbic sera include two active substances, one existing before immunization (alexine), the other a specific antibody created by vaccination. Bordet introduced the method of diagnosing microbes by sera. In 1898 he discovered hemolytic sera and showed that they act on foreign blood by a mechanism comparable to that by which an anti-microbic serum acts on microbes. He also demonstrated that the reactions of all these sera are colloidal in nature. Bordet threw light on the process of formation of coagulin. He studied the formation of analyphylactic poisons. And, with Gengou, he cultivated *B. pertussis*, and laid the basis for the generally accepted opinion that this organism is the cause of whooping cough.

laboratory are filled with test tubes, glass beakers and bottles of various sizes and shapes, syringes and pipettes. On a side counter there is a Bunsen burner on which a large white casserole with a tipsy black lid has been placed. The windowsill at one end of the laboratory contains two simple microscopes under bell jars, and another assortment of pipettes and test tubes in beakers. It is late evening. The shades of the windows have been raised, so that one sees the first sliver of a new moon rising over the tiled, gabled rooftops and tidy chimneys of traditional Belgian architecture. In short, the mural is a portrait of a scientist of gentlemanly origins and demeanor, a solo investigator, working in his laboratory at night in the anatomo-pathological and bacterio-logical era of medicine, and equipped only with his sense of vocation, his personal genius, and simple instruments.

Modern medical research differs from this Bordet image in fundamental respects. More than the style of the buildings, the haberdashery of its investi-gators, and the equipment it employs have changed. Modern research is characterized by a progressive division of labor, increasing specialization and professionalization. Biochemistry, rather than anatomy, pathology, or bacteriology, is the reigning basic medical science. The lone researcher is a relatively rare phenomenon. Increased knowledge, specialization, and the intricacy and expense of medical technology require that research be conducted by teams of investigators as a cooperative enterprise. The commit-ment to teamwork, however, is more than a rational recognition of the most practical way to proceed. Collaboration is considered to be morally as well as intellectually superior to an aloof, aristocratic individualism. Established, prestigious, comfortably remunerated status-roles and careers exist. These are primarily in the university, but also in government and industry. They are not the prerogative of amateur gentlemen scholars. Rather, they are open to persons from wide-ranging social class backgrounds, primarily on the basis of their training and accomplishments.

The greater part of modern medical research is carried out within the framework of large, formal organizations that are essentially bureaucratic. These structures accommodate the changing configurations of medical science, including the rise of new disciplines and subfields, and shifts in the content or scope of basic and applied goals. Furthermore, medical researchers are linked to one another by informal scientific and collegial exchanges, mutually read publications, and membership in loosely organized professional societies. These ties go beyond their formal affiliation with a particular university, government office, or firm. Thus, modern medical research is not coordinated and controlled by one centralized political or economic body. Its florescence is encouraged by the steadfast, enterprising support of government agencies, business firms, universities, and professional as-sociations.

It is a historical fact, rather than a chauvinistic assertion by an American scholar, that these social structural conditions were more fully realized in the United States in the 1950s and early 1960s than in any other society in the world. Medical research, along with other scientific investigation, was regarded "as a resource to be developed according to its immanent possibilities and to be marketed as widely and imaginatively as possible" (Ben-David 1968:55). An "entrepreneurial ... system of research and higher education" prevailed, "characterized by a large number of autonomous and competing organizations, the internal structures of which were flexibly adjusted to the changing requirements of scientific collaboration and division of labor" (*ibid*:45–46). The volume and variety of support for scientific research that these organizational arrangements helped to generate, and the bold idealism, as well as pragmatism, that underlay them, attracted many talented researchers from other countries. This further enhanced scientific creativity and productivity in American society during that period.

EXPERIMENTATION WITH HUMAN SUBJECTS

A final, key attribute of modern medical research is the extensive participation of human subjects in its inquiries and experiments. The furtherance of medical knowledge and skill, most particularly, therapeutic innovation, involves a sequence of steps that weave back and forth between the laboratory and the clinic (Fox 1970:5–6). In the earliest stages of testing a concept, procedure, or drug, where uncertainty and risk are at a maximum, investigators work in the laboratory with animal subjects. These preliminary laboratory trials provide new information and understanding, but they are not perfectly applicable to man. Because limitations and difficulties always exist in extrapolating from animal models to the human being, researchers must engage in experimentation with human subjects. These subjects are selected because they are normal and healthy in specified ways, or because they are afflicted with medical conditions that concern the investigators. Adequate laboratory work with animals is an ethical, as well as technical, prerequisite for human trials. But no neat guideposts are established along the experimental road to signal that the time has indubitably come to move from animal to human experimentation. This transition in clinical research is inherently controversial.

When patients are used as subjects for new forms of therapy, the usual procedure is to advance from work with animals to clinical trials with terminally ill patients, and from there to testing with persons in progressively earlier, more benign phases of the malady. This pattern expresses the conviction that only desperately sick persons for whom established therapy offers no hope should serve as subjects in early human trials. They have little to lose, it is felt, and much to gain from the admittedly outside chance that they may benefit from the new therapy they help to test. Through these initial human experiments, investigators achieve what they consider sufficient knowledge and skill to try the new treatment legitimately on patients less drastically ill.

Human experimentation has increased in magnitude, complexity, and potential peril, and has been accompanied by increasing concern for the ethical and legal character of medical research. Systematic study of these matters was given tragic impetus by the crimes of physicians in Nazi Germany. Out of the Nuremberg trials and the thought they evoked, several codes for human experimentation have been promulgated.[6] These have attempted to define the principles and conditions for research with human subjects, while reaffirming the importance of applying "the results of laboratory experiments ... to human beings to further scientific knowledge and help suffering humanity" (Wolstenholme and O'Connor 1966:219).

Certain medical and surgical developments have quickened concern about the increasingly dangerous and subtle abuses that could result from them. The outbreak of infantile deformity (phocomelia) in Western Europe in 1961 and 1962 caused by the drug Thalidomide was one such potent occurrence. In the United States, for example, it precipitated passage of the Drug Amendments Act of 1962, which legally empowered the Food and Drug Administration to exercise specific kinds of controls over the clinical testing of new drugs on human subjects.

More recently, organ transplantation has come to be a paradigmatic case of the problems that have classically accompanied clinical medical research and of new phenomena, premonitory of intricate ethical issues, that future investigators and their human subjects will encounter.[7] Concern about the ethics of human experimentation has focused on the difficulty of obtaining truly informed, voluntary consent from the subject, of striking a proper balance between the potential benefits and risks to him, and of protecting his integrity and privacy. Organ transplantation has added new dimensions to these questions. Obtaining consent for a transplant involves complex interactions between the medical team, potential donors and their kin, and the candidate recipient and his relatives. Transplantation has also brought other issues into prominence, including the justification for inflicting a major surgical injury on a live donor in order to help a dying recipient; the symbolic meaning of the human heart and other vital organs; the allocation of scarce organs; the transcendent meaning of the gift-exchange between the donor and the recipient, versus the mutual tyranny it can

6 The best-known are the Nuremberg Code and the 1964 Declaration of Helsinki of the World Medical Association, which sets forth a Code of Ethics for Human Experimentation. In the United States, a Public Health Service document dated May 1, 1969, and entitled "Protection of the Individual as Research Subject" sets forth the regulations that must be followed in investigations with human subjects, if a project is to be funded by the National Institutes of the Public Health Service. This agency funds approximately 35 percent of all biomedical research conducted in the United States.

7 These insights, contained in my essay, "A Sociological Perspective on Organ Transplantation and Hemodialysis" (1970), constitute the basic premises of the book on the sociology of organ transplants and dialysis that I coauthored with Judith P. Swazey, a historian of medicine (Fox and Swazey 1974). In the last few years, at least three important published symposia on human experimentation and therapeutic innovation have focused on the case of organ transplantation (Wolstenholme and O'Connor 1966; Ladimer 1970; and Freund 1970).

impose on them; the appropriate definition of death; the distinction between the extension of life and the prolongation of death; and the existential and social implications of the physicianly commitment to do everything medically possible for terminally ill persons.

The fact that in a modern society many persons are willing to act as research subjects and, in numerous instances, are even eager to do so, needs explanation. Since this form of participation in medical research achieved a greater degree of acceptance in American society than in any other, identifying the factors that have contributed to its support is instructive (Fox 1960). The institutionalization of the role of research subject involves a widespread belief in the practical importance and moral excellence of scientific research, and medical research in particular. Contributing to it by taking the role of a research subject is thought to be a humanitarian and potentially heroic act. These individuals demonstrate their readiness to endure the discomforts and hazards of pioneering experiments partly for the self-surpassing goals of collective health and well-being. Thus, the motivation of patients who serve as human subjects often has two facets. It expresses their hope that new insights or treatments may be developed that could directly benefit them; it testifies to their disinterested conviction that, as one patient-subject put it, it will be "for the good of medical science and the humane benefit of others in the future" (Fox 1959:150).

Characteristically, the relationship of the physician-investigator to his human subject is both collegial and collectivity-oriented. The participants are bound to one another by an enterprise that they consider highly significant. They are committed to the values on which the enterprise is based. And the norm of informed, voluntary consent reduces the discrepancy in medical knowledge that ordinarily exists between a physician and a layman. Yet, however close, collaborative, and egalitarian in their orientation a research physician and a human subject may become, there is always enough of a competence gap and sufficient ambivalence between them, so that their relationship depends on the institutionalization of uncontingent solidarity and confidence (Parsons 1970). In this regard, the relationship is a fiduciary one, drawing upon and contributing to the sense of trust that binds social relationships throughout the society.

"ADVANCED MODERN" OR "POST-MODERN" MEDICAL RESEARCH?

A few comments on some shifts in orientation that medical research is undergoing in American society will provide an epilogue to this sociological overview. These emerging patterns appear to be microdynamic expressions of changes in the society at large, and they raise vital questions about the magnitude and significance of these changes. Do these trends constitute "advanced modern" developments? That is, are they further extensions of the value system and social structure underlying modern scientific research?

Or will they prove to be "post-modern" in the sense of being sufficiently discontinuous and incompatible with the social and cultural attributes of modern science to represent a break with them? Although it is too early to formulate definitive answers to these questions, it is important to ask them.[8]

Two developing patterns are especially notable.[9] The first is the tendency for modern medicine to become more social in outlook. Greater emphasis is being placed on the extent to which society is responsible for health and illness. Good health and medical care are coming to be viewed as basic human rights. Social arrangements are increasingly referred to in explaining the persistence of certain illnesses and the emergence of others, as well as to account for injustices in the delivery of medical care. And the belief that illness, along with poverty, pollution, overpopulation, and war, can be brought under control by the organized implementation of public conscience is gaining momentum.

One of the consequences of this new orientation for medical research is an augmenting pressure on investigators to address themselves to "relevant" matters. The definition of what is relevant is veering toward massive efforts to eliminate certain diseases. In this respect, cancer has become symbolic of the most recalcitrant, painful, and lethal medical disorder in modern society to be overcome. But even more pronounced is the demand for solutions to social and economic problems that adversely affect health and its care. This development seems to call into question some of the commitments that have given modern medical inquiry moral and material support. After a decade of steady expansion in funds allocated by the United States Government for medical research, the growth rate in Federal support has leveled off, and is now beginning to decline. In addition, particularly among younger people, a crescendo of doubt is being expressed about the intellectual and ethical values of scientific research and its pertinence to social issues.

The second major alteration through which modern medicine seems to be passing is a shift toward greater interest in the moral enigmas and existential questions that confront physicians. The sources of this new awareness are complex. In part, it grows out of the stage in knowledge and technique that modern medicine has reached. Understanding and control of disease and death have been impressively advanced. The potential human life span has been greatly extended. And yet, people still fall ill and die. The juxtaposition of these accomplishments and limitations has reawakened reflection on philosophical and religious questions. Are disease and death inalterably a part of the human condition? If so, why? What does this tell us about the nature of man and the purpose of his existence?

Resuscitative techniques and organ transplantation have contributed

8 I have greatly benefited from several personal exchanges with Talcott Parsons on these questions, most particularly from a letter I received from him dated March 24, 1971.

9 The discussion that follows draws upon a still unpublished paper entitled "Medical Evolution," which I contributed to a forthcoming *Festschrift* for Talcott Parsons, edited by Jan Loubser, Victor M. Lidz, Andrew Effrat, *et al.*

to the fact that the cessation of breathing and heartbeat are being superseded by irreversible coma, or the so-called brain-death syndrome, as the criterion of death. The discussion that has surrounded this process has increased physicians' consciousness of the fact that codified notions of death are approximate and arbitrary, and do not solve philosophical or religious questions about what death really is. The debate about heart and lung death versus brain death has also brought physicians to consider in a new way the ambiguities concerning where the prolongation of life ends and the prolongation of death begins.

Participation in organ transplantation in the role of medical professional, donor, or recipient has increased cognizance of widespread, essentially mystic conceptions about the human body, even in a science-oriented society. Furthermore, participation in the network of giving and receiving established by transplantation can be a religious experience. Many report that it has enhanced their self-understanding and self-worth, and given them a sense of commitment and oneness with humanity unlike any they have known before.

In addition, physicians and biological scientists, in collaboration with lawyers, theologians, philosophers, and social scientists, are trying to foresee the moral and spiritual implications of possible biomedical developments.[10] Notable among the futuristic biomedical phenomena with which they are concerned are the widespread transplantation of all human organs, including the brain; the implantation of various kinds of artificial organs; genetic engineering, including cloning (the asexual reproduction of genetic carbon copies of an adult); and behavior control through neurophysiological or pharmacological manipulation of specific areas of the brain.

The entwined existential and social orientation that seems to be emerging in modern medical research is probably not an ephemeral happening. The best indicator of this is that the young men and women who have entered American medical schools over the past few years are increasingly engaged by this perspective. Their commitment is born out of their protest over what they consider to be the deficiencies of the medicine they have inherited and out of their belief in what it could become. Whether or not we are moving from the modern to a post-modern phase of medical research will be ascertained in the course of their generation.

10 I belong to a group concerned with these problems, The Institute of Society, Ethics and the Life Sciences, of Hastings-on-Hudson, N. Y.

Literature Cited

Barber, Bernard
   1952 *Science and the Social Order*. Glencoe, Ill.: Free Press.
Bellah, Robert N.
   1964 "Religious Evolution." *Am. Sociol. Rev.* 29:359.
   1965 "Epilogue," in Robert N. Bellah, ed., *Religion and Progress in Modern Asia*. New York: Free Press.

Ben-David, Joseph
  1968 *Fundamental Research and the Universities.* Paris: Organization for Economic Cooperation and Development.
Conant, James B.
  1951 *Science and Common Sense.* New Haven: Yale University Press.
Evans-Pritchard, E. E.
  1937 *Witchcraft, Oracles, and Magic Among the Azande.* Oxford: Oxford University Press.
Fox, Renée C.
  1959 *Experiment Perilous.* Glencoe, III.: Free Press.
  1960 "Some Social and Cultural Factors in American Society Conducive to Medical Research on Human Subjects." *Clinical Pharmacology and Therapeutics* 1:423–443.
  1962 "Medical Scientists in a Château." *Science* 136:476–483.
  1964 "An American Sociologist in the Land of Belgian Medical Research," in Phillip E. Hammond, ed., *Sociologists at Work,* pp. 345–391. New York: Basic Books.
  1970 "A Sociological Perspective on Organ Transplantation and Hemodialysis," in Irving Ladimer, ed., *New Dimensions in Legal and Ethical Concepts for Human Research.* Annals N. Y. Acad. Sciences 169.
Fox, Renée C., and Harold I. Lief
  1963 "Training for 'Detached Concern' in Medical Students," in Harold, Victor and Nina Lief, eds., *The Psychological Basis of Medical Practice,* pp. 12–35. New York: Harper and Row, Hoeber Medical Division.
Fox, Renée C., and Judith P. Swazey
  1974 *The Courage to Fail: A Social View of Organ Transplants and Dialysis.* Chicago: The University of Chicago Press.
Freund, Paul A., ed.
  1970 *Experimentation with Human Subjects.* New York: Braziller.
Ladimer, Irving, ed.
  1970 *New Dimensions in Legal and Ethical Concepts for Human Research. Annals N. Y. Acad. Sciences* 169.
Lévi-Strauss, Claude
  1966 *The Savage Mind.* Chicago: University of Chicago Press.
Malinowski, Bronislaw
  1948 *Magic, Science, and Religion and Other Essays.* Glencoe, Ill.: Free Press.
Merton, Robert K.
  1949 "The Self-Fulfilling Prophecy," in *Social Theory and Social Structure.* Glencoe, Ill.: Free Press, pp. 179–195.
  1957 "Priorities in Scientific Discovery: A Chapter in the Sociology of Science." *Am. Sociol. Rev.* 22: 635–659.
Parsons, Talcott
  1951 *The Social System,* Glencoe, Ill.: Free Press.
  1967 *Sociological Theory and Modern Society.* New York: Free Press.
  1970 "Research with Human Experiments and the "Professional Complex"", in Paul A. Freund, ed., *Experimentation with Human Subjects,* pp. 127–128. New York: Braziller.
Wolstenholme, G. E. W., and Maeve O'Connor, eds.
  1966 *Ethics in Medical Progress.* Boston: Little, Brown.

PART III

The Adaptive Significance
of Medical Traditions

The full emergence of cosmopolitan medicine in the twentieth century initiated a revolutionary transformation in the conditions of human life. This is not a revolution that advanced industrial countries have passed through, and that now proceeds with uncertain prospects elsewhere. In one way or another the revolution proceeds in communities throughout the world. Its scope is suggested by reflecting on the consequences for Soviet and American societies of the changes in infant mortality and life expectancy shown in Tables 6 and 7 of Mark Field's essay. A good place to do this is in a nineteenth-century cemetery, where the numerous tombstones for children, for young men and women, and for husbands and wives with growing families remind those of us who have grown up or raised our own families over the past generation how different our lives have been from those of our immediate ancestors because we have not confronted death in the ways they did.

The scope of the revolution is also suggested by speculation: What if the ability to prolong life made dying ordinarily depend upon choice? What if reproduction became an entirely manageable process that we could separate from sexual pleasure and regulate to improve the genetic composition of populations? What if the various forms of ill health were controllable to a degree that the distribution of suffering they occasion was not an "act of God," but a decision of medical policy? These situations are only partly hypothetical. Renée Fox concluded her essay in the preceding section by suggesting that an "entwined existential and social orientation" is emerging in the United States among medical students and researchers who, confronting issues of this kind, are more concerned than their predecessors for social justice in the delivery of medical care, and for the ways that advances in medical technology raise perennial questions about the meaning of life and death. If this orientation is to mature in rational and effective action, it should be informed by comparative historical knowledge of the evolution and variation of medical systems.

For comparative purposes, one way to conceive of medical systems is as

117

modes of adaptation—orders of knowledge and social institutions to avoid injury and illness, and to cope with these events when they occur. This perspective is concerned with functional part–whole and means–end relationships, and its paradigmatic work is in evolutionary biology (Alland 1966). Thus we ask: What has been the significance of great- and little-tradition medicine for the Darwinian fitness of populations? How do changing cosmopolitan medical systems effect natural selection? And how should questions of this kind be formulated in designing new research?

Ivan Polunin opens the present section with a cautionary essay. He doubts the notion that medical systems evolve as adaptive responses to biological patterns of illness and death, pointing out that societies ignore some forms of morbidity, classify others as religious phenomena rather than health problems, and invent syndromes of affliction based upon erroneous theories of disease causation. A scholar at another symposium asserted that "anthropologists underreport and underestimate tendencies toward verification, testings, and empirical approaches" in traditional societies, that "primitive medicine contains a storehouse of empirical knowledge," and that the evolutionary success of the species "is due in no small part to the local solution of medical problems" (Laughlin 1963:116,120); but Ivan Polumin here adopts a different tone. He rejects "moldy-bread-means-they-had-antibiotics" interpretations of medical practices, and is skeptical that "processes of social selection" favored "general disease-preventing behavior" in ways that significantly effected adaptation. He argues that the major changes in disease and mortality have not been caused by medical practices but by changes in diet and ecology related to the domestication of plants and animals, permanent settlements, increasing population size and density, and new forms of social organization.

Fred Dunn follows Polunin's essay by presenting a conceptual model to analyze the adaptive significance of medical systems. Using "web-like thinking," he defines health as a condition with multiple causes that varies as "adaptive training" occurs in group and individual responses to successive "insults." Among these responses, medical systems are the social institutions and cultural traditions that evolve in deliberate efforts to improve health, although these efforts may in fact provoke ill health. Dunn would acknowledge Polunin's point that nondeliberate health-enhancing behavior has had a much greater effect on the Darwinian fitness of populations than their medical systems, but he complicates the picture in a most useful manner by considering the function of medical systems related to "human ideas of comfort, ease, satisfaction, and joy in life." His analysis is further enriched by the distinction between adaptability and adaptedness, and by a pluralistic conception of coexisting local, regional, and cosmopolitan medical systems. Finally, as he outlines "the characteristic and adaptive strengths" of Chinese, Āyurvedic, and Yunānī medicine, Dunn suggests historical trends by distinguishing their past and present structures.

In contrast to Polunin and Dunn, who draw upon bodies of research in paleopathology, epidemiology, medical history, and anthropology, William Caudill's essay is based upon a single intensive comparative study in Japan and the United States. Polunin and Dunn ask primarily about the biologically adaptive functions of medical systems, but in doing so they argue that the social and cultural functions are probably more significant for understanding these systems. One of the first and strongest impressions a stranger gets upon entering a community with cultural traditions different from his own is that the people live in and experience their bodies in a distinctive manner. Caudill asks how these modes of "body management" are learned. In an elegantly designed and executed study of urban middle-class Japanese and American families, he relates his findings to the epidemiology and medical traditions of these societies.

William Caudill was one of the first scholars in the United States to specialize in medical anthropology. He died within the year following the Symposium at Burg Wartenstein for which he wrote the present essay. We learn by the example of his research in this volume and in his other publications one way to be both humane and scientific. This volume is dedicated to his memory.

CHARLES LESLIE

Literature Cited

Alland, Alexander
  1966 "Medical Anthropology and the Study of Biological and Cultural Adaptation." *Am. Anthropologist* 68(1): 40–51.
Laughlin, William S.
  1963 "Primitive Theory of Medicine: Empirical Knowledge," in Iago Galdston, ed., *Man's Image in Medicine and Anthropology*. New York: International Universities Press.

Disease, Morbidity, and Mortality in China, India, and the Arab World

IVAN POLUNIN

Systems of medical practice have developed largely through interactions between sick persons and the people they consult. We might expect, therefore, that disease patterns have influenced the ways medical systems have evolved. My impression is that this has not been the case to any great extent. To support this impression, and to provide a background for the comparative study of medical systems in Asia, I will summarize various ideas and facts about diseases, morbidity, and mortality in China, India, and the Arab World.

Valid thought and action concerning disease is often difficult because the nature and causes of health and illness are incompletely understood. In spite of advances in observation, experiment, technology, and probabilistic thinking, the medicine of recent times has been rich in error. Thus, quinine therapy was abandoned in India following inadequate therapeutic trials (Russel 1955), and B.C.G. vaccination after the Lübeck disaster fell into disuse for invalid reasons. Millions of teeth and tonsils have been sacrificed because of once-fashionable ideas about focal sepsis. I assume that similar mistakes will continue to be made, and have occurred in other systems of medicine, particularly those based on veneration for the teaching of great masters. I am skeptical of the idea that there must be something valid in all traditional practices, which we might call the "moldy-bread-on-wounds-means-they-had-antibiotics" theory. By a valid medical practice, I mean one where the effects claimed for it are exerted by means of its intrinsic properties, though I do not deny the psychological and social benefit of a practice which can exist independent of this kind of validity.

The judgment about what constitutes health or disease varies from group to group. In most societies, disease is probably conceived as a departure from the usual state of health. Thus, a morbid condition which is common may not be perceived to be abnormal and to need a remedy. We are told that some Chinese communities do not recognize trachoma as a disease because it is mild and common, and the resultant blindness is delayed and insidious (Chen 1961). Again, Marjorie Topley (1970) found that Chinese mothers in Hong Kong recognized measles to be dangerous, but they did not consider it a disease. They conceived of it as a developmental stage in which the child's body was freed of a hot maternal poison. Thus, measles was treated as an essential *rite de passage* rather than as a medical problem.

Examples could be multiplied from many societies: smallpox in India is almost universally conceived as a religious rather than a medical event, while taking narcotic drugs has been dealt with largely as a problem of law enforcement in the United States, and in Britain until recently as a medical problem. An example relevant to many societies would be parental attitudes toward high infant mortality. Only in societies where modern medicine and hygiene have demonstrated that almost all infant deaths are preventable does a statement like "I have had ten children and buried five" become a confession of failure rather than a boast of parental success.

A system of medicine provides a conceptual structure by which people are judged to be healthy or sick. Because of the importance of hunting and gathering in man's past, all societies must have gained empirical knowledge of the effects of physical injury, of poisonous plants and animals, and of acute poisoning due to spoiled food. However, the causes of most diseases are not at all obvious, and where known they have mostly been uncovered within the last century. Infective agents of disease other than the larger worms could only be recognized when microscopy was sufficiently developed. A long incubation period between exposure to the pathogenic agent and the development of characteristic disease; a low attack rate in persons exposed to risk; and the existence of multiple or alternative causes of diseases have all obscured their causation.

The question arises as to the status of ideas in traditional medicine which coincide with ideas well grounded in modern scientific research. For example, the idea of the circulation of blood is said to have been expressed in ancient Chinese and Indian texts, and some ancient and contemporary traditional societies have independently developed the idea that mosquitoes cause malaria. How do we evaluate these resemblances? In my opinion, we must examine the body of knowledge which supports the idea. If the idea merely associates malaria with swamps and places likely to have numerous mosquitoes, it is a lucky guess that is scarcely more significant as a scientific concept than the idea that malaria is caused by "bad air," as its name implies. Common-sense deductions from observed facts can be misleading. For example, since disease often caused wasting, it is reasonable to suppose that to be fat is to be healthy, though most modern evidence points to the contrary.

Finally, concepts within a medical system may generate a morbid entity, or effect the way a morbid condition is expressed. In the present volume, Gananath Obeyesekere uses the term *cultural disease* for this phenomenon. The forms which hysterical manifestations take are largely presentations of the patient's ideas about symptomatology. In 1967 a short epidemic of *koro* occurred is Singapore. Chinese men suffering from this malady were brought to clinics and hospitals in fear of imminent death due to their penis shooting into the body.

Varying ideas about diseases can be expected to influence what is considered significant or worth describing by medical men, or worth taking to the doctor in the case of laymen. Different practitioners have different experience of disease, and Maxwell (1929) pointed out that in China there were classes of disease that were rarely brought for treatment to modern doctors, who had a reputation for curing other diseases. Such differences probably occur whenever different therapeutic systems coexist (Read 1966).

EVIDENCE FROM THE PAST

The most direct evidence for the history of disease comes from ancient human remains, but their value is largely limited to disease affecting the skeleton and to parasites. While descriptions of disease in ancient documents yield fuller information, they deal largely with the patient's complaints, and are seldom complete. A single complaint like cough, diarrhea, or headache may be the expression of many possible diseases, and a confident diagnosis is often unjustifiable even with modern facilities. It follows that only a few descriptions of disease in ancient texts allow us to make a diagnosis with reasonable certainty. Furthermore, the description of a recognizable disease in an old text does not mean that the disease constituted an important part of the morbidity load in the society. Literate healers saw an unrepresentative sample of sick people, and an individual practitioner confronted with his patients reported little more than clinical impressions about them. An accurate picture of the disease situation in populations can only be obtained through epidemiological surveys, and such studies have not been done until recently. Epidemiological information for ancient societies mainly concerns major lethal epidemics and major geographical variations (Ackerknecht 1965).

There remains our vast body of knowledge of present-day diseases. I believe that this, together with our knowledge of past and present conditions of life, provides the best evidence for reconstructing the probable disease patterns of the past. The small and so-called primitive contemporary communities provide especially useful though potentially misleading models of the past situation (Polunin 1967).

Biological agents of disease are the products of evolution, so they must have undergone changes in the past. In the last few decades of intensive investigation, there has been limited evidence for such change except for the emergence of strains of bacteria resistant to antibiotics and of insect vectors resistant to insecticides, and it is likely that many agents of infection have undergone little significant change since classical times.

POPULATION CHANGES, DIET, AND INFECTIONS

The transition from sparse mobile hunter–gatheres to denser, more settled populations of cultivators affected the transmission and evolution of agents of infection.

During the greater part of human history, population increase was slow. The rate of annual increase was about 0.002 percent before the invention of agriculture, while now, at 2 percent, it is 1,000 times greater (Ehrlich and Ehrlich 1970:9). Data on series of ancient skeletons suggest that a high proportion of those populations died in childhood (Welles 1964:176–177). Until very recently, death rates at all ages were higher than they are now, especially for the young. Up to one-third of all children born died before their first year, and sometimes only a minority survive into adulthood in present-day populations (Polunin 1967). Even so, the development of agriculture probably caused infant mortality to decline, simply because it led to a more stable and protective settlement pattern and a larger and generally more secure food supply. Among hunter–gatherers, the wide range of animal and plant food-stuffs ensured a well-balanced diet. The danger was shortage of calories, though evidence from present-day hunter–gatherers suggests that they do not suffer much from undernutrition (Lee and DeVore 1968:6).

Unfortunately, the cereals, which formed the greater part of the increased food supplies of the cultivators, are deficient in many essential nutrients. Unless supplemented with other foods, their consumption would give rise to deficiencies of proteins, vitamins, and minerals. Pellagra among maize eaters reached a peak about a hundred years ago (Hirsch 1883), while beri-beri among rice eaters probably peaked later. Deficiences of certain essential nutrients are still widespread among Asian peasants.

Cultivation has always carried with it the risk of famine from crop failure or warfare, for which extended opportunities were provided by the accumulation of food surpluses. Famine is selective in affecting the poor, particularly the young and the aged, but also typically involves a general undernutrition. Hungry people may eat poisonous "famine foods," and there have been serious epidemics of paralysis from Lathyrus sativus, and of dropsy from Argemone oil in India (Patwardhan 1961) and from Atriplex leaves in China (Maxwell 1929). Dietary deficiencies aggravate infections, particularly in tuberculosis, dysenteries, typhus, and measles; while infections always aggravate dietary deficiency and may precipitate keratomalacia and protein–calorie malnutrition (Scrimshaw *et al.* 1968).

According to T. Aidan Cockburn (1971), before the invention and spread of agriculture men were like other large mammals in producing only a limited modification of the environment. The parasites that infect mankind probably evolved from those of pre-human ancestors, and a limited number of infections would have been contracted through contact with wild animals (Hare 1968). But with agriculture, human communities entered into new kinds of biotic relationship:

Man lost his mobility and became tied to his land, and many animals moved into his ecological niche to be supported by him, willingly or otherwise. Population increased and spread, bringing long-separated human groups into contact. All of these changes, as well as the agricultural practices themselves, tended to increase certain infectious hazards. (Cockburn 1971:48)

Infections which could be maintained in small pre-agricultural populations were those which conferred no effective immunity and which as a result were long-lasting. With progressive increase in the size of populations, infective agents with progressively shorter infectivity and lengthened immunity could maintain themselves. The extreme is reached by viruses causing "childhood diseases," in which infectivity lasts for a few days and is followed by lifetime immunity. They require very large host populations because susceptibles are quickly used up. They are most likely to have arisen among the great Asian civilizations, because they were the first to develop sufficiently large populations. Additional evidence for this inference is that they were unknown in the American continents until they were introduced from the Old World by European conquest (Cockburn 1971; Hare 1968). The civilizations of the Central Andean and Middle American regions lost an estimated 70 or 80 percent of their populations through these epidemics.

It is unlikely that newly-introduced infections played such a cataclysmic role in the history of Asian civilizations as they did in the New World and the Pacific Islands; Asian groups had sufficiently large populations to maintain the infections once they had evolved *in situ*, or spread from other areas in early times. Nevertheless, Siberian tribes have been devastated by smallpox (Hirsch 1883); and the Black Death, which spread from Asia, killed between 25 and 75 percent of the population of Europe (Hinman 1966). Such infections are nearly always absent in small, isolated populations exemplified by island or forest-dwelling tribes. When introduced from outside, they produce explosive epidemics affecting most of the people, with high fatality rates, and are followed by complete disappearance of the infection, since the infected survivors become immune.

Although genes must be important determinants of human susceptibility to infections, we lack good evidence that such epidemics are due to unusually high genetic susceptibility. Rather, they have been ascribed largely to the infection of vulnerable age groups, the serious disorganization produced when the majority of a community is affected, and the absence of simple nursing measures (Polunin 1967).

Increasing population density leads to the increase in density of parasites, and of peri-domestic hangers-on which may be reservoirs or vectors of infection. Whether human crowding is associated with more or less infection depends on whether concomitant cultural changes with hygienic effects outweigh the crowding effect. The specific infections probably reached a zenith in the mid-nineteenth century in the West and somewhat later in tropical Asian cities, due to unhygienic crowding in the early stages of industrialization and to improved means of transportation (of pathogens, along with people).

It is difficult to generalize about the effects of crowding on vector-borne diseases. In general, the more the environment is modified by man, the fewer the species of animals and plants which survive, and the greater the population density of those opportunistic species which can adapt. Environmental modification may have the effect of controlling infection where the vector is a "wilderness" species, or of promoting it where the vector is an opportunist. In malaria, where many vector species are capable of transmitting infection, an operation such as clearing the forest may control or promote the infection, according to whether the local vector species breeds in shady or sunny waters.

When large numbers of people come together from different local communities, ideal conditions occur for the transmission of infections and their dissemination when people return to their homes. Such conditions arise among refugees from wars, famines, and floods, where hygienic breakdown is inevitable. Even more common are great religious gatherings, like the pilgrimages and fairs which are a prominent part of Indian religion, where vast numbers, makeshift arrangements, and a feeling that they are under supernatural protection, have conspired to increase risks. This historical pattern must have been an important source of epidemics in the past. The Great Pilgrimage to Mecca played an important part in the worldwide dissemination of cholera in the nineteenth century.

Modern textbooks of medicine usually begin by describing the diseases due to specific microbial infections. These diseases best fit the current concepts of disease. They were until recently the principal causes of death, and their control has been the greatest success of modern medicine. Some of the deadliest survive in small, diminishing areas of the less developed world, and are minor causes of death. The decline in mortality from specific infections is a main cause of the current increases in population. However, infections, particularly respiratory infections due to viruses, still cause about 1.5 sickness episodes per person per year in the United States, and pneumonia is probably the greatest single mode of death in the world (Le Riche 1967).

Mutant strains of influenza have twice in this century given rise to pandemics. The first caused the greatest die-off the world has ever known. In the second, the "Asian" A2 influenza virus first appeared in Kweichow in 1957. A pandemic of cholera has affected Asian countries during the last ten years. It probably resulted from the dessemination of the El Tor type of cholera bacillus from isolated endemic foci in Celebes, which has displaced the classical organism in most of its original habitats. Also, blood fluke infection (schistosomiasis) is spreading in the Arab lands wherever permanent irrigation works have led to a multiplication of vector snails and people contaminate water channels with feces.

Nevertheless, in this century, considerable improvement in morbidity and mortality has occurred in Asia. The crude death rate, or percentage of the population dying each year, was 3.4 percent in India between 1901 and

1910 (United Nations 1966). In China it was reduced from between 2.7 and 3 percent in 1929–31 (Winfield 1948) to 0.7 percent in 1959 (Chen 1961). In India and Egypt, the expectancy of life at birth doubled during this century to more than 50 years (United Nations 1966). The specific infections are becoming less important in the disease patterns of these societies, and people survive to an age where degenerative diseases and cancers predominate.

Before turning to several specific regions, I want to comment on the relationship between the large and long-established populations in China and India and the medical systems that evolved in these areas. I believe that the populations expanded and were maintained by the comparatively advanced agriculture, technology, and domestic skills, rather than through special medical knowledge or efforts. Small differences in survivorship can make massive differences to the ultimate population size in the long time available. Thus, if we consider two populations differing only in that 50 percent of live births survive to reproductive age in one and 51 percent in the other, there would be a 2 percent difference in the size of the breeding populations after about one generation.

The avoidance of unboiled milk by Indians, or unboiled "cooling" water by Chinese, or their consumption of a diet in which foods with "heaty" or "cooling" properties were balanced, doubtless protected life and health. But the extent of disease and death which was preventable by nontechnical methods available in the past suggests that the process of social selection of disease-preventing behaviors was not very effective. Though technological "mutations" like wet-rice cultivation or antibiotics can spread rapidly through the world's communities, this was not usually the case with general disease-preventing behavior. This behavior and the associated morbidity and mortality probably showed little improvement between, say, 500 B.C. and 1500 A.D.

CHINA

Ancient hygienic and preventive medical measures have been discussed by Joseph Needham and Gwei-djen Lu (1959). They quote the Confucian Analects of about 500 B.C., which proscribe eating damaged food, along with the proverb "Anything thoroughly boiled or cooked cannot be poisonous." The disinclination for cold food which characterized cuisine was likely to prevent food-borne infections. The practice of drinking only boiled water must also have been a potent factor in preventing water-borne infections, though fuel shortages in overpopulated, deforested areas may have led to inadequate cooking (Worth 1963). Another practice that would have promoted health was frequent, at least regular, bathing. Bath-houses are often mentioned in old texts, though foreign travelers in more modern times have frequently judged the common people to be dirty.

In normal times, the caloric intake of adults was probably nearly adequate, but floods and the destruction of crops were a recurrent part of the Chinese scene until the present time, and are themselves, in part, the indirect result of high population density. In a bad year, as in 1956, a quarter of the cultivated land may be affected (May and Jarcho 1961).

Pellagra was scarcely mentioned in the ancient literature (Ta'o Lee 1940), but it was common in modern times in maize-eating areas in the provinces northeast of the Yangtze (May and Jarcho 1961). Night blindness was reported nearly 1500 years ago, and has been common in recent years (May and Jarcho 1961). In Ch'ao's "General Treatise on Diseases," which is about 1200 years old, several beri-beri syndromes were described for the rice-eating South, but not in the North. More recently, beri-beri was a major killing disease in the cities. It was promoted by machine milling wherever rice eaters lacked other sources of thiamine. Also, rickets has been described from time to time for over a thousand years (T'ao 1940). Its adult form, osteomalacia, was reported to be common in women in some provinces during this century, and to have caused many deaths in childbirth (Snapper 1941). In China (as in India and the Arab lands), there is abundant sunshine, which can prevent rickets, so this disease depends on behavior.

The use of human feces as agricultural fertilizer was universal in China, so that soil-transmitted helminth infections were occupational diseases of farmers. In the recent past, about 25 percent of deaths were ascribed to fecal-borne infections (Winfield 1948). Feces discharged into water helped cultivation of water plants and animals, but made China the principal reservoir of lung, liver, and intestinal flukes and the Oriental schistosome, all of them serious causes of chronic illness. However, China's huge population could not have survived without the use of human feces as fertilizer, and recent progress has been made in reducing the risks of this practice.

Cholera was probably introduced from India, and for a long period epidemics occurred at approximately four-year intervals. These epidemics would spread from the south, and about half the cases died (Maxwell 1929). The killing diseases of China were classified in order of importance as fecal infections, tuberculosis, measles, smallpox and diptheria, tetanus neonatorum, and insect-borne diseases such as malaria, plague, and kala-azar (Winfield 1948).

Since 1949, great improvements in the communicable-disease situation have been reported (Chen 1961; Worth 1963). Cholera, plague, and smallpox are said to have been eradicated, and typhus and relapsing fever brought under control. In addition, many areas have been freed of schistosomiasis.

INDIA

The Indian subcontinent is another area where an ancient civilization has been associated with the development of a large population and risk of famine. The increase in famines between 1860 and 1908, though precipitated by failure of monsoon rains, had as underlying causes an unbalanced economic development and the stagnation of agricultural enterprise (Bhatia 1967). Indian communities, unlike most other contemporary populations, have an excess of males at all ages, due to higher female mortality rates at all ages which reflect the explicit disposition in Indian culture for males to receive preferential access to nourishing food and health care.

A recent study of South Indian villages showed that the poor spend approximately 90 percent of their income for food, but are often clearly near famine level (Rao et al. 1959; Rao 1962). In this situation foods were often valued as a symbol of prestige rather than for ideas about their nutritional value. A general review of diet and health described rice as the main staple in the South and wheat in the North, as in China; but leguminous pulses replace soya bean (Patwardhan 1961). Cereal and legume protein contain essential amino acids in different proportions, and when taken at the same meal they produce a mixture little inferior to animal proteins. Unfortunately, consumption of legumes and foods of animal origin is limited and very unevenly distributed by caste and social class, though nearly 20 percent of the world's cattle and goats, and half the world's buffaloes, are estimated to be in India.

Milk, curds, and ghee are highly prized foods among all classes, and only a small minority, mainly of richer people, are vegetarians. Though religious rules and food preferences aggravate the situation, the most important social factor causing undernutrition is poverty, as food supplies are inadequate. May and Jarcho (1961) estimated that the intakes of calories, protein, and foods of animal origin were declining. Despite the "green revolution" which has greatly increased productivity in recent years, many places are still designated famine areas by local governments.

The principal nutritional deficiency diseases are beri-beri, in regions where thiamine is not diffused through the rice grain by parboiling before milling; kwashiorkor, due to weaning onto a protein-deficient high-calorie diet; marasmus, where there is also calorie lack; and protein-deficiency edema. Osteomalacia and rickets were formerly common among some prosperous segments of society, because of the seclusion of women and children from the sun's rays (Chandrasekhar 1959).

Most deaths are due to infections. Fevers with rashes are the province of a goddess who resents the giving of drugs, and this may lead to inadequate treatment (Singh et al. 1962). Tetanus is a major cause of death, probably because of the extensive use of cow dung. Malaria has been reduced from about one hundred million attacks and one million deaths a year to 56,000 deaths in 1966–67 (Morris 1945; India 1967). Gastroenteritis is a major cause of death among infants and small children. The low-lying and densely inhabited plains of Bengal are probably the original home of cholera, whence it surged to other regions.

THE ARAB WORLD

Paleopathological knowledge is more complete for the ancient Egyptians than for any other early people. Schistosome eggs and atheromatous change in arteries have been found in a three-thousand-year-old mummy (Ruffer 1910). Tuberculosis and leprosy, tapeworms, filarial elephantiasis, and various ectoparasites were known (Sandison 1967). Dental disease was roughly similar to that of other ancient and modern peoples with abrasive diets. Gum disease was the most common cause of loss of teeth, and caries was uncommon, especially in the predynastic period (Ruffer 1920).

Standards of living have improved little in the present century. About 2 percent of the total calories are of animal origin, although religious traditions place no value on a vegetarian diet. Rickets, iron-deficiency anemia associated with parasitism, and pellagra in the maize-growing areas are the chief nutritional diseases. Most of the population is undernourished (May and Jarcho 1961). Childhood protein-deficiency syndromes are common and show a seasonal peak, following those of gut and respiratory infections which trigger them (Darby 1966). Gastrointestinal and eye infections, especially trachoma, are important, as are malaria and parasitic infections, including dracontiasis. Gastroenteritis is responsible for over half the infant deaths in the United Arab Republic, and shows a striking peak of incidence during the dry, hot fly season (Labib 1971). Other specific infections important in the Arab World are tuberculosis, hookworm, smallpox, rickettsioses, relapsing fever, cutaneous leishmaniasis, rabies, tetanus, anthrax, and brucellosis (Simmons et al. 1954).

CONCLUSION

Some important differences exist in the disease patterns of China, India, and the Arab world, particularly for infections with intermediate hosts—e.g., schistosomiasis is absent from India. But the point I wish to make is that a bewildering variety of sickness has always existed in these areas, and most episodes of sickness are due to diseases common to all areas. We should look elsewhere for explanations of the way in which the different systems of medicine have developed. I do not believe that medical scholars in the past looked at the pattern of diseases before them and asked themselves what new ideas might explain the facts. On the contrary the process was one in which the spectrum of sickness was largely observed and explained in terms of the current culture. Thus, "Medical history is an inseparable component of general and cultural history" (Thorwald 1962). Commenting on the *Nei Ching*, one medical historian wrote that medicine was but a part of philosophy and religion, both of which propounded oneness with nature (Veith 1949). Of course, cutting for stone would be an unlikely skill where bladder stones were rare, and it is very difficult to imagine the development of surgical reconstruction of the nose without the practice, formerly prevalent in North India, of cutting off people's noses. But only occasionally, and in this limited sense, does a special morbidity pattern appear to be an important element in determining a part of a traditional medical system.

Literature Cited

Ackerknecht, Erwin H.
  1965 *History and Geography of the Most Important Diseases*. New York: Hafner.
Bhatia, B. M.
  1967 *Famines in India*, 2nd ed. Bombay: Asia Publishing House.
Brothwell, Don, and A. T. Sandison, eds.
  1967 *Diseases in Antiquity*. Springfield, Ill.: Charles C. Thomas.
Chandrasekhar, Sripati
  1959 *Infant Mortality in India, 1901–1955*. London: George Allen and Unwin.
Chen, W. H.
  1961 "Medicine and Public Health," in S. H. Gould, ed., *Sciences in Communist China*, pp. 323–408. Pub. No. 68, Am. Assn. for the Advancement of Science.
Cockburn, T. Aidan
  1971 "Infectious Diseases in Ancient populations." *Current Anthropology* 12: 45–62.
Darby, W. J.
  1966 "Advances in Nutrition in the Middle East." *Jordan Medical J.* (Special Number).
Ehrlich, Paul R., and Anne H. Ehrlich
  1970 *Population, Resources, Environment; Issues in Human Ecology*. San Francisco: Freeman.
Hare, Ronald
  1968 "The Antiquity of Diseases Caused by Bacteria and Viruses," in Don Brothwell and A. T. Sandison, eds,, *Diseases in Antiquity*. Springfield, Ill.: Charles C. Thomas.
Hinman, F. H.
  1966 *World Eradication of Infectious Diseases*. Springfield, Ill.: Charles C. Thomas.
Hirsch, August
  1883 *Handbook of Geographical and Historical Pathology*, trans. from 2nd ed. London: New Sydenham Society.
India, Government of
  1967 *India, a Reference Manual*.
Labib, Ferdos M.
  1971 *Principles of Public Health*. Cairo: Sherif.
Lee, Richard B., and Irven DeVore
  1968 "Problems in the Study of Hunters and Gatherers," Lee and DeVore, eds., *Man the Hunter*, pp. 3–12. Chicago: Aldine.
Le Riche, W. Harding
  1967 "World Incidence and Prevalence of the Major Communicable Diseases," in G. E. W. Wolstenholme and Maeve O'Connor, eds. Ethics in Medical Progress, pp. 1–50. Boston: Little, Brown.
Maxwell, James L.
  1929 *Diseases of China*, 2nd ed. Shanghai: A. B. C. Press.
May, Jacques Meyer, and Irma S. Jarcho
  1961 *The Ecology of Malnutrition in the Far and Near East*. New York: Hafner.

Morris, Jeremy Noah
 1945 "Health of Four Hundred Millions." *Lancet* 1: 743–748.
Needham, Joseph, and Gwei-djen Lu
 1959 "Hygiene and Preventive Medicine in Ancient China." *Health Educ. J.* 17: 170–179.
Patwardhan, Vinayak Narayan
 1961 *Nutrition in India*, 2nd ed. Bombay: Indian Journal of Medical Science.
Polunin, Ivan Vladimirovitch
 1967 "Health and Disease in Contemporary Primitive Societies," in Don Brothwell and A. T. Sandison, eds., *Diseases in Antiquity*, pp. 69–97. Springfield, Ill.: Charles C. Thomas.
Rao, K. Someswara
 1962 "Malnutrition in South India," *in* A. Burgess and R. F. A. Dean, eds., *Malnutrition and Food Habits.*, pp. 29–39. London: Tavistock Institute.
Rao, K. S., M. C. Swaminathan, S. Swarup, and V. N. Patwardhan
 1959 "Protein Malnutrition in South India." *Bull. World Health Organization* 20: 603–639.
Read, Margaret
 1966 *Culture, Health, and Disease*. London: Tavistock Institute.
Ruffer, Marc Armand
 1910 "Note on the Presence of "Bilharzia Haematobia" in Egyptian Mummies of the Twentieth Dynasty, 1250–1000 B.C." Brit. Medical J. 1:16.
 1920 "Studies of Abnormalities and Pathology of Ancient Egyptians' Teeth." *Am. J. Physical Anthropology* 3: 335–382.
Russel, Paul F.
 1955 *Man's Mastery of Malaria*. London: Oxford University Press.
Sandison, A. T.
 1967 "Parasitic Diseases," in Don Brothwell and A. T. Sandison, eds., *Diseases in Antiquity*, pp. 178–188. Springfield, Ill.:Charles C. Thomas.
Scrimshaw, Neville S., Carl E. Taylor, and John E. Gordon
 1968 *Interactions of Nutrition and Infection*. Geneva: World Health Organization Monograph Series, No. 57.
Simmons, J. S., T. F. Whayne, G. W. Anderson, H. M. Horack et al.
 1954 *Global Epidemiology*, 3 vols. Philadelphia: Lippincott.
Singh, Sohan, John E. Gordon, and John B. Wyon
 1962 "Medical Care in Fatal Illnesses of a Rural Punjab Population." *Indian J. Medical Research* 50: 870–880.
Snapper, Isidore
 1941 *Chinese Lessons to Western Medicine*. New York: Wiley Interscience.
T'ao Lee
 1940 "Historical Notes on Some Vitamin Deficiency Diseases in China." *Chinese Medical J.* 58: 314.
Thorwald, Jurgen
 1962 *Science and Secrets of Early Medicine*. London: Thames and Hudson.
Topley, Marjorie
 1970 "Chinese Traditional Ideas and the Treatment of Diseases: Two Examples from Hong Kong." *Man* (N.S.) 5: 421–437.
United Nations
 1966 *Demographic Yearbook*.
Veith, Ilza
 1949 *Huang Ti Nei Ching Su Wen* (*The Yellow Emperor's Classic of Internal Medicine*). Baltimore: Williams and Wilkins.

Wells, Calvin
  1964 *Bones, Bodies, and Diseases*. London: Thames and Hudson.
Winfield, G. F.
  1948 *China, the Land and the People*. New York: Sloane.
Worth, Robert M.
  1963 "Health in Rural China: From Village to Rural Communes." *Am. J. Hygiene*
      77: 228–239.

Traditional Asian Medicine and Cosmopolitan Medicine as Adaptive Systems

FRED L. DUNN

This paper offers a preliminary and tentative assessment of the adaptive significance of three major traditional systems of medicine in Asia. I shall approach this assessment by reviewing the general characteristics of medical systems, and by outlining the problems that intrude in attempts to measure the adaptive value or efficacy of such systems.

DEFINING A MEDICAL SYSTEM

A generic definition of medical systems, or systems of health-care delivery, may usefully being with the concept of health. The World Health Organization has defined health as a "state of complete physical, mental, and social well-being, and not merely the absence of disease." This utopian definition has several disadvantages. It implies that the condition of being healthy is static and absolute, and it does not provide for differences in perspective. Such provision is desirable, since conditions may be regarded as healthy in one society and unhealthy in another. Rene Dubos (1965:344–351) considered these issues in discussing "the mirage of health," and despaired of efforts to formulate a satisfactory abstract definition of health. R. N. Wilson (1970:12) also considered the problem and proposed a relativistic definition by outlining the "idea of health as functional competence in enacting social roles."

The approach which I favor conceives of health as a dynamic, constantly varying condition of the individual or the group (Audy 1971:Audy and Dunn, 1974). This approach emphasizes the idea that the "level" of health may change from one point in time to the next, and that the quantity *and* quality of health changes as the level changes. Health is therefore viewed as a scalar quantity, subject to measurement (Audy 1971). Such a scale is illustrated in Figure 1. A middle zone on this scale represents the transition for any individual (or group) between health and ill health. Thus ill health corresponds to a substantial diminution in health. In semi-quantitative or qualitative terms, current health can be measured against such a scale for an individual, group, community, or whole society.

133

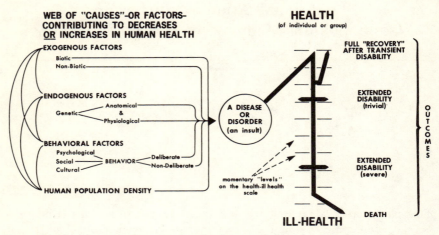

FIGURE 1. Health as a scalar quantity: the intervening insults (diseases and disorders) that influence the level of health, and the causal web that "controls" these insults.

A dynamic, scalar conception of health carries with it the idea of adaptive training as the organism (or group) experiences and responds to successive "insults." Thus, infection by polio virus early in life may be an inapparent or minor insult, but the adaptive result—immunity to reinfection—is a contribution to the long-term health of the host. On the other hand, when initial exposure to the polio virus occurs later in life, the result is often a permanent diminution of health through crippling paralysis. The consequence of infection in infancy is an incremental increase in the level of the host's health, and the same result is achieved through artificial immunization procedures. We may also learn to cope with many forms of psychological and social stress as we experience them and are scarred (and "immunized") by them.

Clearly an insult is *not* the same thing as ill health; it may lower the level of health, permanently or transiently; it may have little effect; it may result in a permanent increase in health. All insults, collectively, constitute the diseases and disorders of human experience. They can be categorized in many ways, and one taxonomy of major determinants of ill health and mortality is summarized in Table 1. This classification is derived from some of the ideas of V. C. Wynne-Edwards (1962) on the factors of social control that influence mammalian population regulation (see also Dunn 1968). A few alternatives in the spectrum of "outcomes" of diseases and disorders are suggested in Figure 1.

Figure 1 also displays a web of causes or factors which can modify diseases and disorders and thus influence the health scale. Changes, however subtle, of relationships within the web are likely to shift the level of health downward *or* upward. The categories "biotic," "non-biotic," "genetic," and so on, encompass all of the factors that are normally considered to be of epidemiologic importance. The perspective that considers the web as a whole—"web-

A Classification of Diseases and Disorders as Determinants of Human
Ill Health and Death

---

1. Socially "uncontrollable" and "unacceptable" determinants:

Food deficits
Accidents
Predation
Exogenous agents: biotic (e.g., parasites)
                    non-biotic (e.g., chemicals)
Endogenous factors: genetic
                      degenerative (aging)

2. Socially "controllable" and (sometimes) "acceptable" determinants:

"Stress" disorders; psychological, social, and psychosocial disorders.

Abortion, infanticide, suicide, homicide, geronticide, sacrifice,
territoriality, head-hunting, warfare, etc.

NOTE: Diseases and disorders in category 1. are often 2. *independent* of population density, while
those in category are often density-*dependent*. However, this distinction is frequently
blurred. Predation, for example, is clearly density-independent in certain respects, and
contributes to uncontrollable loss; but it is also density-dependent insofar as the prey may
"cooperate" in making its surplus members available to predators.

like thinking"—is usually designated "medical ecological." The category of
health-related behavior is divided between "deliberate" or "non-deliberate,"
and in relation to the outcomes this yields four alternatives: deliberate
health-enhancing; deliberate ill-health-provoking; non-deliberate health-
enhancing; and non-deliberate ill-health-provoking behavior. Using this
scheme, I prefer to define a medical system as *the pattern of social institutions
and cultural traditions that evolves from* deliberate behavior *to enhance health,
whether or not the outcome of particular items of behavior is ill health.*

TYPES AND GENERAL CHARACTERISTICS OF MEDICAL SYSTEMS

Medical systems can be conveniently classified by reference to their geographical and cultural settings. Thus there are *local medical systems*, a category
which can accommodate most systems of "primitive" or "folk" medicine;
regional medical systems, such as Ayurvedic, Unani, and Chinese medicine;
and the *cosmopolitan medical system* (often referred to as "modern," "scientific,"
or "Western" medicine). A dictionary definition of "cosmopolitan" conveys
the ideas "worldwide rather than limited or provincial in scope or bearing;
involving persons in all or many parts of the world." Local and regional
systems are almost invariably indigenous and traditional; and they are

normally intracultural, although by no means insulated from exchange with other systems. The traditionalism of the local system tends to be popular and nonscholarly, while that of the regional system tends to be scholarly.

This paper is primarily concerned with regional systems; where the term "traditional" is used it should be understood to mean "scholarly-traditional." The cosmopolitan system is a transplant in most parts of the world, in the sense that it arose in the "West" and retains "traditional" elements which betray its regional origins. Still, with each succeeding decade in the present century, these elements have been transformed, or have become more heavily overlaid by new elements contributed to the system from every part of the world. Obviously, cosmopolitan medicine is subject to considerable regional and local variation—it is not globally homogeneous. Obviously, also, much regional variation exists in the degree to which these three categories of medicine overlap and interpenetrate.

I have abandoned the terms "modern," "scientific," and "Western" in favor of "the cosmopolitan medical system." This system is often termed "scientific medicine," but if we accept a broad definition of science it can be readily demonstrated that scientific elements are present in local and regional medical systems. Many medicinal plants used in systems of "primitive medicine" are now recognized to have specific beneficial pharmacological effects. Indeed, much of the basic armamentarium of pharmacology today has been built up by investigating the properties of traditional herbal remedies. Traditional use of such remedies evolved through countless trials and errors—in short, through human experimentation.

The methods of investigation employed by traditional herbalists are not qualitatively different from those employed in modern clinical chemotherapeutic investigations. The difference lies principally in time. While the clinical investigator today may evaluate a new remedy in the course of a few days by testing it in subjects and giving a placebo or some other remedy to controls, the traditional herbalist, or a line of herbalists through several generations, reaches a decision about a remedy through decades of experience in treating his fellowmen with it, and his "controls" are others of his fellows with similar disorders who are treated with other remedies or not treated at all. A. L. Basham, M. Porkert, and P. U. Unschuld have indicated that, in addition, documentary evidence exists of early experimentation, in the conventional modern sense, in Indian and Chinese traditional chemotherapy. Medicinal plants exemplify the rational scientific element that we scientists and outsiders can detect in someone else's system of medical care. But we must also consider the perspective of the practitioner or client within a traditional system. Acupuncture, for example, is not generally considered "scientific" in cosmopolitan circles—but since it is considered to have a scientific basis within traditional Chinese medicine, it falls within the broad definition of science at the heart of Joseph Needham's (1954) wide-ranging exploration of science and civilization in China.

Whether or not local and regional medical systems are considered to be at least partially scientific, it will be readily accepted that the cosmopolitan system relies on art as well as science. For example, cosmopolitan medical practice is clearly much more scientific than any particular variety of "folk" medicine, but both systems rely heavily on tacit communication between practitioners and clients, and thus on factors that are usually regarded as beyond the fringe of science.

Finally, any traditional medical system in 1971 is as "modern" in its own terms as is the cosmopolitan system in 1971.

I believe that cumulative research findings will show that all medical systems span the spectrum of health-care delivery, although they vary in emphasis. The spectrum of health-care delivery includes the following elements:

1. Health education, broadly conceived, of both practitioners and their clients.
2. Public health sanitation and control.
3. Risk assessment for the individual and the group or community.
4. Prevention for the individual and the group or community.
5. Case-finding in the group or community.
6. Diagnosis.
7. Establishment of prognosis.
8. Therapy: acute, terminal, and supportive, including the very broad field of psychosocial, pastoral, or comfort-supplying care.
9. Rehabilitation.

All elements in this list are represented in the cosmopolitan system, although it is clear that emphasis in terms of numbers of practitioners and allocation of resources is focused on the curative portions of the spectrum, and elements such as risk assessment have been strikingly neglected until very recently (Sadusk and Robbins 1968). In local and regional medical systems, too, emphases seem to center in the curative area, but we are beginning to appreciate that the degree of emphasis has often been exaggerated. Gunnar Myrdal, for example, is surely incorrect in stating that "indigenous medicine is in principle merely curative" (1968:1576). The narrow range of information about traditional systems that has been assembled over the years by scientists and scholars is probably responsible for statements of this kind. Anthropologists have focused almost exclusively on the curative aspects of ethnomedicine. At least 95 percent of the ethnographic literature on health-enhancing behavior and on the values and beliefs that underlie such behavior is concerned with curing. This is partly because much curing activity is dramatic and focused on events that can be observed during the relatively short span of time that the ethnographer is in the community. Other elements of the spectrum—health education, public health, risk assessment, prevention, rehabilitation—have yet to receive much attention from ethnologists and other students of traditional systems.

TABLE 2

A Comparison of Some Characteristics of Three Categories of Past and Present-Day Medical Systems, With Emphasis on Actual Practice Rather than Theoretical Ideals

	Local Medical Systems	Regional Medical Systems	The Cosmopolitan Medical System
	("folk medicine")	(e.g., Ayurvedic, Unani, Chinese)	(i.e., "modern," "Western," or "scientific" medicine)
	indigenous popular-traditional	*indigenous scholarly-traditional*	*transplanted* (in most parts of the world)
Geographical emphasis	usually local, rural, or urban	regional, rural or urban	global, largely urban, slowly expanding rural emphasis
Diseases and disorders of concern	limited range of locally distributed + universals	broader range of regionally distributed + universals	all of man's diseases and disorders
Emphasis on: Conventional health education (of clients)	little	little to moderate	moderate
Public health	little	*past*: strong (parallel development especially urban, and not necessarily linked to other medical institutions) *today*: little	strong

Preventive medicine	moderate	*past*: moderate (strong in theory) *today*: declining	moderate
Curative medicine	strong	*past*: moderate in China (theory strong), strong in India	very strong
Access to care	variable, all adults often have equal access (esp. in small-scale societies), children may have less access (*benefits of care more or less less equally distributed in the population*)	*today*: strong highly variable, usually sharp differentials, in access related to age, birth order, sex, religion, economic status, etc. (*benefits of care usually quite unequally distributed*)	*past*: urban elite had greatest access *today*: the ideal is *equal access for all*; the reality is *access proportional to income*
Practitioner characteristics	male or female practitioners practitioners not elitist, often part-time	usually male (some females today) *past*: often close to or members of elitist circles (sometimes social stratification related to specialization) *today*: often marginal in urban areas (sometimes middle-class); among the elite in rural areas	*past*: male *today*: male or female secondary elite (before the elaboration of professional and paraprofessional specialties) *past*: *today*: a range from secondary elite to intermediate and low social status

TABLE 2 (*Contd.*)

	Local Medical Systems ("folk medicine")	Regional Medical Systems (e.g., Ayurvedic, Unani, Chinese)	The Cosmopolitan Medical System (i.e., "modern," "Western," or "scientific" medicine)
	little to moderate specialization	*past:* considerable specialization *today:* little specialization	*past:* little specialization *today:* very strong specialist fragmentation
Informal training and formal education of practitioners	spirit intermediator often "self-trained following inspiration" herbalist and/or ritual-magic specialist; father–son or master–pupil education	today usually a scholarly master-pupil relationship or scholarly education at a school; self-training uncommon	scholarly education at a school
Mode of entry into "practice"	self-designation as a practitioner or by inheritance	usually informal or formal examinations, often some form of licensing	formal examinations, licensing

Charles C. Hughes (1963) and Joseph Needham and Lu Gwei-djen (1962) are exceptions to the preceding generalization. Hughes' essay, "Public Health in Non-Literate Societies," and Needham and Lu's "Hygiene and Preventive Medicine in Ancient China" are based on historical records and scattered observations by field workers. As Hughes shows, no one up to 1963 had made an intensive field study of a traditional preventive medical system. In 1971 the only comprehensive investigation I know about is a study of prevention in a Malay village by A. C. Colson (1969). Other investigators (e.g., Chen 1970) are beginning to explore the non-curative elements of traditional medical systems, however, and this area of research should expand in the future.

Still other data need to be considered in any comparative analysis of medical systems. Practitioner characteristics are particularly significant, for they differ profoundly even between systems of the same type. Practitioners in a particular system should be described with respect to their age and sex; socioeconomic status; caste, religious, political, and other affiliations; educational experience and method of entry into practice; degree of specialization. We need to learn who, in theory and in fact, can and do become practitioners. Also, the social characteristics of clients or recipients of medical care require analysis. Again, such characteristics as sex, age, birth order, race, religion, and political affiliation need to be ascertained to adequately describe the structure and function of a particular medical system.

This descriptive information bears on this question: Within a particular population, who has greatest access, who has less, and who perhaps lacks access to the available medical care? What are the alternatives for a member of the population who has little or no access to one or all of its systems of medicine? Also, W. J. McNerney has pointed out that "creating access does not necessarily elicit use" (1971:226). Thus a description of access should distinguish the ideal and the actual, or the ideational and the phenomenal (Goodenough 1964).

This discussion of types and general characteristics of medical systems is summarized in Table 2. This tabulation attempts to compare the characteristics of medical systems in terms of actual practice rather than theoretical ideals. Thus, for example, a preventive perspective is strongly evident in classical Ayurvedic literature, but in practice in ancient India preventive medicine was probably slighted in favor of curative medicine. Of course, my definition of a medical system excludes non-deliberate health-related behavior, so that the concern for ritual purity in Hindu religion and caste organization is not considered to be part of the medical system, even though it probably affects the level of health.

HEALTH-ENHANCING BEHAVIOR OUTSIDE ANY MEDICAL SYSTEM

Non-deliberate health-enhancing behavior has made an enormous contribution to improvements in health for which professionals within medical systems have been inclined to take credit. An example is the dramatic fall in the death rate for respiratory tuberculosis in England and Wales during the last century and a half. About 1840, the mean annual death rate was nearly 4,000 per million. About 1880, when the tubercle bacillus was identified, the rate had fallen to 2,000, and before 1920 the figure dropped below 1,000. The rate had declined to about 500, and the trend was still strongly downward, when specific chemotherapy finally became available in the late 1940s. T. McKeown and C. R. Lowe conclude "that medical measures made no contribution to the course of tuberculosis before the twentieth century" (1966:9). They assert that no evidence exists for changes in virulence of the organism or resistance of the host during this time, and conclude that the fall in death rate must be ascribed to miscellaneous "environmental influences, with the exception of medical measures."

Rene Dubos (1965:422) has commented: "Comparison of disease patterns in prosperous countries fifty years ago with what they are today brings to light the puzzling fact that several medical problems have all but disappeared without benefit of scientific understanding." In the same vein, W. J. McNerney claims it is a myth that "most health services make a big difference in the health of the population—thus, with enough money, health can be purchased" (1971:225). He points out that "in countries where infectious diseases are no longer among the predominant causes of death, it is often difficult to demonstrate a strong relationship between longevity and the amount spent on health services. The amount spent on health resources can vary as much as 100 percent, and morbidity and mortality rates will vary on the order of 5 percent" (1971:225).

Examples of non-deliberate health-enhancing behavior that affects rates of mortality are given by Carl E. Taylor and M. F. Hall, who claim that: "In some Asian countries child mortality for females is considerably higher than for males, largely because mothers and families take more conscientious care of sons than of daughters. The quality of a mother's care has been shown to be the most important identifiable factor influencing child health" (1967: 651). Taylor and Hall also write: "In Ceylon, after World War I, mortality rates fell approximately equally in the non-malarious third of the island and in the much-publicized malarious area where mosquito control was dramatically effective. In both cases, general economic and nutritional improvement were probably the dominant forces." Assessment of the adaptive efficacy of a medical system is enormously complicated by the difficulty in measuring the impact of these health-improving forces.

THE ADAPTIVE EFFICACY OF MEDICAL SYSTEMS

I consider in this section some problems in measuring the efficacy of behavior directed to maintaining and enhancing health. Each medical system evolves to meet a people's conception of their health needs. It does not follow from this that a system meets their needs very well, either as they see their needs or as an outside scientist might define them. We do have evidence, however, to suggest that a long-standing, indigenous, traditional system may be more efficacious in meeting certain health needs than a recently transplanted system, *and vice versa*.

In discussing adaptive efficacy, a clear distinction is required between health needs that are directly related to Darwinian fitness and those that primarily influence the quality of life. The first category concerns diseases and disorders that lead to manifest ill-health or death. They can be conveniently referred to as biological needs. Their prevalence, incidence, and other epidemiologic characteristics can often be determined with some degree of accuracy. The second category of needs is less readily measurable, and generally related to human ideas of comfort, ease, satisfaction, and joy in life. Mark Field and others refer to the need for pastoral or supportive care, but I shall use the term "psychosocial needs." Ascertainment of a medical system's success in meeting psychosocial needs is difficult, because individual or group perceptions of health are difficult to measure, but I believe that they *can* be measured and that this is a task which behavioral epidemiologists and medical ethnographers should undertake.

The first step toward assessing the adaptive efficacy of a medical system must be an attempt to measure the biological and psychosocial health needs of the society. Then we must measure the degree to which the system successfully responds to each broad category of need, and to each of many subcategories. We have attained some proficiency in measuring biological needs and the success of responses to such needs in living societies, but our measurements for societies of the past are crude and fragmentary. Measurements of psychosocial needs and system responses are impressionistic for modern societies, and our knowledge of this aspect of past systems requires interpretive social and cultural historical research.

At this point I should like to distinguish between adaptability and adaptedness with respect to health-related behavior. "Adaptability" refers to a capacity for response to change, while "adaptedness" refers to a concept of equilibrium or homeostasis. Thus, high adaptability is a great capacity for adjusting to biological or sociocultural change; high adaptedness, on the other hand, implies biological or sociocultural stability. The terms are not polar: at theoretical extremes a population, society, or medical system could be highly adapted and highly adaptable, poorly adapted and non-adaptable, highly adapted but non-adaptable, or poorly adapted but very adaptable.

When, therefore, we say a medical system is effective or has great adaptive efficacy, are we referring to its capacity to sustain biological or psychosocial stability by adjustments of equilibrium? Or are we describing its efficacy in meeting change? Are both concepts involved? These questions must be answered by attempts to clarify an understanding of adaptive efficacy.

Other questions and hypotheses then emerge. For example, is a medical system more likely to be adaptable—capable of responding to new insults—if it is closely associated with other medical systems? Or is it likely to become rigid and unresponsive in such circumstances, to protect its integrity? Again, which medical system is better able to sustain psychosocial equilibrium in a society: a local system which is the only option in a traditional village society, or a traditional system which is oriented to meeting psychosocial needs, but is simply one of an array of medical systems open to members of a more complex society? How, in general, are degrees of cultural homogeneity and heterogeneity related to the biological adaptive value of a medical system, to the capacity of a system to respond to new conditions, and to its ability to maintain psychosocial equilibrium?

I have noted that objective and reliable measurements of adaptive efficacy are available only for a limited range of biological needs. Even in this category, the health statistics for most physically manifest diseases and disorders in most societies are grossly inadequate. Definitive statements about the comparative efficacy of medical systems simply cannot be made at the present time. Fortunately, another approach to the problem allows us to make tentative comparative assessments of the efficacy of medical systems. This indirect approach analyzes the characteristics of medical systems along the lines outlined and summarized in Table 2. In this approach we assess efficacy by estimating elements in the spectrum of health-care delivery receive special emphasis in different systems, and by the known characteristics of practitioners and clients.

We can at least identify health needs that are probably most adequately met by a particular medical system. Also, we can determine the general character of differential access to the system, and who is most likely to profit or suffer from the differential. Of course, these questions must be asked to ascertain what the system does in theory, and then repeated to ask what it accomplishes in practice. In the final part of this essay I shall use this indirect approach to assess the adaptive efficacy of several traditional Asian medical systems. Before proceeding, however, I must briefly examine the issue of cosmopolitan medicine's adaptive efficacy in modern Asia.

The cosmopolitan medical system appears to have had a profound impact on the health of Asian populations in only a few specialized fields such as mass control of certain infectious diseases. As Figure 1 shows, since any determinant of ill health is linked to a causal web, it is in varying degrees biophysical, psychological, and sociocultural in origin. This is true even when we are accustomed to think of the disease or disorder only in its markedly biological aspect. An example would be smallpox. The medical response to this biophysical–psychological–sociocultural event that we call an episode of ill health due to smallpox should also be a multifaceted biophysical–psychological–sociocultural one if it is to be fully adaptive. While an indigenous and traditional medical system may include responses of this kind to some health problems, and may therefore be efficacious, the cosmopolitan system may respond only biologically—for example, by the proferral of smallpox vaccine and little else in the face of an epidemic—and thus cannot be considered fully adaptive, even if the epidemic is controlled.

The limited spheres of health touched by cosmopolitan medicine in some regions today seem to be those most closely tied to the specific health problems which provided the original stimulus for introducing the system. For example, the health problems which led in South Asia to the introduction, more than a century ago, of the cosmopolitan system were: demand on the part of expatriate Europeans for health care similar to that in the homeland; demand for similar care on the part of some elements of the local elite; care of plantation or industrial laboring populations to increase labor efficiency and economic productivity; control of diseases of mass epidemic potential associated with high case-fatality rates, such as smallpox, cholera, and plague, because these are diseases that can be readily spread to and kill in any other part of the globe. The cosmopolitan medical system in India and other South Asian countries has provided fairly satisfactory solutions for these well-defined and specialized needs, but it has not yet become fully accessible to most of the people.

TRADITIONAL ASIAN MEDICINE IN THE ·PAST

In this section I shall outline some of the characteristics and adaptive strengths in ancient and medieval times of each of the three great regional medical systems of Asia: Chinese, Ayurvedic, and Arabic-Persian or Unani. This discussion provides the background for a similar assessment in the next section of the three systems today. The general format for the discussion of each system corresponds to that in Table 2.

Chinese Medicine
The geographical setting of traditional medicine in China is, of course, diverse. Environmental conditions ranging from cool temperate to subtropical, from riverine and coastal to montane and plateau, from wet to arid, from high latitude to low latitude, guarantee an exceptional diversity of diseases and disorders. Some of the principal health problems of the far north must have been substantially different from those in the far south in ancient times, as today. Yet the Chinese medical tradition has apparently maintained considerable homogeneity in beliefs and practices throughout the land and through a long span of time since the late Chou or Han dynasties, when a class of secular physicians emerged distinct from priests and sorcerers (Croizier 1968:14). Local differences in patterns of disease may have been associated with a great diversity of local or folk medical systems which existed alongside and overlapped with the evolving regional tradition, but descriptions of such systems were not recorded or have not survived, as far as I know.

In ancient Chinese medicine the elements of the spectrum of health-care delivery that received special emphasis appear to have been the education of practitioners, public health (especially sanitary measures), prevention, diagnosis, and curative medicine. Conventional health education, risk assessment, case-finding, and rehabilitation probably received little attention. Prevention was a highly valued concept, and was a concern of the elaborate bureaucracy of medical and health officials attached to the Han imperial staff (Needham and Lu 1962). Han sanitary officials were responsible for water and food hygiene, and for such matters as the condition of latrines in the homes of the elite. The claim that a formal examining and grading system existed for physicians in the Chou dynasty is in doubt (Croizier 1968:28); but such formalities, along with medical schools, were well-established by the Sung dynasty.

The central concern of ancient Chinese medicine was curing. Through its eclecticism, Chinese curative medicine developed, especially from Chou through T'ang times, into a strong and highly complex subsystem with a rich materia medica, considerable specialization, and a wide array of theories and practices based on an elaborate philosophy of disease (Wong and Wu 1932). Many substantial therapeutic achievements have been recorded: for example, substances containing iodine to cure goiter, ergot to hasten difficult labor, ephedrine to lower blood pressure and control asthma, and pomegranate rind to expel tapeworms (Huard and Wong 1968:142). Variolation was in use as a protection against smallpox in the sixteenth century if not the eleventh (Needham 1954:58), and chaulmoogra oil was employed in treating leprosy at least as early as the fourteenth century (Wong and Wu 1932:96). Midwifery was developed as a highly skilled specialty. Although the management of fractures and dislocations was elaborated into an art in itself, the practice of ophthalmology and surgery, together with any systematic study of anatomy, was disdained. Psychological as well as biological disorders were managed through acupuncture, moxibustion, and other measures to restore internal harmony (Croizier 1968:19). It is abundantly clear that ancient Chinese medicine could relieve symptoms and alleviate ill health in many ways.

Access to bureaucratized medical care in ancient China appears to have been relatively open, at least in theory, and the concept of state responsibility for medical welfare existed even in the Chou dynasty (Croizier 1968:28). In the Sung dynasty, state-supported hospitals and dispensaries were well established, and physicians of the State Bureau of Medical Care visited the poor in their homes or in the hospitals (Eberhard 1967:58). Clinics and other facilities for "social relief" during the Sung dynasty are described in some detail by Hsü (1956).

Although it appears that the elite of most dynasties were especially favored, the general population, including the indigent, also had access to state-supported health services. Pediatric, obstetrical, and gynecological specialties had developed by the T'ang dynasty (Wong and Wu 1932), which suggests that in theory there were at that time no major differentials in access to government medical care for women compared to men or for children compared to adults. One gains an impression of egalitarianism in access to care from reading the descriptions of early Chinese medicine. Even the urban-rural differential in access may have been overcome to some extent, as it continued to be early in the twentieth century, by the evolution of areas of medical care coinciding with the hinterlands of market towns (Yang 1945). Rural people within each market area could consult physicians and purchase medicines in the town, combining these activities with their normal trading rounds.

The practitioners of state-supported medicine in ancient China were men, and at least until Sung times, most of them were among the honored members of the society. During the Sung period four classes of practitioners evolved, according to Paul Unschuld (personal communication). At the top were the Confucian medical theoreticians (*ru-i*), below them certain famous part-time specialists (*ming-i*), then a class of full-time specialists (*chuan-i*), and at the bottom those wandering doctors (*ling-i*) who offered primarily symptomatic and supportive therapy. All classes but the *ru-i* have survived to the present. Specialization probably reached its zenith during the T'ang dynasty (Wong and Wu 1932:48–52), when four categories of full-time specialists—physicians, acupuncturists, masseurs, and exorcists—were recognized. Each category was ranked and each type of specialist could apparently sub-specialize in one of the recognized branches of medicine.

The adaptive strength of Chinese medicine in the past would appear to lie in (1) its eclectic diversity, which provided a wealth of diagnostic and prognostic alternatives, several sanctioned therapeutic options for any health problem, and a coherent philosophical foundation which could be applied to psychological and psychosocial disorders; (2) the strong emphasis on public health measures and preventive approaches; and (3) the centralization and bureaucratization which resulted, at least in theory, in open access to the system for the poor as well as the rich, for females as well as males, for children as well as adults, and perhaps for rural people as well as those of the cities. The greatest weakness of the system appears to have been in the neglect of surgery.

Ayurvedic Medicine
Traditional medicine in the Indian subcontinent evolved in a somewhat less diverse geographical setting than that of China. The region is largely tropical and subtropical; rainfall differences provide the principal climatic contrasts. The diseases of the subcontinent associated with specific exogenous agents are, and presumably also were in the past, rather uniformly distributed throughout the land. The vector-borne infectious and parasitic diseases are relatively more important than in most of China. Thus the broad pattern of disease and disorder in India differs considerably from that in China;

in this light, one might expect to find that the medical systems in the two regions also differ.

The principal emphasis of ancient Indian medicine seems to have changed several times, first as the Harappans gave way to the Aryans, and later as the Vedic medical literature gave way to the classical literature of Ayurveda. The archaeological record provides evidence of a strong concern with public health in the Indus valley cities of 4500 to 3500 years ago. At both Mohenjodaro and Harappā, excavations of the houses of well-to-do citizens have exposed bathrooms, privies, elaborate drains, sewage soakpits, rubbish chutes, and brick-lined wells that must have minimized contamination of drinking water. Stuart Piggott remarked that "the whole conception shows a remarkable concern for sanitation and public health without parallel in the Orient in the prehistoric past" (1952:168). After the collapse of the Harappan culture, which presumably coincided with the Aryan invasion about 3500 years ago, this preoccupation with public health seems to have diminished. However, a concern with public health does survive in Ayurveda of the classical period (A. L. Basham and C. Leslie, personal communications).

In the Vedic medical literature of 3000 years ago or more, the focus was on curing through magical means. Heinrich Zimmer (1948:2) found in the concern with magical, supernatural, and religious ideas the beginnings of a psychosomatic approach to the task of healing which continued as a strong element of classical Ayurveda, especially in the first major Ayurvedic text, the Caraka Samhita, which dates from the first century in its present form. Religious and magical practices continue to be recommended in Caraka, but a new healing approach is elaborated that is rational, humoral, and centered on drug therapy and diet. Prevention is emphasized in theory, especially through attention to proper diet and household arrangements. However, preventive medical acts other than personal hygiene and diet are not conspicuous in the Ayurvedic classics. The second authoritative text of Ayurveda, the Susruta Samhita, dating from about the fourth century, described surgery in more detail than other texts. Under the influence of the Susruta, surgical practice flourished in India; but in recent centuries this wing of Ayurveda has withered. The third authoritative Ayurvedic text, the Vagbhata Samhita, compiled about the eighth century, continued and strengthened the rational and secular traditions of the system. Throughout the history of Ayurveda until recently, the education of the practitioner was in the hands of a master. As in traditional Chinese medicine, general public health education, risk assessment, case finding, and rehabilitation were apparently not stressed in the classical texts.

Perhaps the greatest contrast with ancient Chinese medicine lies in the matter of access to care. Access to the Chinese system seems to have been more open than to the Ayurvedic system. Greatest access to care was apparently given to the urban adult male of one of the three upper classes of Indian society. Classical Ayurvedic care was to be available first to the king, second to the army, and third to those of the twice-born castes (Zimmer 1948:86). Although a few references exist to charitable facilities supported by Ayurvedic practitioners (Sastri 1960:7–8), to social medicine (Zimmer 1948:86), and to public medical service (in the seventh century— A. L. Basham, personal communication), there is little in the historical records on Ayurveda resembling the records of a centralized, state-supported, bureaucratized system of medicine in ancient China.

Practitioners of ancient Ayurveda were invariably male, and were drawn from the Brahmin, Ksattriya, and Vaisya varna (Zimmer 1948:76). Entry into Ayurvedic practice was therefore open in theory to members of many different castes. It is known that, in fact as well as theory, Ayurvedic physicians were drawn from many castes in the eighteenth and nineteenth centuries (Leslie 1968:564)—as they are today. Except for very low castes, and physician castes in Bengal and Kerala, caste appears never to have been a major factor governing entry into practice, and it seems also that vaids have always accepted clients from many different castes (Charles Leslie, personal communication). On the other hand, the barrier to female admission to Ayurvedic practice appears to have survived until quite recent times. (Charles Leslie tells me that some female vaids are now trained in the Ayurvedic colleges.) As in China, specialization by practitioners reached a peak in the classical period of Ayurveda during the first millenium of the present era.

Ayurvedic medicine in its classical period seems to have provided curative medical care of considerable adaptive significance to a limited range of recipients. The remainder of the Indian population apparently had little access to learned practitioners, and continued to rely on local medical resources. Classical Ayurvedic surgery and internal medicine surely contributed significantly to the health of kings and court leaders, soldiers, and male members of elite castes. Any genetic benefits in terms of fitness resulting from ancient Ayurvedic care must have been unequally distributed, favoring this small segment of the population. Later, after the classical period, the scope and therapeutic significance of Ayurveda apparently diminished, especially with the disappearance of surgery. Whether the therapeutic efficacy of Ayurveda in psychosocial realms was also reduced in later centuries is a moot question. The answer to this question is linked to the following research problems: How have the social characteristics of those receiving Ayurvedic care changed between the classical period and modern times? Has the proportion of the total population receiving Ayurvedic care at any moment in time remained about the same since classical time, or has it steadily increased?

Arabic-Persian (Unani) Medicine
This ancient medical tradition, with its origins in the Mediterranean world and its development in the Middle East, was brought to India with the spread of Islamic civilization (Leslie 1968:565). Thus in India it was originally

a transplanted medical system, although over the centuries it has become indigenous and traditional. The geographical region of Arabic-Persian medicine's development is more circumscribed and homogeneous than that of Ayurveda, and much more so than that of Chinese medicine. Mainly arid and subtropical to temperate, across a narrow latitudinal span, the region supports a smaller range of tropical—especially vector-borne—diseases than does India or China.

As the geographical setting was circumscribed and ecologically homogeneous in comparison to China, so also the classical Arabic-Persian system of medicine was rather narrow in scope and limited in complexity compared to that in China. Strong emphasis was given to rational internal medicine which, however, followed Galenic humoral doctrines implicitly. Magical and supernatural approaches had little place in this system of medicine. On the other hand, considerable attention was given to mental disorders, and one authority claims that Arab physicians were the first to practice psychotherapy (Menninger 1963:424; Whipple 1967). Innovation in classical Arabic-Persian medicine was limited largely to pharmacology, medical education—especially the introduction of bedside teaching in a teaching hospital—and hospital construction (Whipple 1967). The development of surgery was severely stunted by reliance on Galen's anatomical ideas and by prohibitions against dissection and autopsy (Whipple 1967:77; Robinson 1943:192). Prevention and public health received some limited attention, principally in urban areas.

Practitioners in the classical period were largely established in the cities, and one gains the impression that their clients were principally members of elite circles. The majority of patients who came to the attention of the Arabic-Persian physicians were probably urban and male. Although Avicenna was clearly not a typical physician, his life at least exemplifies the preoccupation of the most competent practitioners of the time. Avicenna began his career by curing a prince, soon received a post with a sultan, and later traveled widely, curing various rulers and other patrons (Krueger 1963). He and men like Rhazes, al-Tabari, and Haly Abbas attended patients of lower status as well, but their first responsibility was always to their patron. Nevertheless, at least in the great cities, facilities for the indigent poor were provided—for example, a twelfth-century hospital for the poor in Baghdad was described by Benjamin of Tudela. This hospital, supported at the Caliph's expense, included a unit for patients requiring psychiatric care (Anonymous 1970).

For the population as a whole, the activities of Arabic-Persian public health workers were of greater adaptive significance, but these activities also appear to have been confined to great cities such as Baghdad. A muhtasib or inspector general was charged with hygienic regulation of city water supplies, foods offered for sale, slaughterhouses, and public baths (Whipple 1967:73).

Viewed as a system, classical Arabic-Persian medicine seems to have provided sophisticated care in the field of internal medicine, or pharmacothera-peutics, to a limited range of patients, probably primarily male. In principle, medical care must have been available to all, regardless of class, but in fact such care was probably almost nonexistent outisde the larger towns and cities. Various folk systems presumably existed throughout the classical period in the Middle East, and would have been the only sources of health care in the villages and towns. Public health sanitation must have provided some benefits for those residing in the larger towns and cities. As in India, and perhaps China, little or no attention was given to village public health work in the ancient Middle East. Although mental disorders attracted some attention, this highly rational medical system cannot have had much to offer toward the alleviation of psychological and psychosocial disorders. For support in this sphere, the society undoubtedly turned to religion and to the local medical systems. J. Christoph Burgel's essay for the present volume asserts that the Islamically-inspired local medical systems of the Middle East in the medieval period were so homogeneous that they comprised a second regional system, which he labels "Prophetic medicine," and which competed with Arabic-Persian or Galenic medicine.

TRADITIONAL ASIAN MEDICINE TODAY

The modern descendants of the three regional traditions of Asian medicine are examined in this section as independent entities and as systems interacting with the cosmopolitan medical system. I restrict the discussion to China and India, in the latter case treating Ayurveda and Unani as the Indian representa-tive of the Arabic-Persian tradition. The Arabic-Persian medical tradition also survives in Southeast Asia and in the Near and Middle East, but in more tenuous form than in Pakistan, India, and Sri Lanka. Certainly there has been no conscious movement toward revival of the ancient tradition, as there has been in South Asia and in China. Ralph Croizier has suggested that Arabic-Persian medicine played no great role in modern Arab nationa-lism, because it is closely related to early European medicine and thus cannot be asserted to have a unique value unknown to the West (1968:7).

The traditional medical system thrives in modern China because the system has real therapeutic or adaptive value, because the professionals and para-professionals trained in the cosmopolitan system have never been sufficiently numerous to provide even minimal care for all of China's people, and because a blend of traditionalism and "cultural nationalism" is supported by China's intellectual leaders (Croizier 1968). Ilza Veith has referred to "the dynamic revival of traditional medicine in present-day China" (1966:ix), and Ralph Croizier's essay in the present volume describes its ideology. I shall identify outstanding traits of the modern traditional system and examine briefly its adaptive efficacy.

What survives or has been revived in Chinese medicine is: (1) the formal education of practitioners; (2) the hardy subsystem of curative medicine; (3) strong central bureaucratic control of the system; and (4) egalitarianism in access to care. The physician, including the paraprofessional practitioner, is a graduate of a standardized course in traditional medicine, as were his predecessors in the Sung dynasty. Curative medicine survives in its traditional and eclectic diversity, offering therapeutic options, apparently with special emphasis on acupuncture and use of herbal remedies, founded on ancient theoretical principles. The encouragement that traditional medicine receives comes from the state, perhaps to an even greater degree than in the Han, T'ang, or Sung dynasties. On the other hand, public health and preventive medical activities have long been separated from traditional medicine. Since the nineteenth century these activities have been increasingly "cosmopolitanized" (Wong and Wu 1932). While the traditional practitioner may be asked to assist in some aspect of a local preventive or public health program, or perhaps in health education (Worth 1963), his direct responsibilities apparently do not include these matters. Most significant, perhaps, from the adaptive point of view is the reinforcement of an egalitarian principle which can be found in medical texts dating back to the Chou dynasty (Croizier 1968:28). At least in the ideal, any citizen of China can consult and receive treatment from a traditional practitioner.

Open access to traditional care is probably the rule, especially in rural areas, partly because other practitioners may be in short supply or nonexistent, and also because in 1958 traditional medicine was granted status equal to or superior to cosmopolitan medicine (Sieh 1967:382). However, the reliance upon and encouragement of traditional practitioners has failed to meet all needs for health care. A category of "middle doctors" has been created to provide assistants to doctors. In country areas such assistants, who have usually received two years of practical training in basic medicine, may set up clinics and function essentially as qualified practitioners (Sieh 1967:383). They probably use a blend of cosmopolitan and traditional skills and remedies. In addition, "barefoot doctors" have been introduced to the countryside in large numbers since 1965. They are chosen by their fellow collective-farm members to receive about three months of formal training, and return to their home communities to divide their time between medical and other work (Sibley 1971). Thus, four categories of state-supported medical practitioners exist in China, and many other local or folk resources persist, overlapping with and supplementing the government-sanctioned systems of care. The blurring of lines between popular-traditional and scholarly-traditional Chinese medicine in Hong Kong is stressed by Marjorie Topley (1970), and may also exist in the rest of China.

That traditional medicine in modern China is perceived to be a valuable health-care resource is demonstrated by its strong state support and by its evident popularity. This does not constitute evidence for its adaptive value in biological terms, but it does indicate that it is adaptive in the supportive or psychosocial sense. The complexity of the system suggests that it meets many needs in many realms of ill health. It could be argued, however, that its complexity may inhibit adaptive responses to certain needs. Areas of weakness in the tradition such as surgery and ophthalmology provided areas in which the cosmopolitan system was rapidly accepted (Wong and Wu 1932). This division of labor between the traditional and cosmopolitan systems has been fostered by the state in the past two decades, so that today a blend of systems is beginning to emerge (Sieh 1967). The systems are no longer wholly distinct, and in the future a "traditional Chinese–cosmopolitan" hybrid system may indeed evolve, a possibility critically discussed by Ralph Croizier (1968:237–238). Because the blending has already begun, it is even now impossible—or at least I find it so—to estimate the adaptive efficacy of traditional Chinese medicine in modern China.

Both scholarly medical traditions of India's past—Ayurveda and Unani—continue to flourish in India. Much that can be said about the condition of either system today can also be applied to the other; thus I shall examine the two systems together. One important difference exists, however: "With notable exceptions, Vaids, or Ayurvedic physicians, rather than Hakims [Unani practitioners], have been the more persistent and active proponents of professionalization" (Leslie 1968:565).

Although I have suggested that Ayurvedic medicine lost some of its classical therapeutic efficacy by the eighteenth and nineteenth centuries, its total adaptive impact as a system would not have diminished if the proportion of the population with access to Ayurvedic care increased. It is my impression, in fact, that such a broadening of access existed and has continued to the present time. However, access to care still appears to be more restricted than is the case for Chinese traditional medicine today. Although Ayurvedic care is available in rural and urban areas throughout India, and probably cuts across lines of social and economic status as never before, the vaid is still usually a male, and strong governmental support for the system is lacking. Female access to Ayurvedic care, at least for certain disorders, will inevitably be limited as long as the practitioners remain primarily male. The extent to which members of marginal socioeconomic groups meet difficulties in seeking this form of care because of economic and social barriers is an important current research problem. Finally: "Before and after independence, most of the official backing for Ayurveda has come from provincial governments, and this has varied widely" (Croizier 1968:232).

What has been said above about access to Ayurveda holds also for Unani medicine. The practitioner is male, and in Muslim communities especially, a female is unlikely to seek some kinds of medical aid from a male physician. Little centralized support has developed for Unani medicine, and hakims have not united and pushed strongly for professionalization. On the other hand, the Muslim egalitarian tradition in theory opens access to Unani care to persons in any economic condition.

Data are available from the Khanna studies in India on differential access to medical care. These studies in villages of the Ludhiana District, Punjab, have documented differentials in mortality that are clearly linked to differences in sex, age, and caste (used as an index of social and economic status). Higher death rates were discovered in infants, preschool children, females, the elderly, and in persons of lower social and economic status than in other categories of people. An analysis of use of all resources for medical care, including vaids and hakims, auxiliary health workers, spiritual healers, and physicians in the city of Ludhiana found that categories of the population with excessive death rates received the least attention from and were the least liable to seek assistance from health specialists (Singh et al. 1962; Gordon et al. 1963, 1965). These studies provide one measure of the adaptive value of health care in the study villages, but the findings cannot be used to identify the *relative* value of the local, regional and cosmopolitan components of medical practice. Of course the Khanna studies did not attempt to measure the adaptive efficacy of Ayurvedic and Unani medicine in the domains of their presumed greatest strength, i.e., symptomatic and psychosocial support. Nor are there any studies, to my knowledge, that attempt to quantify the contributions of regional and local systems of medicine to health in Indian villages.

Qualitative assessments have been attempted, and several deserve brief attention. Harold Gould (1957), writing about a village in Uttar Pradesh, did not directly concern himself with scholarly traditional medicine, but he did identify a broad "division of labor" in the community: thus the cosmopolitan system "serves critical and incapacitating dysfunctions" while the local medical systems serve the "chronic non-incapacitating dysfunctions." He also noted, as did the Khanna studies, the importance of socioeconomic status as a factor in choice of type of care. McKim Marriott (1955), Morris Carstairs (1955), and Stephen Fuchs (1964) have all brought out the diversity of indigenous options for medical care that exist in Indian villages, and emphasize the blurring—as did Marjorie Topley (1970) in writing about traditional Chinese medicine in Hong Kong—that exists between the scholarly and popular medical traditions. Marriott's study provides a fine understanding of the functional roles of hakims and vaids who practice alongside magicians, exorcists, priests, and snakebite curers in the villages of northern India. He demonstrated that vaids, despite high socioeconomic status in the villages, can be consulted by village members of any status. Fees adjusted to economic status, free clinics for the poor, and charges only for proven results are some of the mechanisms that serve to increase access to this form of medical care. In the present volume, too, the essays by Alan Beals, Edward Montgomery, and Carl Taylor document and analyze the pluralistic structure of the medical system, with Beals particularly addressing the problem of how villagers decide whether they should resort to one or another kind of health specialist.

In modern India, the indigenous systems remain enormously important as providers of medical care, not only in the villages but also in the cities, and there can be no doubt that Ayurveda and Unani contribute substantially to the cumulative impact of these systems on Indian health and ill health. Cosmopolitan medicine is also at home in India and will no doubt continue to extend its adaptive influence, especially as it becomes more effective in rural areas and as rapid changes occuring in the whole society bridge the cultural gap between villagers and cosmopolitan medical workers. While there can be little doubt that popular traditional medicine will indefinitely survive, whatever the level of development of cosmopolitan health care, the future of scholarly traditional medicine in India is obscure. In China the extinction of the scholarly medical tradition is not an issue. It will survive in independent form or in the sort of traditional Chinese–cosmopolitan hybrid system that Croizier has described. In India, on the other hand, Ayurveda and Unani are not today on a par with cosmopolitan medicine. There are three alternatives for the future rather than the two that face traditional Chinese medicine. The Indian traditions may hybridize with the cosmopolitan transplant, or survive in their present independent forms. They may also wither and disappear as effective adaptive systems, losing their identities in the complex and diverse matrix of popular traditional medicine.

Literature Cited

Anonymous
  1970 "Mental Hospital and Psychiatric Care in Bagdad as Described by Benjamin of Tudela (12th Century)," *Israel J. Med. Sci.* 6:616, 654.
Audy, J. R.
  1971 "The Measurement and Diagnosis of Health," in P. Shepard and D. McKinley, eds., *Eviron/mental*, pp. 140–162. Boston: Houghton Mifflin.
Audy, J. R., and F. L. Dunn
  1974 "Health and Disease" (Chapter 15), and "Community Health" (Chapter 16, in F. Sargent, ed., *Human Ecology*. Amsterdam: North-Holland Publishing Co.
Carstairs, G. M.
  1955 "Medicine and Faith in Rural Rajasthan," in B. D. Paul, ed., *Health, Culture, and Community*, pp. 107–134. New York: Russell Sage Foundation.
Chen, P.C.Y.
  1970 "Indigenous Concepts of Causation and Methods of Prevention of Childhood Diseases in a Rural Malay Community." *J. Tropical Pediatrics* 16: 33–42.
Colson, A. C.
  1969 "The Prevention of Illness in a Malay Village: An Analysis of Concepts and Behavior." Doctoral diss., Anthropology Dept., Stanford University.
Croizier, R. C.
  1968 *Traditional Medicine in Modern China: Science, Nationalism, and the Tensions of Cultural Change*. Cambridge: Harvard University Press.
Dubos, R.
  1965 *Man Adapting*. New Haven: Yale University Press.

Dunn, F. L.
    1968 "Epidemiological Factors: Health and Disease in Hunter-Gatherers,"
        in R. B. Lee and I. DeVore, eds., *Man the Hunter*, pp. 221–228. Chicago:
        Aldine.
Eberhard, W.
    1967 "The Structure of the Pre-Industrial Chinese City," in *Settlement and Social
        Change in Asia* (Collected Papers of W. Eberhard, vol. 1), pp. 43–64. Hong
        Kong: Hong Kong University Press.
Fuchs, S.
    1964 "Magic Healing Techniques Among the Balahis in Central India," in A. Kiev,
        ed. *Magic, Faith and Healing: Studies in Primitive Psychiatry Today*. London:
        Free Press, Collier-Macmillan.
Goodenough, W.
    1964 "Introduction," in *Explorations in Cultural Anthropology*. New York: McGraw-
        Hill.
Gordon, J. E., S. Singh, and J. B. Wyon
    1963 "Demographic Characteristics of Deaths in 11 Punjab Villages." *Indian
        J. Med. Res.* 51: 304–312.
    1965 "Causes of Death at Different Ages, by Sex, and by Season, in a Rural Popu-
        lation of the Punjab, 1957–1959: A Field Study." *Indian J. Med. Res.* 53:
        906–917.
Gould, H. A.
    1957 "The Implications of Technological Change for Folk and Scientific
        Medicine." *Am. Anthropologist* 59: 507–516.
Hsu, I.-T.
    1956 "Social Relief During the Sung Dynasty," in E. Z. Sun and J. DeFrancis,
        eds., *Chinese Social History: Translations of Selected Studies*, American Council
        of Learned Societies: Studies in Chinese and Related Civilizations, no. 7.
        Reprinted New York: Octagon Books, 1966.
Huard, P., and M. Wong
    1968 *Chinese Medicine*. New York: World University Library, McGraw-Hill.
Hughes, C. C.
    1963 "Public Health in Non-Literate Societies," in I. Galdston, ed., *Man's Image
        in Medicine and Anthropology*. Monograph IV, Institute of Social and Historical
        Medicine, N. Y. Acad. Medicine. New York: International Universities Press.
Krueger, H. C.
    1963 *Avicenna's Poem on Medicine*. Springfield, Ill.: C. C. Thomas Co.
Leslie, C.
    1968 "The Professionalization of Ayurvedic and Unani Medicine." *Trans. New
        York Acad. Sci.*, series II, 30: 559–572.
    1969 "Modern India's Ancient Medicine." *Trans-action* (June 1969): 46–55.
    1973 "The Professionalizing Ideology of Medical Revivalism," in Milton Singer,
        ed., *Entrepreneurship and Modernization of Occupational Cultures in South Asia*,
        pp. 216–242. Durham: Duke University.
Marriott, McKim
    1955 "Western Medicine in a Village of Northern India," in B. D. Paul, ed.,
        Health, Culture, and Community, pp. 239–268. New York: Russell Sage Founda-
        tion.
McKeown, T., and C. R. Lowe
    1966 *An Introduction to Social Medicine*. Oxford: Blackwell Scientific Publications.
McNerney, W. J.
    1971 "Health Care Reforms—The Myths and Realities" (tenth Bronfman lecture).
        Am. J. Public Health 61: 222–232.

Menninger, K.
  1963 *The Vital Balance*. New York: Viking Press.
Myrdal, G.
  1968 "Health," in *Asian Drama—An Inquiry into the Poverty of Nations*, Vol. III, pp.1553–1619. New York: Twentieth Century Fund.
Needham, J.
  1954 *Science and Civilization in China*, vol. I, *Introductory Orientations*. Cambridge: Cambridge University Press.
Needham, J., and Lu G.-D.
  1962 "Hygiene and Preventive Medicine in Ancient China." *J. History of Med. and Allied Sci.* 17: 429–478.
Piggott, S.
  1952 *Prehistoric India*. Harmondsworth, Middlessex: Penguin Books.
Robinson, V.
  1943 *The Story of Medicine*. New York: New Home Library.
Sadusk, J. F. Jr., and L. C. Robbins
  1968 "Proposal for Health-Hazard Appraisal in Comprehensive Health Care." *J. Am. Med. Assoc.* 203:1108–1112.
Sastri, K. A. N.
  1960 "Facets in the History of Indian Medicine." *Indian J. History of Med.* 5: 1–8.
Sibley, J.
  1971 "Community-Health Specialist Here, Return from China, Praises the Barefoot Doctors." *N. Y. Times*, Nov. 21.
Sieh, M.
  1967 "Doctors and Patients," in W. T. Liu, ed., *Chinese Society Under Communism: A Reader*, pp. 381–394. New York: Wiley.
Singh, S., J. E. Gordon, and J. B. Wyon
  1962 "Medical Care in Fatal Illnesses of a Rural Punjab Population: Some Social, Biological, and Cultural Factors and Their Ecological Implication." *Indian J. Med. Res.* 50: 865–880.
Taylor, C. E.
  1968 "The Health Sciences and Indian Village Culture," in W. Morehouse, ed., *Science and the Human Condition in India and Pakistan*, pp. 153–161. New York: Rockefeller University Press.
Taylor, C. E., and M. F. Hall
  1967 "Health, Population, and Economic Development." *Science* 157: 651–657.
Topley, M.
  1970 "Chinese Traditional Ideas and the Treatment of Disease: Two Examples from Hong Kong." *Man* (N.S.) 5: 421–437.
Veith, I.
  1966 *The Yellow Emperor's Classic of Internal Medicine*, new ed. Berkeley and Los Angeles: University of California Press.
Whipple, A. O.
  1967 *The Role of the Nestorians and Muslims in the History of Medicine*. Princeton: Princeton University Press.
Wilson, R. N.
  1970 *The Sociology of Health: An Introduction*. New York: Studies in Sociology, Random House.
Wong, K.-C., and Wu L.-T.
  1932 *History of Chinese Medicine*. Tientsin: Tientsin Press.
Worth, R. M.
  1963 "Health in Rural China: From Village to Commune." *Am. J. Hygiene* 77: 228–239.

Wynne-Edwards, V. C.
  1962 *Animal Dispersion in Relation to Social Behaviour*. Edinburgh and London: Oliver and Boyd.
Yang, M. C.
  1945 *A Chinese Village—Taitou, Shantung Province*. New York and London: Columbia University Press. (Paperback ed. 1965).
Zimmer, H. R.
  1948 *Hindu Medicine*. Baltimore: Johns Hopkins Press.

The Cultural and Interpersonal Context
of Everyday Health and Illness
in Japan and America

WILLIAM CAUDILL

INTRODUCTION

Culture and social structure are interrelated with the occurrence of disease
and its treatment. This is true for both major and minor illnesses, and for the
attitudes, beliefs, and behaviors that make up the everyday care of the body.
My focus in this paper is on how patterns of everyday "body management"
are learned by young children in interaction with their parents in Japan
and America. Attitudes toward and the day-to-day care of the body influence
the course and treatment of the particular states of the body that come to be
labeled illness. They also influence the nature and organization of both
traditional and modern medical systems, as indicated in the present essay and
elsewhere in this volume.

Japan and the United States provide a good comparison for exploring these
matters. Both countries are highly urban and industrialized, both have
well-developed medical systems, and both are plagued with the myriad
problems of modern societies: urban deterioration, overcrowding, environmental pollution, the ennui of increasing leisure time, a lengthening lifespan
with an attendant shift from infectious to chronic diseases, and the bleakness
of retirement and old age. At the same time, however, the two countries have
quite different cultural backgrounds and modern social structures (see
Caudill ms.; and Nakane 1970), and these differences are related to differences
in the patterning of illness and its treatment.

In matters of general health, the United States and Japan have been
about the same for several years. As an illustration of the impact of cultural
differences on medical matters, however: The crude birth rate in Japan in 1966
showed a precipitious drop to 13.8 live births per 1,000 population, compared
with the more normal levels in contiguous years of 18.6 in 1965 and 19.4
in 1967. Sixty years earlier, in 1906, the same dramatic decrease occurred.
Azumi (1968) helps us to understand this curious matter: Each of these years
marked the beginning of a cycle of the old lunar–solar calendar when, once
in sixty years, the sign of the fire and the horse are in conjunction. Girls born

159

in such a year, so the belief goes, will be of harsh temperament and invite misfortune. To avoid this, the Japanese apparently falsifield the registration of the year of birth in 1906, at the start of the earlier cycle; and actually restricted the number of births, by legal abortion and other means, in 1966, at the start of the current cycle. Yet the motivation was the same in both instances, linking the feelings of parents across three generations of time and over the even wider gulf of two world wars, fantastic scientific progress, and social change.

If traditional beliefs have served to influence the birth rate in Japan, scientific advances have lowered infant mortality to a point well below that for the United States. For example, in 1967 the crude infant mortality rate (deaths under 1 year of age per 1,000 live births) in the United States was 22.4, whereas in Japan it was only 14.9 (United Nations 1970).

As in the United States, the leading causes of death in Japan have shifted from infectious to chronic illnesses. Cancer and heart disease are high on the list of causes of death in both countries. The location of cancer in the body is, however, quite different. In Japan the incidence of lung cancer in males and of breast cancer in females is low, but the incidence of stomach cancer in both sexes is high, and is probably related to Japanese food habits (Japan Information Service 1970). Japan has one of the lowest rates of coronary heart disease in the world, and the United States one of the highest; but the situation is the reverse for rates of cerebral hemorrhage (Matsumoto 1970). At present the causes of these differences between the two countries are medical puzzles. The same may be said for the greater rate of suicide in Japan, especially among young people between 15 and 24 years of age (Kato 1969). These youthful suicides are popularly attributed to the great pressures for passing examinations to enter colleges or business firms, but I feel that behind such reasons lie deeper problems in making the shift from reliance on parents and family to establishing separate lives in marriage and the occupational world.

An intriguing difference relative to body management in the early years of life is that the death rate due to accidental falls is lower for children under 5 in Japan than in the United States. At less than 1 year old the rates for 1967 are 2.5 and 4.6, and for ages 1 to 4 they are 1.6 and 2.0 (World Health Organization 1970). Similarly, Japanese-American children in California have a lower accident rate than white or black children (see Kurokawa 1966). Japanese mothers seem to pay greater attention to preventing accidents than American mothers, and since Japanese mothers sleep and bathe together with their children, differences in these arrangements in the two countries could affect the chances for serious falls. On the other hand, the death rate for children under 5 who are hit by motor vehicles is much higher in Japan. For children between 5 and 14 the American rate is higher, and this may be due to both the greater physical independence allowed the American child and the greater supervision of Japanese children in going to and from school.

Finally, for adults, the average number of days taken off from work because of sickness is considerably greater in Japan than in the United States. Since the general health of the populations in the two countries is roughly the same, this indicates a more lenient attitude by Japanese employers about time off for sickness, and a greater amount of self-indulgence concerning minor illnesses on the part of Japanese. I will return to this matter of hypochondriacal concerns in the two countries.

Turning to systems of treatment, traditional Chinese medicine has been practiced in Japan for over a thousand years and has to a degree developed its own Japanese flavor. Dr. Otsuka, in his paper in this volume, provides us with many details about the history and practice of traditional medicine in Japan. Hashimoto has written a little book on Japanese acupuncture which helped me understand how closely traditional medicine in Japan is tied to the everyday ideas and feelings of people. For example, Hashimoto writes that the concept of "*ki*" is the "essence which sustains the body, which causes it to move and to live"; she goes on to say that "this essence has a mysterious power which works invisibly and which exists within everything in the universe" (1966:22). The *ki* to which she refers is the word, or strictly speaking the Chinese character, which is usually translated as "spirit," or "nature," or "feeling." This word, and the concept to which it refers, combines with hundreds of other words which together refer to a wide range of behaviors and feelings in everyday Japanese life: for example, *genki* (cheerful, vigorous, full of pep); *kimochi* (feeling, mood); *kichigai* (crazy, mad—or more softly and literally, of a different or disturbed spirit); *ki o tsukeru* (to be careful. to pay attention to what one is doing); *ki no doku* (pitiful, sad, regrettable—or literally, "the spirit is poisoned"); and so on and on.

Equally, when Hashimoto discusses the "causes of disease" in terms of the five exterior perverse climates (wind, heat, moisture, dryness, cold) and the five interior emotions (anger, joy, worry, grief, fear), the explanation is not only important for understanding traditional medicine, but also refers to matters which are an everyday part of Japanese belief and feeling. Japanese are inordinately sensitive to climatic changes and emotional disturbances which may exert an adverse influence on bodily functions. When adversely affected, a person is very likely to try to restore his balance with nature or with other persons by taking a traditional or currently popular medicine, retiring to bed to rest, going to a hot spring to bathe, or having a massage.

Thus, traditional medicine and general cultural belief blend into one another, and both are strongly influenced by very old ideas stemming from Shintoistic and Buddhistic thought about the position of man in the environment. For people in the modern world, the origins of many of these ideas are lost, but they still exert their influence covertly through the culture. The same thing may be said for the West in terms of the relation of Christianity and older systems of religious thought to attitudes toward the body; but in the West, illness is less a matter of imbalance and more an affliction for improper behavior.

Both Japan and the United States have well-developed modern medical systems (Okuyama 1970; Yamamoto and Sawaguchi 1970; Bowers 1965). Relative to population, there are more hospital beds available in Japan than in the United States, but somewhat fewer physicians. For Japan in 1966, there were 90 persons per bed and 910 persons per physician; while in the United States in 1967, the figures were 120 persons per bed and 650 people for every physician (United Nations 1970). Japan has a national health insurance system with extensive coverage including, for example, up to three years of hospitalization for mental illness in private hospitals, and cheap, easily available abortion, while the United States largely relies on an antiquated and costly system of private health insurance. Medical education has been in great upheaval in recent years in Japan, as a result of the protests of medical students and young doctors against what they considered the "feudalistic" practices of medical schools (Brooks 1970).

Let me turn now to how Japanese illness and treatment fit with everyday customs of body management.

BODY MANAGEMENT AND CHARACTER STRUCTURE

When I first went to Japan in 1954, I was struck, both from reading and from direct relationships, by what seemed to me to be an overconcern about minor physical imperfections, and a great use of sickness and bodily weakness as excuses for not getting things done. For example, the "trace of a dark spot over Yukiko's left eye" which came and went with her menstrual periods, as described by Tanizaki (1957) in *The Makioka Sisters*, was a source of agitation in the family and seriously jeopardized the arrangement of her marriage. More personally, I had a close friend whose attractive daughter was reaching marriageable age. I knew this daughter for something over a year and never noticed that one nostril was slightly larger than the other until this was pointed out to me by her mother, who was concerned about this being a problem in trying to find a suitable husband. The daughter herself was sensitive about it—and partly for that reason, she eventually married an American army officer rather than a Japanese.

As my first year in Japan progressed, I found myself increasingly bewildered and irritated by the number of times research assistants or friends would not carry out work or would miss engagements because they were "suffering from being sick." Subsequently, over the following 17 years, I have come to accept this sensitivity about the body and its minor ailments as part of ordinary Japanese character structure. Indeed, people are often rather proud of having a somewhat "weakly body," as this sets them a bit apart from ordinary folk. Such people are usually described in common language as being *shinkeishitsu*—that is, as being of a nervous temperament, with the implication that for physical reasons they are more sensitive than other people and hence they are more subject to sickness and disturbances arising from anxiety in human relations.

Our studies of psychiatric patients in Japan show that the most typical form of neurosis is one which Morita therapists have called *shinkeishitsushō*, or nervous temperament illness (Caudill and Schooler 1969). Such patients are very tense in interpersonal relations; they sweat, blush, and stammer, and often withdraw to home and even into bed for long periods of time. These symptoms are coupled with numerous phobias about parts of the body such as ears, eyes, stomach, heart, body odors, or about almost anything else one could think of. The Japanese quality to these phobias is that they are phrased in terms of the possible offense or bad impression they may cause for *other* persons with whom one is in contact (Kasahara 1970). Naturally, in the United States one also finds patients who are suffering from anxiety reactions, but the cluster of symptoms going with these reactions is not nearly as distinctive as it is in Japan. Around 1917 Dr. Shōma Morita devised a specific type of psychotherapy for such patients (Kora 1965; Iwai and Reynolds 1970; Doi 1962a). Morita believed that they were suffering from a constitutionally based "hypochondriacal tendency" which, in combination with environmental events, caused them to become *shinkeishitsu*.

Other studies have also pointed to a strong hypochondriacal tendency among Japanese. For example, Kato (1964) analyzed the results of a nation-wide estimate of severe psychoneurotics and labeled the main symptom-cluster as "hypochondriasis." Masuda and Holmes (1967) studied how normal populations in Japan and the United States would react to life crises, and found that the two samples were similar in their reactions, but that the Japanese were more concerned with major personal injury or illness. Lazarus (1966) caried out experimental studies on stress with groups of college students in the United States and Japan, using a sub-incision film and a bland film as stimuli. The Americans showed higher levels of anxiety on viewing the sub-incision film, but the Japanese showed equally high levels of anxiety for both films. It appears that the Japanese students were reacting to the unfamiliar testing situation *per se*, and this is in line with *shinkeishitsu* behavior. Finally, although I find it hard to believe, Lynn (1968) has correlated national levels of anxiety and economic growth rates for the period 1950–1965. His scores for anxiety are taken from Cattell's Personality Factor Test in various countries, and what Lynn means by anxiety are people who tend to be "tense, highly strung, irritable, and moody." Among the 11 countries which he uses, Japan is close to the top of the list on both anxiety and economic growth rate, whereas the United States is near the bottom on both of these measures.

A study I made provides further insight into the context of minor illness in Japan. I wanted to learn more about the emotions occurring in the ordinary events of daily life, and so I had a set of pictures of such events drawn and used them as the basis for interviewing a sample of persons (Caudill 1962). One of the pictures shows a man lying in Japanese bedding (*futon*) and being taken care of by a woman. The main interpretation of this picture was that the man had a cold or had been drinking a bit too much the night before, and his wife or mother was taking care of him with sympathetic concern while he relaxed and enjoyed the attention. Thus, the responses to this picture suggested that minor illness in Japan has a very ego-syntonic quality. People rather welcome the chance to be mildly sick if this involves staying at home and being cared for by others.

Beyond this, there was also the suggestion in the responses that illness serves as a "form of communication." Japanese are less prone than Americans to express their feelings directly in words, and illness provides an opportunity both for the ill person and the caretaker to express their emotions in actions. One of our subjects clearly indicated this in her response to the "sick" picture:

Japanese won't express their feelings such as "I love you" or "I like you" or "I dislike you" or that sort of thing in words. Rather than using words, they often show their feelings in their behavior, and sick time is a very good time for this. It is the one time you can show in action how much you love the other. Often with young couples just after getting married, the wife will feel very lonely since the husband comes home late all the time, and she feels that he does not love her any more, and then he happens to become sick and she will take care of him nicely, and that's her way of saying that she is in love with him. Then he will understand what she is doing, and what sort of feeling she has toward him. That is a good chance, for both of them, to communicate not with words, but in another way.

Both the enjoyable and communicative aspects of mild illness rest on the assumption that family members consider themselves as an interdependent group in which the needs of one member will be taken care of by another. Such interdependency and, again, the emphasis on physical rather than verbal communication can also be seen in a study of sleeping arrangements in Japan (Caudill and Plath 1966). This work was done as part of a preliminary survey concerning the daily life of young children, prior to a more intensive longitudinal study. Using a sample of several hundred families in Tokyo and Kyoto, we examined the sleeping arrangements in these households; and the most general conclusion is that Japanese parents, not of necessity because of overcrowding but rather because they want to, tend to sleep together with their children from birth until about 12 years of age. After that age siblings will sleep together in the same room. And if there are grandparents in the home, they will often take one of the children to sleep with them. Few persons sleep alone by preference in Japan, because to do so is to be "lonely" (*sabishii*).

In general, our results on sleeping arrangements have been confirmed by Morioka (1968), Kuromaru (ms.), and Nainan (ms.). Studies of sleeping arrangements in other countries such as Italy (Gaddini and Gaddini 1970) show results similar to those for Japan; and it would appear that the United States is rather peculiar in its early and rather drastic separation of parents and children at night.

Enough evidence has been given, I think, to show that the Japanese have a somewhat different set of attitudes toward and behaviors concerning body management than Americans. These differences occur within the context of rather different personality structures in the two countries—the emphasis in Japan being on the interdependency of people, the use of physical rather than verbal communication, and the expectation that it is legitimate "to rely and presume upon the benevolence of others" (Doi 1962b; Caudill 1970). I wished to learn how such attitudes came to be held by people, and therefore in 1961 I started a longitudinal study of children over the first six years of life in Japan and the United States. This study is concerned with the development of behavior and personality among Japanese and Americans, but in the flow of day-to-day events, matters of health, illness, and body management necessarily came up. I will describe this longitudinal study, focusing on the development of attitudes toward body management.

BEHAVIOR IN INFANCY AND CHILDHOOD, AND BODY MANAGEMENT

To begin our study we chose 30 first-born infants, equally divided by sex, all living in intact, urban, middle-class families in Japan. We observed the everyday lives of these infants when they were 3 to 4 months of age. Our observations were made in the homes on two consecutive days. We then matched the families of these infants with the families of 30 white American infants, and observed them in the same way we observed the Japanese babies. As the first 20 infants in each country reached the age of $2\frac{1}{2}$, we again observed them in their homes, and repeated this process for the third time at age 6. At each age level we also interviewed the mother. At infancy most of the Japanese observations were done by a psychologist, Mrs. Seiko Notsuki, and in America by an anthropologist, Mrs. Helen Weinstein. I participated in the observations at infancy in a number of cases in each culture, in order to gain a firsthand knowledge of the lives of the infants and to provide data for a reliability check and the standardization of scores on variables across cultures.

While the data were collected at three age levels, we have done most of our analysis on the material from infancy (Caudill and Weinstein 1969). We are in the process of coding the data from the later ages, and I have a good general idea of what is in the interview and observational material. In this paper I will make use of some preliminary analyses of the data from $2\frac{1}{2}$ years of age. For the most part, the data at infancy and at $2\frac{1}{2}$ have been analyzed through the analysis of variance, and results given here for these age levels are statistically significant in terms of these procedures.

At infancy we made our observations on the morning of one day and the afternoon of the next day. Data were obtained by time-sampling, one observation being made every fifteenth second over a ten-minute period, and recorded by using a predetermined set of categories concerning the behavior of the mother or other caretaker and the behavior of the infant. The resulting observation sheet contained 40 equally spaced entries recording the occurrence of the behavioral categories. There was a five-minute break between observation periods, and ten observation sheets were completed on each of the two days, giving a total of 800 observations for each case.

The general findings show a basic similarity in the biologically rooted behavior. The infants in the two countries spent about the same time in sucking on breast or bottle, and about the same time sleeping. The data also show a basic similarity in the behavior of mothers in the time spent in feeding, diapering, and dressing infants. Beyond these similarities, however, the American infants show greater amounts of gross bodily activity, play with toys, hands, and other objects, and happy vocalization. In contrast, the Japanese infants seem passive, and only have a greater amount of unhappy vocalization. The American mothers do more looking at, positioning the body of, and chatting to their infants; the Japanese mothers do more carrying, rocking, and lulling of their infants.

Interpreting these general findings, I feel that the mothers in the two cultures are engaged in different styles of caretaking: the American mother seems to encourage her baby to be active and vocally responsive, while the Japanese mother acts in ways which she believes will soothe and quiet her baby. Secondly, I believe the infants in the two cultures have become habituated by the age of 3 to 4 months to respond appropriately to these differences. I am struck by the fact that the responses of the infants are in line with general expectations for behavior in the two cultures: in America, that the individual should be physically and verbally assertive; and in Japan, that he should be physically and verbally restrained. If the infants in the two cultures have already, by 3 to 4 months of age, "learned" certain rudiments of body management in line with the expectations of their mothers, then they are already well on their way toward developing culturally different attitudes and behaviors in connection with the use and care of their bodies.

Very few cross-cultural observational studies of infancy are reported in the literature. However, Rebelsky (1967) obtained similar results in her study of Dutch and American infants. Like the Japanese mothers, the Dutch mothers did less talking to, and stimulation of, their infants; and the Dutch infants seem similar to the Japanese infants both in the degree of physical passivity and in the greater amount of unhappy vocalization. One important caution is necessary: studies carried out on infants in the United States indicate that middle-class mothers do more "talking to" their infants than do working-class mothers, and middle-class infants are more responsive to the mother's talking in that they do more happy vocalization than do working-class infants (Messer and Lewis ms.; Kagan ms.; Tulkin and Kagan ms.). Thus, our results should for the present be limited to middle-class families, rather than used for inferences about working-class families.

There also is one possible unanticipated consequence of the Japanese mother's tendency to soothe her infant by carrying and rocking him. Korner and Thoman (1970) found that infants who are given greater vestibular stimulation by their mothers (holding the infant or picking him up in arms) show a greater amount of alertness and awakeness than do infants who are given less of such stimulation. Since, as will be seen shortly, the Japanese mother uses such techniques to help her baby go to sleep, the result may be the opposite of what she intends.

I was particularly interested in the greater happy vocalization of the American infant, because it is significantly correlated with the mother's looking at and chatting to her baby. In contrast, the lesser amount of the Japanese infant's happy vocalization does not show any clear pattern of relationship with the mother's behavior. This patterning of correlations is intriguing, and it does suggest a different use of vocal communication between infant and mother in the two cultures. However, findings phrased as correlations do not answer the question of how the flow of vocal communication actually proceeds in daily life in each culture. It is possible to enter further into this problem by making use of the sequential property of the data over the 800 observations in each case at infancy. We can construct a logical set of environmental situations such as, for example, the situation in which the infant is awake and alone. We can then ask, within the limits of our 40 observations on each sheet, what happens in a particular situation when the infant begins a string of unhappy, happy, or mixed vocalizations. That is, we can ask how quickly the mother responds to each of these types of vocalizations— or alternatively, what happens when the mother does not respond and the infant must himself resolve the matter.

The most usual response for the infant when he handles the situation himself is for him to go to sleep. When this happens there are no differences between the cultures in the amount of time that it takes the Japanese or the American infant to go to sleep. This argues for the essential biological similarity of the infants in the two cultures. Yet great cultural differences exist in the responses of the mothers to the logical set of environmental situations, and these differences go a long way to help answer the question of why the American infant should have a greater amount of happy vocalization, while the Japanese infant has a greater amount of unhappy vocalization.

First, from the sequential analysis we found that the pace of the American mother is livelier. She is more in and out of the room, thus providing more naturally-occurring opportunities to speak to her baby and for him to respond vocally as she comes to care for him. Secondly, we found that the American mother in general responds more quickly to her baby's vocalization, regardless of whether these are happy or unhappy. Thirdly, the American mother differentiates more sharply between kinds of vocalizations, coming to care for the baby in a shorter time in answer to his unhappy than to his happy sounds. In this latter regard, the American mother appears to be teaching her infant to make a more discriminating use of his voice. Fourthly, the

American mother has more vocal interaction with her baby, especially by chatting to him when he is happily vocal. These findings help describe the American mother's style of caretaking—which we believe serves to increase her infant's happy vocalization and, more broadly, to emphasize the importance of vocal communication.

In contrast, the pace of the Japanese mother is more leisurely and, although she does not spend any more total time in the care of her baby, her periods of caretaking are fewer and longer. Secondly, she is more involved in the process of her baby's going to sleep and waking up. Part of the Japanese mother's style of caretaking is to carry, rock, and lull her baby to sleep, with the result that when the sleeping baby is put down he tends to awaken and cry, and the process begins again. Here, obviously, is one reason for the greater unhappy vocalization of the Japanese baby. In checking on the sleeping baby, the Japanese mother is more likely to go beyond glancing in at him to also doing other care which brings her into physical contact with the baby, and this added care often results in the baby waking and crying for a brief period. While the American mother tends merely to glance into the room where the baby is sleeping, the Japanese mother goes beyond this to adjusting the baby's covers, wiping the sweat off the baby's forehead, and so on. These additional actions have the effect of interfering with the baby's normal rhythm of sleep.

Thirdly, and directly related to the greater intervention by the Japanese mother, the Japanese baby is in and out of sleep more frequently and is more unhappily vocal during these transitions. Fourthly, the Japanese mother is slower in general in her response to her infant's vocalizations; and fifthly, she does not discriminate between his unhappy and happy sounds by responding more quickly to one than to the other. Finally, the Japanese mother has less vocal interaction with her baby during caretaking, and this is particularly true for the situation where the mother is chatting to a happily vocalizing baby. These aspects of the Japanese mother's style of caretaking point to a lesser reliance on and refinement of vocal communication between mother and infant, while at the same time emphasizing the importance and communicative value of physical contact (Caudill 1971).

We might ask why the Japanese mother persists in a style of care that leads to her baby being fussier than American infants. Since much of the Japanese baby's fussiness occurs within the context of the management of sleep, such conditioning in infancy may well be related to the greater anxiety expressed at later ages by Japanese children about going to sleep (Iwawaki et al. 1967), and the greater occurrence of sleep disturbances among adult Japanese psychiatric patients (Schooler and Caudill 1964). In attempting to answer this question, let me outline what I feel are the cultural contexts of the relation of mothers to their babies in the two cultures.

In America, the mother views her baby, at least potentially, as a separate and autonomous being who should learn to do and think for himself. For her, the baby is from birth a distinct personality with his own needs and desires which she must learn to recognize and care for. She helps him to learn to express these needs and desires through her emphasis on vocal communication, so that he can "tell" her what he wants and she can respond appropriately. Obviously here, in psychological terms, we have the beginnings of a greater separation between mother and infant, and the development of sharper ego boundaries, than in Japan. The American mother deemphasizes the importance of physical contact such as carrying and rocking, and encourages her infant, through the use of her voice, to explore and learn to deal with his environment by himself. As noted, the American mother does more encouraging of her baby to reach out for toys, and to be more physically active. Indeed, one of our mothers was encouraging her baby, at 3 or 4 months of age, to use a spoon by himself.

Just as the American mother thinks of her infant as a separate individual, so also she thinks of herself as a separate person with her own needs and desires, which include time apart from her baby in order to pursue her own interests, and also to be a wife to her husband as well as a mother to her baby. For this reason, the pace of her caretaking is quicker, and when she is caretaking, her involvement with the baby is livelier and more intense. Partly this is true because she wishes to stimulate the baby to activity and response so that when it is time for him to sleep, he will remain asleep and give her a chance to do other things—both during the day and at night.

In Japan, in contrast to the situation in America, the mother views her baby much more as an extension of herself, and psychologically the boundaries between the two of them are blurred. A striking example of this is that almost all of our Japanese mothers were given their baby's umbilical cord at the time they left the hospital. In Japan the mother usually stays in the hospital until the ninth or tenth day when the umbilical cord shrivels and drops off. The remnant of the cord is placed in a pretty wooden box tied with ribbon and presented to the mother. Half of our mothers said that they thought this was an important symbol of their tie to the child, and the other half said that it was just an old custom. None of the mothers, however, threw the cords away. It is true that American parents save baby shoes, locks of hair, and other odds and ends to remind themselves of their infant, but the symbol used in the Japanese custom is a much more direct statement of the tie between mother and child. (On other Japanese customs in childhood, see Sofue 1965.)

Because of the great emphasis on the close attachment between mother and child in Japan, the mother is likely to feel that she knows what is best for the baby, and there is no particular need for him to tell her what he wants because, after all, they are virtually one. Given this orientation, the Japanese mother places less importance on vocal communication and more on physical contact. Also, there is no need for her to hurry because she expects to devote herself to her child without any great concern for a time away from him, even for a separate time to be with her husband. This expectation extends throughout the night, because Japanese parents and children sleep together in the same room.

We can see that a considerable amount of culturally patterned behavior has already come into being by 3 to 4 months of age, including the forerunners of attitudes toward the body and its management. In America, even the infant is encouraged in some ways to care for his own needs, whereas in Japan the infant has learned that his needs will be taken care of by others if he complains hard enough.

Before comparing the children at later ages, I want to refer to evidence we have gathered recently which clearly indicates that the differences in behavior between the Japanese and American infants are more due to conditioning than to group genetic factors. Using the same observational methods, we obtained data during 1970 on a sample of 21 Japanese-American infants—all from the third generation to be born in the United States. These infants are genetically Japanese, but by this time their parents are culturally much more American than Japanese. If group genetic factors are influencing the kinds of differences we find at infancy, then the Japanese-American infants should be more like the Japanese than like the white American infants. But the reverse turns out to be the case: the Japanese-American and white American infants are alike in having high levels of happy vocalization and physical activity in response to greater stimulation from their mothers. In these respects, the Japanese-American infants have learned to be like other American infants (Caudill and Frost ms.).

The basic line of thought in our predictions from the findings at infancy to the behavior of children and caretakers at later ages was that the differences noted at infancy would continue to develop in a fairly straightforward manner. We expected that at age $2\frac{1}{2}$ the American children would be more vocal, more physically active, and more independent in various areas of behavior than the Japanese children; and similarly, that the American caretakers would be doing more talking to their children, would be more physically active with their children, and would be encouraging their children to do things for themselves more than would the Japanese caretakers.

The method of data collection at the ages of $2\frac{1}{2}$ and 6 was somewhat different from that used at infancy. At these later ages we made more continuous, rather than time-sampled, observations over a total period of approximately eight hours—four hours on one afternoon, and an additional four hours on the subsequent evening, staying until the child went to sleep. Our observational time unit during these eight hours was two minutes in length. In our set of dependent variables concerning the behavior of the child and others in the environment, a variable could occur or not occur during a two-minute unit. If a variable did occur, then by definition it could not reoccur until the next unit. Over an eight-hour period we would have 240 observations, but in fact our time spent in observation varied from approximately seven to nine hours, or roughly between 200 and 300 observations for a particular case. The occurrence of each of the dependent variables is converted into a rate relative to the total observations in a particular case, and then these rates are used in an analysis of variance in which the main independent variables are culture and the child's sex. We controlled for the effects of one independent variable while looking at the effects of the other. Levels of significance at 0.05 or better are always determined by use of a two-tailed test, which means the conservative position is taken that the direction of a result is not predicted.

At the later ages, the full analysis of the data involves working out the interrelations of several hundred dependent variables concerning the behavior of our child, other children, and adults in the environment. We are only at the beginning of this work, but for purposes of this paper we did some preliminary analysis on a limited set of variables at $2\frac{1}{2}$ years of age. This preliminary analysis is still relatively crude because the data are not as yet controlled on numerous matters, such as whether the behavior occurred indoors or outdoors, but I do not expect the final results to change very much from what is presented here.

In this paper, results are presented for age $2\frac{1}{2}$ in terms of the total amount of caretaking done by adults and the amount of time spent by both caretaker and child in verbal, physical, and emotional behavior and in body management. All variables used in the research have precise definitions and rules for coding. Let me at least indicate the nature of those variables for which results will be given.

Total caretaking behavior is simply the rate obtained from the number of observations in which the caretaker is actively engaged in any way with the child. *Verbal behavior* is divided into chatting, lulling, and expressive vocalization, and these component parts are additive to give a composite variable of total verbal behavior. *Physical behavior* is divided into high, moderate, and low levels of behavior. *Emotional behavior* includes two kinds of positive emotion—happy, and manicky or overexcited—and three kinds of negative emotion—unhappy, angry or aggressive, and fearful or apprehensive; these component parts are additive to give a composite variable of total emotional behavior. *Body management* is divided into dressing; going to the toilet (including diapering); bathing in tub; washing hands, face, and other parts of the body in a basin; caring for hair (and similar activities); caring for minor cuts and bruises; and going to sleep at bedtime. Each of these component parts is scored as either being done by the child alone or with the assistance of the caretaker. All parts are additive and are combined into three composite variables: total child does body management alone, total caretaker assists with body management, and total all body management. (Just for the reader's information, feeding and eating are part of other variables and are not included in the analyses for this paper.)

For the series of dependent variables just outlined, no interactions between the independent variables of sex and culture are significant. The main effects of sex of child are of minor importance. In line with what seems to be a universal tendency from other studies, girls are more chatty than boys in Japan, and the means are also in this direction in the American data. In both cultures, girls are doing more care of their hair than boys, even at $2\frac{1}{2}$ years of age. The main effects of the independent variable of culture, on the other hand, are highly important in discriminating between behavior in the two groups.

As was true at infancy, the total amount of time spent in interaction with children by the caretakers at age $2\frac{1}{2}$ does not show a difference between the cultures. In both cultures, mothers were in interaction with their 3 to 4 month-old infants about 40 percent of the time, and at age $2\frac{1}{2}$ this percentage rises to about two-thirds of the time (the mean rates are A 63.8, J 68.5, not significant). However, the patterning of what mothers do with their children in each culture is different in many ways.

American caretakers and their children are more totally verbal at age $2\frac{1}{2}$ than are their Japanese counterparts (the mean rates for caretakers are A 84.7, J 76.6, F ratio 7.6, p < .01; and for children, A 66.0, J 54.7, F ratio 10.5, p < .01). In general, these results correspond with those at infancy. Despite the significant differences in these rates, I am impressed with the great amount of verbalization that goes on in both cultures. It is interesting that in either country the adults are doing more verbalization than the children, but it is equally interesting that even the children are verbal over 50 percent of the time, on the average. Human beings simply do a lot of talking as part of their behavior. It happens that Americans do more of it, but this does *not* mean that the Japanese are silent; they just do less of it.

Chatting makes up the bulk of verbalization in both countries; but relatively, American caretakers and children are doing more of it (the mean rates for caretakers are A 84.4, J 72.8, F ratio 13.5, p < .001; and for children, A 61.7, J 50.4, F ratio 10.1, p < .01). When we look at lulling, just as was true in infancy, the Japanese mothers do more of it; but in both cultures this is a relatively infrequent event (A 0.1, J 2.0, F ratio 14.0, p < .001). In Japan verbal exchange is punctuated by a wide range of expressive sounds which have no literal cognitive meaning but are meant to convey agreement, surprise, disbelief, and so on, and Japanese mothers make more use of such sounds (A 0.3, J 1.8, F ratio 13.6, p < .001). It is interesting that at age $2\frac{1}{2}$ the children in both cultures use more expressive sounds than do their caretakers, but for the children there is no cross-cultural difference in this regard (A 4.3, J 4.2, not significant).

Japanese caretakers and children are greater in low physical activity (mean rates for caretakers are A 2.6, J 11.2, F ratio 11.9, p < .01; and for children A 17.0, J 22.5, F ratio 4.3, p < .05). Also, a finding that almost reaches an acceptable level of significance indicates high physical activity for the American caretaker (A 16.8, J 12.2, F ratio 3.5, p < .07), but this is not true for the child's high physical activity (A 25.8, J 25.6, not significant). When, however, high and moderate rates of physical activity are combined in a composite variable (which may be called "not low" activity), then the means are significantly greater for both the American caretaker and American child. Thus, the results for physical behavior at age $2\frac{1}{2}$ are consistent with those at infancy, just as this has also been shown to be true for verbal behavior.

Somewhat surprisingly, because we thought the Americans would be more openly emotional, there are no differences between the cultures at age $2\frac{1}{2}$ in the total emotionality shown by caretakers (the mean rates are A 17.4, J 15.2, not significant) or children (A 19.5, J 18.7, not significant). The kind of emotion expressed, however, does reveal differences. Both the American caretakers and children express more anger or aggression. The Japanese children, on the other hand, show more unhappy emotion, and this is in line with the greater amount of unhappy vocalization among the Japanese babies at infancy. Emotionality needs further, and more refined, analysis by controlling for targets of the emotion, the context in which the emotion is expressed, and whether the mode of expression is primarily physical or verbal.

In body management at $2\frac{1}{4}$ years, there is not a difference in the total amount of time spent by caretakers in assisting their children (the mean rates are A 9.1, J 11.3, not significant), and this is also true for each of the detailed kinds of body management. However, American children clearly do more total body management for themselves than Japanese children (the mean rates are A 8.1, J 2.7, F ratio 21.6, p < .001); and in the details, this is so for the American children with regard to dressing, going to the toilet, bathing, and going to sleep at bedtime.

Thinking about these results in a somewhat different way, they mean that whenever body management in general occurs, in Japan the caretaker is assisting the child over 80 percent of the time (caretaker's rate is 11.3, while child's rate is 2.7), whereas in America this is so only about 50 percent of the time (caretaker's rate is 9.1, while child's rate is 8.1). Moreover, in Japan the caretaker is significantly doing more to assist the child than the child does for himself in *each* of the seven kinds of activity that make up the general variable of body management. In America, on the other hand, the caretaker only does more to assist in dressing, and in the care of minor wounds; the child does more going to sleep by himself, and the rates for the other activities are evenly balanced.

The main conclusion to be drawn from these results is that, at age $2\frac{1}{2}$ the Japanese child expects that things will be done for him in the area of body management, while the American child is more engaged in learning to do these things for himself. These opposite tendencies are particularly clear in the activities of going to the toilet (which includes diapering), bathing, washing, and going to sleep. Let me briefly illustrate these tendencies from some of the more qualitative aspects of our observations at 2½ and 6 years.

By 2½ years of age most of the Japanese children in the study were fairly well toilet-trained, but many of the American children were still wearing diapers. The Japanese mothers did not achieve this result by harsh measures; instead, they were very attentive to any signs that their children might want to urinate or defecate, and then helped them to do so. In the observations, the Japanese mothers are continually asking their children if they wish to go *oshikko* (to urinate) or *unko* (to defecate) or *unun* (the sound one may make in trying to have a bowel movement), and then physically helping the children to do so. The American mothers are more relaxed about these matters, and are less concerned that their children may be wearing wet diapers either when awake or asleep. The Japanese mother is also more concerned about the quality of the waste product, and more given to casually discussing this with her child—for example, "*Mā yoroshii, ii unko deta!*" ("That's fine, you had a good bowel movement!") The American mother shows less close involvement in these processes, and her goal is that the child should learn to go to the toilet by himself and gradually learn to exercise control over his own bowel and bladder functions.

Similar variations between the two cultures occur in the interpersonal situations of bathing and washing. The Japanese mother does more for and with the child because she bathes with him in the tub, whereas the American mother is more likely to put the bubble-bath soap into the tub and then leave the child alone to play by himself before coming to wash him from outside the tub. The physical nature of the Japanese house also plays a part in body management around washing. In Japan, shoes are taken off before entering the house; and if a child has been outside and his feet are dirty, the Japanese mother is likely to come to the entrance with a bucket of water and wash her child's feet before he comes into the house. Such a situation is less likely to occur in America, except for concern over tracking mud into the house; and if this happens, the American mother is more likely to tell her child (especially by 6 years of age) to wash his own feet, instead of getting down and washing them for him.

Finally, the American mother does less body management in helping the child to go to sleep than does the Japanese mother. The American mother (or father) will read the child a story ending with an affectionate goodnight and leave the room, whereas the Japanese mother will usually lie in the bedding with the child until the child is asleep.

CONCLUSION

I began this essay by pointing out that Japanese tend to be hypochondriacal and to have permissive and sympathetic attitudes about the occurrence and treatment of minor illnesses. The behavior patterns in infancy and early childhood seem to presage and lay the groundwork for these adult attitudes toward the body and the treatment of its ills. In infancy the Japanese baby, in contrast to the situation in America, is more physically passive and more unhappily vocal, and is being carried, rocked, and soothed more by his mother. At age $2\frac{1}{2}$ the Japanese child is still behaving within much the same pattern, and his mother is doing more management of his body for him than is the American mother, who encourages her child to care for himself. Because the mother and child rely less on verbal communication in Japan, it is likely that the greater interdependency in matters of body management becomes in itself a more meaningful form of nonverbal communication. This would be true for the Japanese mother and child not only during the everyday activities they share together, such as going to the toilet, bathing, and sleeping, but also during periods of minor illness.

The evidence in this paper indicates that future research should focus not only on formal systems of medical care, whether these are traditional or modern, but also upon everyday recurring activities concerning body management. These commonplace activities constitute the context within which a person develops, almost from birth, attitudes about his body and its treatment. If we increase our understanding of such everyday care of the body, then we will also gain additional insight into those correlations between disease and culture and social structure which at present often seem incomprehensible.

Literature Cited

Azumi, Koya
    1968 "The Mysterious Drop in Japan's Birth Rate." *Trans-action* 5 (May): 46–48.
Bowers, John Z.
    1965 *Medical Education in Japan.* New York: Harper and Row, Hoeber Medical Division.
Brooks, Thomas J.
    1970 "Medical Education in Japan, 1969." *J. Medical Education* 45: 510–524.
Caudill, William
    1962 "Patterns of Emotion in Modern Japan," in Robert J. Smith and Richard K. Beardsley, eds., *Japanese Culture: Its Development and Charcteristics.* Chicago: Aldine.
    1970 "The Study of Japanese Personality and Behavior," in Edward Norbeck and Susan Parman, eds., *The study of Japan in the Behavioral Sciences.* Houston: Rice University Press. (published as a separate number in a series: Rice University Studies 56. (4: 37–52.)
    1971 "Tiny Dramas: Vocal Communication Between Mother and Infant in Japanese and American Families," in William P. Lebra, ed., *Mental Health Research in Asia and the Pacific*, vol. II, Honolulu: East-West Center Press.
Caudill, William, and Lois Frost
    MS "A Comparison of Maternal Care and Infant Behavior in Japanese-American, American, and Japanese Families."

Caudill, William, and David W. Plath
    1966 "Who Sleeps by Whom? Parent–Child Involvement in Urban Japanese
        Families." *Psychiatry* 29: 344–366.
Caudill, William, and Carmi Schooler
    1969 "Symptom Patterns and Background Characteristics of Japanese Psychiatric
        Patients," in William Caudill and Tsung-yi Lin, eds., *Mental Health Research
        in Asia and the Pacific*. Honolulu: East-West Center Press.
Caudill, William, and Helen Weinstein
    1969 "Maternal Care and Infant Behavior in Japan and America." *Psychiatry*
        32: 12–43.
Doi, Takeo
    1962a "Morita Therapy and Psychoanalysis." *Psychologia* 5: 117–123.
    1962b "'Amae': A Key Concept for Understanding Japanese Personality Struc-
        ture," in Robert J. Smith and Richard K. Beardsley, eds., *Japanese Culture:
        Its Development and Characteristics*. Chicago: Aldine.
Gaddini, Renata, and Eugenio Gaddini
    1970 "Transitional Objects and the Process of Individuation: A Study in Three
        Different Social Groups." *J. Am. Acad. of Child Psychiatry* 9: 347–365.
Hashimoto, Masae
    1966 *Japanese Acupuncture*. Letchworth, England: Garden City Press.
Iwai, Hiroshi, and David K. Reynolds
    1970 "Morita Psychotherapy: The Views from the West." *Am. J. Psychiatry*
        126: 1031–1036.
Iwawaki, Saburo, Kojiro Sumida, Shigeo Okuno, and Emory L. Cowen
    1967 "Manifest Anxiety in Japanese, French, and United States Children."
        Child Development 38: 713–722.
Japan Information Service
    1970 "Scientists and Citizens Fight Cancer in Japan." *Japan Report* 26 (Dec. 1): 4–6.
Kagan, Jerome
    MS "On Cultural Deprivation." Available through Kagan, Dept. of Social
        Relations, Harvard University.
Kasahara, Yomishi
    1970 "Fear of Eye-to-Eye Confrontation Among Neurotic Patients in Japan."
        Working Paper published by the Culture and Mental Health Program,
        Social Science Research Institute, University of Hawaii.
Kato, Masaaki
    1964 "Taijin kyōfu o megutte" ("On the Problem of Anthrophobia"). *Seishin
        Igaku (Clinical Psychiatry)* 16: 107 ff.
    1969 "Self-Destruction in Japan: A Cross-Cultural, Epidemiological Analysis
        of Suicide." *Folia Psychiatrica et Neurologica Japonica* 23: 291–307.
Kora, Takehisa
    1965 "Morita Therapy." *Internati. J. Psychiatry* 1: 611–640.
Korner, Anneliese F., and Evelyn B. Thoman
    1970 "Visual Alertness in Neonates as Evoked by Maternal Care." *J. Experimental
        Child Psychology* 10: 67–78.
Kurokawa, Minako
    1966 "Family Solidarity, Social Change, and Childhood Accidents." *J. Marriage
        and the Family* 28: 498–506.
Kuromaru, Shoshiro
    ms. "Separation Anxiety of Japanese Children and Youth." Paper presented
        at the Third Conference on Culture and Mental Health in Asia and the Pacific,
        East-West Center, Honolulu, March 15–19, 1971.

Lazarus, R. S.
  1966 *Psychological Stress and the Coping Process.* New York: McGraw-Hill.
Lynn, R.
  1968 "Anxiety and Economic Growth," *Nature* 219 Aug. 17: 765–766.
Masuda, Minrou, and Thomas H. Holmes
  1967 "The Social Readjustment Rating Scale: a Cross-Cultural Study of Japanese
    and Americans." *J. Psychosomatic Research* 11: 227–237.
Matsumoto, Y. Scott
  1970 "Social Stress and Coronary Heart Disease in Japan: A Hypothesis." *Milbank
    Memorial Fund Q,* 47: 9–36.
Messer, Stanley B., and Michael Lewis
  ms. "Social Class and Sex Differences in the Attachment and Play Behavior of
    the Year-Old Infant." Available through Messer, Dept. of Psychology,
    Rutgers University.
Morioka, Kiyomi
  1968 "Dare to dare ga issho ni neru ka" ("Who Sleeps Together?"). *Seishin (Mind)*,
    1 (June 1): 18–23.
Nainan, Yasuko
  ms. "Independence Training of Selected Preschool Children in the United States
    and Japan."
Nakane, Chie
  1970 *Japanese Society.* Berkeley and Los Angeles: University of California Press.
Okuyama, Kenji
  1970 *Nihon no iryō (Medical Treatment in Japan).* Tokyo: Shin Nippon Shuppansha.
Rebelsky, Freda Gould
  1967 "Infancy in two cultures." *Psychologie* (Nederlands Tijdschrift voor de Psy-
    chologie en haar Grensgebieden) 22: 379–385.
Schooler, Carmi, and William Caudill
  1964 "Symptomology in Japanese and American Schizophrenics." *Ethnology*
    3: 172–178.
Sofue, Tokao
  1965 "Childhood Ceremonies in Japan: Regional and Local Variations." *Ethnology*
    4: 148–164.
Tanizaki, Junichirō
  1957 *The Makioka Sisters.* New York: Knopf.
Tulkin, Steven R., and Jerome Kagan
  ms. "Mother-Infant Interaction: Social Class Differences in the First Year of
    Life." Available through Tulkin, Dept. of Psychology, State University of
    New York at Buffalo.
United Nations, Statistical Office
  1970 *Statistical Yearbook, 1969.* New York: United Nations.
World Health Organization
  1970 *World Health Statistics Annual, 1967,* vol. I, *Vital Statistics and Causes of Death.*
    Geneva: World Health Organization.
Yamamoto, Mikio, and Susumu Sawaguchi
  1970 "The Development of the Social and Health Sciences in Japan." *Social
    Science and Medicine* 3: 639–652.

PART IV

The Culture of
Plural Medical Systems

The anthropologists whose essays appear in this section describe societies that range from villages in Sumatra so remote from the centers of learning and government that they possess a degree of cultural autonomy resembling that of tribal societies, through peasant villages in India—one in a traditional rural area and the other near the city of Bangalore—to the professional and popular cultures of urban Sri Lanka and Hong Kong. Humoral concepts are prominent in all of these societies, though they vary considerably within and between communities. For example, Alan Beals writes that the Indian peasants he studied "give different names to the humors, and it is impossible to determine whether there are three, four, five or six humors." Yet the hot–cold opposition is a recurrent humoral concept in all of these societies. Describing the practice of a folk doctor in Sumatra, M. A. Jaspan says that "Man Aher's first step in any diagnosis was to determine whether the ailment or disease belonged to the hot or cold variety." Peasants in Sri Lanka are said to believe that increases of the fiery element during the hot season cause excessive bile in the body and "heaty, infectious diseases," while the rain and lower temperatures of the monsoon "cool" the body, exposing people to "illnesses caused by excessive phlegm." And among city-dwelling health specialists and laymen in Sri Lanka and Hong Kong, Gananath Obeyesekere and Marjorie Topley both report the importance of metaphysical hot and cold attributes of foods, situations, individual temperaments and illness syndromes.

I draw attention to these phenomena because a study of the literature on Southeast Asia and Latin America observed that anthropologists have frequently described them "as if they were a distinction of a particular culture or region." The author urged that new research be undertaken to show the "interaction between the great and little traditions ... and the *oikoumenè*, possibly world-wide distribution, of such notions" (Hart 1969:74–75). The present section demonstrates some of the complexities and rewards that may be found in ethnographic research of this kind.

Medical pluralism is a topic of essays in other sections of this book, as well as

181

the focus of the present section. In earlier sections, for example, J. Christoph Bürgel described the historical conflicts between Galenic tradition and Prophetic medicine, and Fred Dunn distinguished between local, regional, and cosmopolitan traditions to analyze the adaptive significance of medical practices. The relationships between coexisting traditions and forms of practice are also emphasized in essays on the ecology of medical practice and on revivalism in later sections of this volume, where Edward Montgomery and Charles Leslie discuss conceptual models for pluralistic structures of medical specialists.

Laymen and curers in all of the communities described in the essays in this section admire cosmopolitan medicine and want to learn more about it. Access to its practitioners is quite limited for the villagers in Sumatra, and it is more limited for one of the Indian villages Beals studied than for the other, while city people in Sri Lanka and Hong Kong seem to have as great access to cosmopolitan medicine as to other kinds of therapy. In these situations a division of labor has evolved between different forms of curing. Thus, in the simplest case, the villagers in Sumatra depend primarily on folk medicine; but the master physician, Man Aher, encourages some of his patients to consult government doctors. In the Indian villages and in urban Sri Lanka and Hong Kong, many laymen resort to other forms of therapy than cosmopolitan medicine, because concepts coded in their world-views and religious rituals form "metamedical concepts" that give rise to "cultural illnesses" cosmopolitan practitioners do not acknowledge to exist. In addition, Beals shows the ways that family structure, economy, and other variables enter these decisions.

While laymen in all of these communities treat the different forms of medicine as complementary or supplementary resources, Obeyesekere analyzes clinic and hospital records, along with questionnaires to medical students and practitioners, and demonstrates that in Sri Lanka specialists as well as laymen allocate particular kinds of problems to professionalized Āyurvedic practice. He also reports that Āyurvedic physicians themselves occasionally consult cosmopolitan doctors. Nevertheless, the curiosity and respect these specialists have for other practices, and their willingness to refer patients to other kinds of therapy, put them in an asymmetrical relationship with cosmopolitan practitioners, who maintain a closed, competitive attitude toward other specialists.

The Western literature on medical subjects in Asian countries has been largely written by specialists in cosmopolitan medicine whose purpose was to advance the effectiveness of their own institutions. Except for China, where recent events have brought traditional medicine to the world's attention, these specialists have ignored the institutions of great- and little-tradition medicine, or observed them only in a peripheral or condescending manner. One might expect a more evenhanded approach by anthropologists, but this has not been the case, for they have been disproportionately concerned with supernatural curing, particularly shamanism. And when they have considered other ways that people cope with health problems, they have usually adopted the perspective of cosmopolitan medical specialists by treating their subject in a selective manner derived from questions about how to improve health care. Against this background, the essays in the present section point the way for new research in medical anthropology. This, of course, is not to denigrate the significance of shamanism and of improving the delivery of cosmopolitan medicine; but broader and more objective perspectives are needed for the comparative study of medical systems.

CHARLES LESLIE

Literature Cited

Hart, Donn V.
1969 *Bisayan Filipino and Malayan Humoral Pathologies*: *Folk Medicine and Ethnohistory in Southeast Asia*. Data Paper No. 76, Southeast Asia Program. Ithaca: Cornell University.

Strategies of Resort to Curers in South India

ALAN R. BEALS

Earth, my own mother; father Air; and Fire,
My friend; and Water, well-beloved cousin;
And Ether, brother mine: to all of you
This is my last farewell. I give you thanks
For all the benefits you have conferred
During my sojurn with you. Now my soul
Has won clear, certain knowledge, and returns
To the great Absolute from whence it came.

Bhartrhari (From Brough 1968:235)

As an anthropologist concerned primarily with cultural change, ecology, and conflict in a small number of villages in Mysore State, my information concerning strategies of medical resort is based upon casual observation. Using information acquired in two villages, I will indicate the varieties of information available concerning the diagnosis and treatment of disease and suggest the major outlines for more systematic research concerning strategies of resort to curers. Of the two villages, Namhalli is close to the city of Bangalore and has a long history of experience with sophisticated and urbanized medical practitioners; Gopalpur, in the northern part of Mysore State, is far from any city and has only limited access to urban medical traditions.[1]

In modern Namhalli and traditional Gopalpur, there are a wide range of practitioners including unpaid local healers, saints and religious figures, priests, drug and herb authorities, midwives, astrologers, government doctors, missionary doctors, private doctors, and foreign-returned doctors. Most of these practitioners are sincere and honest men who believe in what they are doing and are trusted in return. A few practitioners in every category are insensitive, dishonest, or incompetent. The decision-making strategy leading to resort to one or several of these curers depends upon (1) the general concept

1 Field trips to these two villages were made in 1952–53, 1958–60, and 1965–66 under the sponsorship of the Social Science Research Council, The National Science Foundation, and the American Institute of Indian Studies.

184

of the nature of things and the proper strategies of life; (2) the kinds of diseases and afflilictions that are present; (3) the folk interpretation of these diseases and their causes, cures, and curers; (4) the economic and social status of the patient and his family; and (5) the kinds of advice and information available at the time a particular strategy is adopted.

1. THE NATURE OF THINGS

In the poem cited above, the Poet maintains harmonious relationships with the world about him, attains to perfect knowledge, and merges with the Absolute. The ordinary man lacks the knowledge and sensitivity which would permit him to maintain such harmonious relationships. When he dies, his soul is dragged unwillingly from his body and taken to the realm of Death. There, his sins and virtues are weighed in a balance, and the punishments and rewards which he is to undergo in his future life are written on his forehead. In the next life, the individual may avoid the fated punishments and increase the fated rewards by engaging in actions which compensate for his sins and indiscretions. In arranging for such compensation, the individual is free to employ any number of stratagems, singly or toegether. These stratagems range from what we would think of as prayer or worship to practical techniques which might be classified as magical or scientific. Virtually any technique, whether it appears to be moral or immoral, can be employed in the attempt to balance the scales and to avert misfortune.

The ordinary man lacks the equipment which would permit him, single-handedly, to attain the clear and certain knowledge of the Poet or the wise man. To avert misfortune, he must examine the knowledge handed down from the ancestors and the knowledge made available by those who appear to have greater wisdom. Because the available knowledge comes from many sources, all authoritative, the basic strategy must be to select from a variety of alternatives those which seem most likely to promise success.

Owing to his lack of knowledge, the ordinary man cannot attempt to resolve conflicting theories or conflicting advice into a single organized structure. He is likely to assume that the information available to him is on the order of what we might think of as a few pieces of an enormous jigsaw puzzle. If a given piece fails to fit, it is not because it belongs to a different puzzle or because it is fraudulent; more likely the contradictions and inconsistencies within his information are due to his lack of understanding and to the fact that the possesses only a few pieces of the puzzle. Differing statements about the nature of things, differing medical philiosphies, differing diagnoses and treatments—all of these are to be collected eagerly and to be made a part of the individual's collection of puzzle pieces. Ultimately, after many lifetimes, the pieces will fit together and the individual will attain clear and certain knowledge.

From this perspective, the presence of plural medical philosphies is a reflection of a generally pluralized conception of the Universe. There are many gods, many roads to Heaven, many scriptures, many intellectual traditions, and many kinds of people. That unity arises out of this plurality is an article of faith. It is not for the ordinary man to attempt to reconcile diversity or to find it surprising when his neighbor holds different views of the nature of things.

2. KINDS OF DISEASES

Although strategies of resort to curers may be regarded as special cases of generally applied survival strategies, they have the characteristic of being triggered for the most part by identifiable disease entities. While a particular illness may be attributed to natural and/or supernatural causes, almost all existing research points to clear psychological or physiological conditions as the precipitating factors leading to identified illness and the search for curers. Definite sources of illness even appear to lie at the root of such esoteric phenomena as spirit possession (Opler 1958; Harper 1963).

To the extent that folk medical practice attributes different causes to different diseases and suggests different strategies of resort to curers for each class of disease, the actual incidence of particular diseases is a major factor in determining the strategy to be undertaken. Practically nothing is known concerning the kinds of diseases which individuals in any particular village are likely to encounter. For the village of Gopalpur, the major source of information concerning diseases common in the region is a missionary-operated dispensary two miles from the village. In 1958, this dispensary reported trating 506 cases of malaria, 505 cases of skin infection, and 344 cases of scabies. Also listed were 174 cases of undulant fever, 179 of dysentery, 104 of other digestive diseases, 137 of influenza, 110 of anemia, 114 of eye inflammation, 87 of otitis media and mastoiditis, 70 of pneumonia, 90 of bronchitis, 53 of veneral disease, 27 of tuberculosis, 21 of poisoning, 20 of smallpox, 14 of skull fracture, 9 of cancer, 13 of heart trouble, and 1 of diabetes, as well as 98 normal deliveries. The above list covers diseases which were reported with some frequency or seem interesting for other reasons. Similar lists are given in Carstairs (1955:123) and Pai (1963:207–217), and serve to indicate the extent of regional variation in the distribution of disease.

A hospital located in a large town twelve miles to the east of Gopalpur treats many more patients, often for critically severe ailments, but reports relatively few cases of malaria, influenza, undulant fever, dysentery, or scabies—suggesting, among other things, that strategies of resort to curers for endemic or chronic diseases tend to involve restricted investments of time or money. In addition to differences in diagnostic technique, identification of illnesses present is made difficult by variations between medical institutions in the kinds of diseases they treat and by considerable differences in the incidence of diseases even in closely neighboring villages.

Causes of death given in census materials from the Gopalpur region reflect a picture more or less in harmony with that given by dispensary and hospital statistics. Diseases listed in census materials include fever, vomiting, cough, diarrhea, stomachache, lack of blood, old age—and, more specifically, malaria, tuberculosis, spirit attack, plague, smallpox, cholera, and influenza. The vagueness of some of the census labels appears to indicate that ease of diagnosis, and correlation between folk and professional diagnosis, have an important bearing on medical strategies.

Because Namhalli is close to Bangalore and has a wide choice of practitioners and treatments, there is no convenient source of disease statistics. A greater familiarity with Western medicine is indicated in the English or Latin labels given to diseases and in the use of soap, vaccination, and separate wells for drinking water. There appears to be almost no scabies, smallpox, cholera, plague, or tuberculosis in Namhalli. As of 1966, following the national malaria eradication campaign, both the Namhalli and Gopalpur regions appeared to be free of malaria.

The range of diseases present would appear to include something for everybody. There are swift and deadly epidemic diseases, hard and easy to identify chronic diseases, annoying or painful minor diseases, curable and incurable diseases, and a wide variety of diseases sufficiently rare to lack known diagnostic characteristics or treatment patterns. With such a range of illnesses present, the design of a uniform system for diagnosis and cure would appear to present formidable problems. The pluralistic attitude toward diagnosis, treatment, and choice of curers may well, in the context of a plurality of diseases, reflect a realistic and consistent view of the nature of things.

3. FOLK INTERPRETATIONS

Epidemic diseases, particularly smallpox, chickenpox, cholera, and skin disease are caused by disease goddesses. These goddesses are variously described as forms of Parvati or younger sisters of Hanumantha. Their function is to punish communities that become sinful by bringing disease, childlessness, flood, crop failure, and cattle disease. To the extent that punishment is not intended or that appropriate strategies are adopted to remove sin, the goddesses may be regarded as protective figures who prevent misfortunes. Although the goddesses are specifically identified with particular ailments, responsibility for any misfortune may sometimes be attributed to them.

People in Gopalpur were in general agreement concerning the above, but there was great disagreement concerning details. One man, Saibanna, described Maremma, the oldest of the sisters, as a helpful deity who cured fever and stomachache and drove out all spirits who had taken possession of people. A woman, coincidentally named Maremma, referred to the goddess as "above all, the most ferocious; she comes every four or five years, and if she wants to she can destroy a whole village." None of the informants asked to identify the goddesses in formal interview settings mentioned the fact that Maremma was the cause of cholera. Maremma's ferocity may be judged by the fact that her image, born in Gopalpur and married into a neighboring village, was thought to bring death to anyone who looked upon it. Nevertheless the goddesses were believed to prevent the diseases they brought: Lacmamma was described as the destroyer of cattle diseases; Masemma brought good crops and kept water in the tank; and Deevamma cured childlessness. Hanumantha, the older brother of the goddesses, and many other supernatural figures and medical practitioners were said to play a hand in curing childlessness.

Through appropriate sacrifices of fine rams or water buffaloes, the goddesses could be prevailed upon to bring good health and good fortune. The source of poor relationships to the goddesses was summed up by Saibanna: "There is no one in our village who makes puja properly or knows the god stories well. Everyone makes puja (prayer, worship, sacrifice) and tells stories by dolt's reckoning."

In the fields or wild places surrounding both Gopalpur and Namhalli, there are particular sites known to be occupied by the spirits of persons who have died violently or before their time. Although it was difficult to elicit much detail concerning such spirits, the overall pattern of their activity was fairly clear. Men who wander about in the dark or even, in one case, at midday in the hot sun, are attacked by the spirits. One man from Gopalpur, who started out to his fields after dark, awoke hours later, having wandered for miles until he came to a temple and was magically cured. Another man was struck down at midday when he wandered in an isolated spot. When he came to the village he was unable to talk and eventually died. Men who came to Namhalli on the late bus were often followed home by spirits whom they resolutely ignored. Although there is no record of any recent death in Namhalli due to spirits, it was assumed that if one looked back or panicked, death would inevitably follow.

In both village, women were also subject to spirit attack. In such cases, the woman, usually a young daughter-in-law, behaved irrationally, refused to work and spoke insultingly and disrespectfully to her mother-in-law. First-stage treatment involved beating the daughter-in-law with a sandal in order to make the spirit uncomfortable; but if this failed, the daughter-in-law could be taken to a shrine where the spirit might be removed. In Namhalli, where marriage took place relatively late and where daughters-in-law were usually close relatives and usually well treated, this disease was comparatively rare. In Gopalpur, where daughters-in-law were often very young and often very badly mistreated, the disease was quite common. Thus, as Opler (1958) and Harper (1963) have suggested, spirit attacks on daughters-in-law represent a more or less culturally sanctioned means of psychological release for oppressed daughters-in-law, which may also have the practical function of securing more humane treatment in the long run. On the whole, although spirit attacks were much more common in some villages than in others, spirits do not appear to be associated with a very wide range of diseases, and relatively few illnesses are directly attributed to them. Among tribal groups such as the Saora, spirits play a far more important role (Elwin 1955).

Outside of spirit attack and the deadly (and disfiguring?) epidemic diseases attributed to goddesses, all diseases seem explicable in terms of known physical causes, some obvious and some rather subtle. Scabies was the only disease commonly attributed both to the supernatural and to the natural world. Several informants attributed it to bad or impure blood. When asked to list the causes of disease (*kaayile* or *rooga*), no informant mentioned the disease goddesses, and only one out of seven listed spirits. There was general agreement that some diseases were the result of obvious and indisputable causes (headache from talking too much, heat exhaustion from working in the hot sun) and that most other diseases were the result of dietary imbalances. Although the words and concepts are perhaps somewhat different, the cultural definitions of illness in Gopalpur and Namhalli, summarized above, resemble those reported elsewhere (Opler 1963).

Although most people in Gopalpur denied any particular access to medical knowledge and almost routinely urged me to take my questions about medicine to someone who knew something, all persons questioned were able to provide extensive lists of diseases together with their causes, symptoms, and cures. No one professed ignorance of causes or symptoms, and only rarely were diseases listed as incurable. The general pattern is clear: There are at least 68 definite diseases. The causes of these diseases are either obvious or attributable to diet. The early treatment of all of these diseases involves the application of drugs or other substances to the site of the disease, if its location is superficial, and the consumption of drugs and other substances if it is nonlocalized or internal. Some diseases are in a series, each one causing or leading to the other. Where the cause is dietary—and it usually is—the cure involves substances designed to correct the dietary imbalance. Excessive consumption of cucumbers or curds leads to cold; cold leads to a head cold followed by a cough, by a chest cough, by whooping cough, and eventually malaria. The cure is to consume such heat-causing foods as garlic, brown sugar, and beeswax. Wind, a source of another series of diseases, may be caused by eating number 24 rice and cured by consuming an infusion of *sooma* (Sarcostemma *viminalis*?).

On the whole, particularly if questioning is restricted to a single individual who has been trained to be consistent and well organized in the anthropologist's terms, an organized and consistent picture of folk medical doctrine emerges. As more persons are interviewed, this consistency and organization dissolves. Each individual is able to supply not one but many causes and cures for each disease, and different individuals attribute different, although not always unrelated, causes and cures to the same disease.

A good example of this situation is given by the example of *tale beene*, or headache. Three out of seven persons interviewed gave headache as the first illness on their lists, one person listed it second, and only two persons failed to mention it. Such a common and psychologically salient disease is one upon which there might well be some sort of agreement. Together, the seven persons interviewed presented the following causes for headache, some listing as many as three: drinking water from a different village, reading too much, talking too much, too much bile, hard work in the heat, and too much cold in the body.

Appropriate treatments were as follows:

Informant # 2. Chop up garlic and put it on the forehead and heat with a flame and put lime near the eyes, and after that wash with water and the head pain will be lessened. If it doesn't get better, go to the hospital.

Informant # 3. Chop up white ginger and put it on the eyes and the headache will be lessened.

Informant # 4. There is a plant called white *gaNajina* (hogweed or Barhaavia *procumbens*?). Take the root of that plant and chop it up with ginger and beeswax and let it fall on the eyes. Then the eye water will fall down, and once that water is gone the headache will be lessened. Alternatively, put lime on the forehead and tie a cloth tightly around it. If it is left like this for three days, it will be cool.

Informant # 5. Put lime on the forehead, then tie a cloth over that and leave it. If that doesn't work, heat some garlic and put it on the forehead. If you do this, whatever head pain came will be better.

Informant # 6. Take ginger and white *gaNajina* root and chop them fine and put them in the eyes and the headache will be less.

Informant # 7. They are using Zindaatilasmit oil (a commercial preparation) and methol ointment and Anacin tablets taken with water or tea.

Although all informants make use of the humoral theory of disease, at least in terms of some diseases, different individuals give different names to the humors, and it is impossible to determine whether there are three, four, five, or six humors. Different individuals ascribe different diseases to different humors, and the same individual may list a mixture of humoral and other causes for the same disease. Fever may be caused by too much cold, too much heat, too much anger, or too much sun. All informants attribute some diseases to obvious associations: idiocy is caused by a failure of intelligence; toothache is caused by holes in the teeth and relieved with salt water; stomachache is caused by bad diet and cured with baking soda; and overexertion in the hot sun leads to fever, cured by resting for two or three days.

Where an individual suspects that the treatment known to him may fail, he advises consultation with a knowledgeable person. Usually this advice is nonspecific—but for a few diseases, individuals advise going to the hospital.

Folk concepts of disease in Namhalli appear to be essentially similar to those in Gopalpur, except that a much wider range of diseases are considered suited to hospital treatment. Although it may not affect the kind of treatment given, many more diseases in Namhalli are viewed as being caused by *hula* (worms and germs).

The knowledge of illness possessed by the individual appears to reflect an almost sponge-like acceptance of medical information, regardless of its source. Consistent with the interpretation of the universe as a complicated place, and with his role in it as a person who lacks the means of arriving at clear and perfect knowledge, the individual often remains prepared to accept all knowledge and to attempt all treatments. Where, as in Namhalli, there has been change in patterns of medical belief and treatment, the change applies to particular treatments for particular diseases. With the exception of a few factory laborers in Namhalli who attempt to conform to modernity in every way, there is no process of conversion from one type of medical treatment to another. Individuals do not become disgusted with folk medicine and adopt Western or Ayurvedic medicine; rather, they gradually shift the assignment of particular types of illness from one type of treatment and practitioner to another. Further, because the different types of treatment are not regarded as inconsistent, there is nothing wrong with trying a variety of treatments simultaneously. The situation has been explored and described by many authors (Carstairs 1955; Marriott 1955).

In attempting to explain this apparently casual and inconsistent attitude, it is worth reflecting upon the fact that the Indian world is complex and plural. There are many kinds of plants and animals, many kinds of people, and many kinds of diseases. The ecology of India is lush, tropical, and complicated. Perhaps simple and uniform theories of disease thrive most successfully where the disease ecology is relatively simple and uniform. Although plural systems of medicine may reflect the presence of a plurality of diseases, further information concerning disease ecology is needed before such a hypothesis can be removed from the realm of idle speculation.

4. ECONOMIC AND SOCIAL STATUS

A strategy of medical resort must, like any other strategy, be based upon the capabilities of the individual and his supporters. Many people in both Namhalli and Gopalpur cannot afford the cash fees or the loss of working time required for visits to medical practitioners in towns or cities. The reluctance to spend time and money in such a fashion is accentuated when there is no certainty of a cure, where a long wait for an appointment is a part of the treatment, or where the fee depends not upon the individual's diagnosis but upon the doctor's diagnosis. It is frustrating to wait all day to be treated for scabies (one rupee), and then to be told that you have some unheard-of illness (invented by the doctor on the spot?), for which it will be necessary to pay ten rupees. In Gopalpur and Namhalli as in Narli-Agrapada (Pai 1963:206), the vast majority of diseases are treated at home through the application of home remedies. Beyond this, great reliance is placed upon those who know spells or treatments for specific diseases and who are willing to make use of their knowledge without charge.

Among 20 families in Gopalpur, 4 have never spent money for medical care. Among the remaining 16 families, heavy expenditures for medical care tend to go to first-born or second-born male children. In one family, for example, thirty rupees was spent on the oldest son, ten rupees on the second son, two rupees on the third son, and no money at all on the four younger daughters. The only exception to this rule is a single Muslim family which has spent whatever it took to keep all ten of its children alive; even here, there are no reported medical expenditures for the eighth, ninth, and tenth children. Among the 19 Hindu families, the amounts reported spent for each male child's most critical illness are given in the accompanying table. Although more detailed information upon the correlation between birth order and medical expenditures would be welcome, the correlation shown in the table is so strong that it is doubtful that additional information would change the picture very much: when a family comes to possess a surplus of male children, medical treatment is denied the superfluous children.

Similarly, female children, although highly valued in some families, receive almost no medical attention. Of the first-born girls in 19 families, only two received medical treatment at the time of serious illness. The total expenditure for 19 first-born girls was thirty-two rupees, and for 18 first-born sons it was eighty-nine rupees. The combination of birth order and sex correlations with medical expenditures results in the virtual absence of medical treatment for late-born female children. Although neglect of children, old people, and women sometimes occurs in dramatic and quite evidently calculated form, the denial of medical care to economically unimportant individuals is probably more casual than deliberate. In some cases, such denial may reflect economic stringencies brought about by the presence of excessive numbers of children within the household.

The type of medical care also appears to be influenced by economic status and position within the family. Except for a few cases treated by the basket-weaver resident in the village, most of the major medical expenses reported in our sample of 20 families took place in the village of Yelher where the missionary dispensary is located. Roughly 50 percent of the families in Gopalpur appeared to have made use of the missionary dispensary at one time or another. There is more than a suggestion that in this very conservative village, Western medicine is actually the most expensive and the most prestigious form of medicine. In Namhalli, with its long history of exposure to Western medicine, this is even more true. This casts doubt upon the assumption that rural people maintain a conservative attitude toward Western medicine or a preference for traditional medicine. Rather, it would appear

TABLE 1

Rupees Spent on Medical Treatment of Critical Illnesses of Male Children
of 19 Hindu Families in Gopalpur Village, Mysore State
(based on materials collected in November, 1959)

Families	1st Son (Total: 18)	2nd Son (Total: 17)	3rd Son (Total: 10)	4th Son (Total: 4)	5th Son (Total: 2)	6th Son (Total: 2)	7th Son (Total: 1)	8th Son (Total: 1)	9th Son (Total: 1)
No. 1	30	10	2						
No. 2	0	0	0						
No. 3	20	0							
No. 4	0	0	5	0	0	0	0	0	0
No. 5	0	0	3	0					
No. 6	0	0	0						
No. 7	0	0							
No. 8	0	0							
No. 9	4	1/4	0	0	0	0			
No. 10	0	10							
No. 11	0								
No. 12	31	0	0	0					
No. 13	0	0							
No. 14	1	0							
No. 15	0	0							
No. 16	0	0	2						
No. 17	0	1	0						
No. 18	4	0	0						
No. 19	0								
Total expense (in rupees)	89	21 1/4	12	0	0	0	0	0	0

193

that the preference lies with the most modern and most expensive forms of medicine, but that economic necessity, procrastination, or faulty diagnosis lead to continuing patronage of alternative systems of medicine.

Assuming that sentiment requires that something be done for the seventh son, for the old person who is likely to die anyway, and for the daughter about to be married off, the presence of alternative forms of medical practice makes it possible to insure that all who suffer from disease can be given some sort of medical treatment. For the head of the family, who must decide which child is to receive which sort of treatment, it must be comforting to believe that all of the possible treatments and practitioners are likely to be effective.

5. ADVICE, INFORMATION, AND RESULTING STRATEGIES

A full understanding of the detailed strategies followed in the search for medical assistance requires the systematic examination of a large number of cases collected for that purpose. Unfortunately, my own information consists of scraps of material winnowed from historical and life-history materials. These permit a few limited generalizations about the types of strategies adopted, but can hardly be regarded as definitive.

The initiation of a strategy of resort begins when a family member or individual exhibits symptoms of severe or chronically debilitating illness. Very often, the reaction to this situation is one of "keeping quiet"; that is, doing nothing beyond a certain amount of nursing, in the hope that the illness will disappear or with the assumption that nothing can be done. If the patient is a valued member of the family and if the possibility of some expenditure can be contemplated, advice concerning treatment is collected from relatives, friends, and neighbors. Much depends upon the agreement among these advisors concerning diagnosis and the type of treatment suggested.

Where the diagnosis reflects the presence of a common, minor, or temporary condition such as a plain headache or a common cold, relatively little advice is likely to be sought and the advice given is likely to refer to one of several home remedies. The only decision involved will have to do with the choice of home remedies and whether to attempt the remedies serially or all at once. A severe headache may often be handled in dramatic fashion, the patient circulating about the village begging aspirin from the ethnographer, prevailing upon the barber to "let the pain out" with his razor, and attempting a variety of home remedies.

The majority of complaints, for which home treatment or home remedies are ruled out, involve fixed strategies, where the identification of the disease calls for a single well-defined action. For typhoid fever, one goes to the hospital. For snakebite, there is a known curer in a neighboring village:

Last summer, my brother was removing hay in the evening. When he pulled his hand away, a snake caught one of his fingers, but he forcibly removed his hand so that it gave a scratch on both sides of the finger. If he had not done so, the snake would have tilted its head and emitted poison. When the news came to me, I sat down; I was not able to talk or stand up. Basappa was there, he immediately ran for the Revenue Inspector. After his arrival, the Revenue Inspector made some medicines and recited some *mantras* (incantations). He told us not to let my brother sleep all night. The next day, he was well.

Because fixed-strategy diseases reflect a common agreement on treatments and curers, resulting from such repeadly demonstrated successes as the above, it seems reasonable to conclude that changes in patterns of treatment would occur slowly if at all. In modern Namhalli, a wide variety of serious ailments, such as typhoid, pneumonia, and hepatitis, have become fixed-strategy diseases treated by instant recourse to a known doctor or hospital in Bangalore. These appear not to have been fixed-strategy diseases previously.

Epidemic diseases in particular—although there have been no recent serious epidemics in Namhalli—appear to call for eclectic strategies in which everything is done that anyone can think of to do. During the time when the village was subject to severe epidemics of plague, the advice of public health workers was scrupulously followed. People moved out of the village and set up temporary residence in the fields, windows were made in all of the houses, and they were scrubbed with phenol. Vaccination was readily accepted, and it was believed that injections automatically cured rheumatism and other chronic aches and pains.

During epidemics, doctors are brought from Bangalore by wealthy individuals and from nearby towns by those who are less wealthy:

M. was rich enough to bring a doctor from Bangalore. Each time the doctor came he billed M. 50 rupees. Those who were not so rich, such as myself, went to town and asked the doctor there to come in a cab. He gave injections and medicines to a number of families in the village. He told me to make my own arrangements for collecting fees and the cost of the medicine, and sent his bill only when he knew that all the patients were safe.

Because epidemics are believed to represent divine punishment for sins, a variety of traditional and innovative religious techniques are also likely to be attempted:

Every house sent coconut and camphor with the washerwoman. Besides, four goats were released in each of the four directions. The goats were paraded through the village and people from each house placed jewelry and coins in a sack tied to the neck of the goat. We thought that the plague goddess would take the offering and the goat and not enter into the village. Besides this, we had religious dramas and worship at the temple and processions with palanquins. Glass bangles were broken on the ground, that plague insects living on them might not fall into the food.

During one epidemic, an old lady seen walking in the fields not far from Namhalli was thought to be the plague goddess. She was placed on a palanquin and carried from village to village receiving offerings of goats and money, so covered with garlands that she could not be seen. Finally she was identified by a relative and lived the rest of her life in disgrace.

By the 1940s plague and other epidemic diseases had ceased to appear in Namhalli. Although others might attribute this to Namhalli's eclectic experimentation with injections and vaccinations, one of the more sophisticated school teachers in the village attributes it to increased consumption of sugar and the now-routine drinking of heavily sweetened coffee.

Eclecticism also appears in individual strategies of resort where supernatural causes are believed to be active. For example, one man in Namhalli is said to have become wealthy by permitting his sisters, all widows who "show Heaven in their hands," to poison a wealthy elderly woman who was living with him. In consequence, his two children died and he was unable to conceive any additional children. For several years, he and his wife traveled from religious shrine to religious shrine spending large sums of money in the hope that the gods would see fit to release him from the curse of childlessness. Ultimately, he acquired an ancient medical textbook, which he referred to as the *Kokokshastra*. Reading the textbook he was able to discover which days of the month were suitable to the conception of males and females. After carefully following the regimen indicated in the textbook, he and his wife succeeded in producing children. Licensed medical practitioners are apparently not consulted in such cases.

Where there is no fixed strategy which might provide the basis for a religious contribution, consultation with a licensed medical practitioner, or a trip to the hospital, the most common recourse is the adoption of a progressive strategy. The cheapest and easiest treatment or treatments are attempted first; and when those fail to produce immediate results, one of the alternatives already suggested is attempted. When suggested alternatives are exhausted, the approach becomes increasingly eclectic, with the patient being taken from place to place and treatment to treatment until he is cured or dies. In this progression, the advice that is followed is not that of medical practitioners but that of authoritative persons within the network of contacts possessed by the family and the village of the patient. What is sought is a known and trusted person who is willing to suggest an infallible recourse. When patience or funds are exhausted, when prolonged treatment is advised, or when the collective wisdom of the individual's social network is exhausted, treatment ends.

In Gopalpur, persons suffering from leprosy or tuberculosis could be prevailed upon to attempt Western medications; but even when these were free, most patients were unwilling to make repeated visits to the dispensary for additional medicine. The resulting experience, then, is that tuberculosis and leprosy are incurable, and this reinforces the unwillingness to seek treatment. Where, as in the following case from Namhalli, there is disagreement concerning the proper treatment, further attempts at cure are often abandoned:

When my female child was about six years old, a licensed medical practitioner in town was treating her for swollen tonsils. He advised me to take her to Bangalore General Hospital for an operation, but my mother refused it. As we had no other children at that time, I spent a lot of money on her clothing, food, and medicines. The tonsils would become a little bigger in winter, but would become small after taking medicines. Just eight days before her death, she came to me where I was working and said, "Older brother, I am dying, are you going to bury me here?" I am hearing those words as if it happened yesterday or today. Exactly on the eighth day, the tonsils swelled too much and she died.

Because the strategies of life depend so much upon obedience to the will of those who are older or more authoritative, a strategy of medical recourse tends to have little reference to the knowledge or beliefs held by a particular patient or his close relatives. A school teacher whose three wives had died, possibly as a result of his sins in an earlier life, was able to provide hospital treatment for only one of them; the other wives received no treatment in one case, and local medicines in the other.

Except in the case of a number of factory workers and members of the "educated class" who regard patronage of Western medicine as something approaching a caste obligation, disease strategies depend to a considerable extent upon diagnostic ability and knowledge of the availability and cost of practitioners qualified to treat the disease as diagnosed. While licensed and Western-oriented medical practitioners are accepted for certain diseases in both Namhalli and Gopalpur, there appears to be no prospect that religious or folk treatments will be abandoned. Nevertheless, over the past forty years or so, an increasing proportion of the illnesses treated in Namhalli have been referred to licensed medical practitioners and hospitals, with a corresponding decline in recourse to other sorts of treatments or practitioners. While in some cases this reflects a general belief in the efficacy of the new medicine, it would appear that the most common sources of this change are improved economic circumstances, personal knowledge of particular curers and hospitals, and the recognition of increasing numbers of ailments in terms of Western diagnostic categories for which a fixed strategy of recourse to the doctor or the hospital is appropriate. There has been a gradual increase in the length of the list of diseases which are believed to be treated cheaply and effectively by licensed medical personnel.

In some cases, even where fixed strategies call for modern medical treatment, such treatment is not given. Although the principle reason for this is expense, including in some cases the lack of immediate and guaranteed cures, other factors are involved as well. The first of these lies in the fact that village networks of kinship and influence often do not reach into modern hospitals. People in Namhalli prefer to visit hospitals where at least some of the personnel are related to the village through marriage or by some other similar means. Two citizens of Namhalli who are employed by the Public Health Service are prime sources of Western medication and treatment.

Appalling food, long waits in an impersonal setting, isolation from relatives in a hospital ward, and a hurried and impersonal diagnosis are more than most people can stand. When my wife contracted hepatitis, we were sent to a particular hospital, because "we know the doorman and he will let you in outside of visiting hours." Needless to say, it was impossible to travel from Namhalli to Bangalore and arrive during visiting hours. There is some support, then, for McKim Marriott's finding (1955:262–265) that the acceptance of Western medicine is partly influenced by customary ways of behaving toward patients that are only vaguely related to strictly medical necessities.

CONCLUSION

The Indian universe is complex, pluralistic, and hierarchical. It has been conceived even by non-Hindus as a "buzzing, blooming confusion." Lacking access to clear and certain knowledge, the ordinary man must place extraordinary reliance upon others. He cannot be overly critical of his sources or develop great expectations concerning his ability to iron out apparent inconsistencies or contradictions.

The quantity and variety of diseases to be found in any village fully supports the idea of a complicated and pluralistic ecology. Folk concepts of disease types, diagnoses, and treatments reflect a similar pluralism. Single individuals embrace a variety of explanations for illness, and different individuals differ considerably in their interpretations of the nature, cause, and cure of illnesses. Folk medical knowledge appears to involve the following assumptions: (1) there are many kinds of diseases; (2) different kinds of diseases have different causes and require different treatments and different practitioners; (3) all diseases are curable if the appropriate practitioner can be found; and (4) appropriate practitioners are best identified through personal contacts and particularly through the advice and counsel of friends and relatives.

Because different individuals are likely to provide different diagnoses or different suggestions for treatment, the first stages of treatment must often be based upon some kind of resolution of conflicting advice. Several different strategies may be suggested and adopted at once—or one of several suggested strategies, often the cheapest, will be adopted. In both traditional Gopalpur and modern Namhalli, recourse to urban medical practitioners is strongly influenced by the costs in time, money, and humiliation. Consequently, urban medicine is likely to be provided to first- and second-born male children rather than to females or to superfluous males. The practice of restricting urban medical treatment to particularly important family members suggests that urban medical treatment is the most desirable kind. On the other hand, urban medical practitioners are often overworked and unfriendly. Rural people, except in modern villages like Namhalli, normally lack personal or kinship ties which would form a basis for exerting control over such practitioners. With the exception of certain ailments, the cost and prognosis of urban medical treatment is unpredictable. Under these circumstances it is not surprising that malaria and scabies are the two diseases most frequently treated at the dispensary near Gopalpur. Both are easily diagnosed and can be cheaply, effectively, and promptly treated.

Epidemic, lingering, incurable, or psychological ailments, which often cannot be treated promptly, cheaply, or effectively by urban practitioners, are likely to be referred to local practitioners or priests (Gould 1957:508–509; Khare 1963:38). Materials available from Namhalli and Gopalpur give no firm indication of the effectiveness of such strategies of resort to a variety of types of curers, and there appears to be no literature on this question. There are cases where faulty diagnosis or lack of faith in prolonged treatment have caused patients with easily curable diseases to abandon urban medical treatments. Where a single medical practitioner may be seeing several hundred patients each day, there seems little point in referring to him patients who cannot afford his treatments or patients suffering from "psychological" ailments such as spirit possession.

While a medical system based upon plural medical traditions may represent an effective adaptation to a complex tropical ecology and a hierarchical social system, its efficiency is almost entirely dependent upon the kinds of diagnosis and advice the patient receives in the process of selecting a practitioner appropriate to his particular illness. Identification of the specific illness serves to identify appropriate strategies of resort, but adoption of particular strategies is dependent upon available estimates of cost of treatment, likelihood of success, and rapidly of cure. Fixed strategies of the form "for disease x take treatment y from practitioner z" appear to develop only when such estimates are available and when the first-level diagnosis is correct.

More accurate referral of diseases to appropriate practitioners appears to involve educational efforts centered about the means of diagnosing particular diseases, or alternatively to be centered about the cost and effectiveness of an available cure for a particular easily diagnosed disease. For the present, useful planned change in the existing plural system of medicine in India is not likely to take place until much more information becomes available concerning such things as folk classifications of disease, diagnostic practices, strategies of medical resort, and distributions of diseases in geographical regions and social groups.

Literature Cited

Brough, John
  1968 *Poems from the Sanskrit*. Harmondsworth, England: Penguin.
Carstairs, G. Morris
  1955 "Medicine and Faith in Rural Rajasthan," in B. D. Paul, ed., *Health, Culture, and Community*, pp. 107–134. New York: Russell Sage Foundation.

Elwin, Verrier
  1955 *The Religion of an Indian Tribe.* Bombay: Oxford University Press.
Gould, Harold A.
  1957 "The Implications of Technological Change for Folk and Scientific Medicine." *Am. Anthropologists* 59: 507–516.
Harper, Edward B.
  1963 "Spirit Possession and Social Structure," in Bala Ratnam, ed., *Anthropology on the March*, pp. 165–197. Madras: The Book Center.
Khare, R. S.
  1963 "Folk Medicine in a North Indian Village." *Human Organization* 22: 36–40.
Marriott, McKim
  1955 "Western Medicine in a Village of Northern India," in B. D. Paul, ed., *Health, Culture and Community*, pp. 239–268. New York: Russell Sage Foundation.
Opler, Morris E.
  1958 "Spirit Possession in a Rural Area of Northern India," in William A. Lessa and Evon Z. Vogt, eds., *Reader in Comparative Religion*, pp. 553–556. New York: Row Peterson and Co.
  1963 "The Cultural Definition of Illness in Village India." *Human Organization*, pp: 32–35.
Pai, D. N.
  1963 "Socio-Economic and Health Survey of Narli-Agripada Village, A Preliminary Report." *Journal of the Gujarat Research Society*, 25: 189–220.

The Impact of Āyurvedic Ideas on the Culture and the Individual in Sri Lanka[1]

GANANATH OBEYESEKERE

Āyurveda is more than a system of physical medicine, because its underlying ideas have permeated religion and ritual. An analysis of these metamedical concepts must begin with the fundamental principles (*mūla dharma*) of Āyurveda, which include the doctrine of the five *bhūtas*, or basic elements of the universe; the *tridoṣa*, three humors; and the seven *dhātus*, or components of the body. The five elements are ether (*ākāsa*), wind (*vāyu*), water (*āp*), earth (*pṛthvi*), and fire (*agni* or *tejas*). Buddhist thought adds consciousness (*cētanā* or *viññāna*) (Filliozat 1964:27), but not in Sinhalese medical tradition.

The five elements are constituents of all life, and as such also make up the three humors and the seven physical components of the body. As the five elements contained in food are "cooked" by fires in the body they are converted into a fine portion (*āhāra-prasāda*) and refuse (*kitta* or *mala*). The body elements are produced by successive transformation of the refined food substance into food juice (*rasa*), blood (*rakta*), flesh (*māinsa*), fat (*medas*), bone (*asthi*), marrow (*majja*), and semen (*śukra*). Semen is said to be the most highly refined element in the body, the "vital juice" that tones the whole organism (Das Gupta 1932:322–324; Filliozat 1964:27).

Physical health is maintained when the three humors are in harmonic balance, but when they are upset they become *doṣas*, or "troubles," of the organism. Since they are also fundamental to body functioning they are also

1 The field research that went into this paper was made possible by a grant from the Wenner-Gren Foundation for Anthropological Research, for which I thank them. I also thank the following informants: Āyurvedic Doctors Marasinghe of Pilimatalava, H.M.D. Banda J. P. of Mavanalla, B. L. Don Pragnaratne of Peradeniya, D. M. Jayasinghe of Kandy, and M. J. Jayasinghe, Chief Āyurvedic physician of the Kandy Municipality. I am also grateful to my colleague Kingsley Ranasinghe, M. D., of the Faculty of Medicine, University of Sri Lanka, for his many suggestions and patient criticism of my paper. I also thank the following persons for their unfailing courtesy and cooperation: Mr. Vimal Navagamuva, Commissioner of Āyurveda, Government of Sri Lanka; Dr. Abeysekera, Acting Principal, College of Āyurveda; and Dr. Ruvan-Pathirana, Medical Registrar, Āyurvedic Hospital, Colombo. In addition I must acknowledge the help of my two research assistants, Percy Liyanage and H. K. Bandara, in administering questionnaires and interviewing physicians.

known as *tri-dhātu*, or the three basic components of the body; but this term must not be confused with the more common use of the word *dhātu* for the seven components of the body.

Such is the substance of the body. The interplay of the three chief elements which enter into its composition, namely, wind, fire, and water, gives it life and movement. But when they are excited or when, on the contrary, their action stops, disease comes in. They are, therefore, simultaneously the three elements, *tridhātus* and the three troubles, *tridosas* of the organism. (Filliozat 1964:28)

The universal element of wind appears in the body as a humor, also called wind (*vāyu*); fire appears as bile (*pitta*), and water as phlegm (*kapha* or *śleṣman*). Illness is due to upsetting the homeostatic condition of these *tridoṣa*. The most serious condition is one in which all three humors are upset (*san-ni-pāta*). When a *doṣa* is "angry" or excited, it increases in proportion to the other humors. The aim of medication is to reduce or control this excess. The excited *doṣa* also damages one or more *dhātu* (blood, flesh, fat, etc.), so that treatment must aim to restore the affected body substance.

FIRE AND WATER

Although the universe consists of five elements (*bhūtas*), from the point of view of peasant societies the most important are fire and water. Increase in fire diminishes the element of water, causing a general depletion of environmental fertility and excessive bile in the human body; this results in heaty, infectious diseases, plagues, and pestilences. The opposite tendency, for heavy rain and low temperature to "cool" the human body, exposes people to illnesses caused by excessive phlegm. Thus, people say that diseases like chickenpox and measles occur during the hot season, and fevers due to phlegm occur during the monsoon period.

Destruction from rain and floods is not a serious threat in Sri Lanka, and people rarely explain it in supernatural terms. Moreover, diseases attributed to humidity and low temperatures are not as serious as those caused by heat. The most notorious heaty disease was smallpox. Though totally eliminated today, it was an affliction that the medical system of traditional Sri Lanka could not allay or control. To a lesser extent this was also true for chickenpox, measles, mumps, and conjunctivitis. Thus, the interpretation of these diseases and the mode of cure became strongly associated with religion and ritual—a metamedical interpretation of illness and its cure. If illness is caused by the anger of one of the humors, the metamedical view postulates that the anger of a deity causes the increase in heat which stimulates the humor. The term for humoral imbalance is *tun-dos-kopa*, "anger of the three doṣas," and the anger of a deity is referred to as *deva-kopa*.

The most common belief among the Buddhists and the Hindus of the east coast is that the excess of heat is due to the anger of Pattini, the goddess whose life is portrayed in the great Tamil epic, the *Silappadikaram*. The myths of Pattini relate the story of the original fire and drought caused by the anger of the goddess. She burned the city of Madura in mythic times, until the gods pleaded with her to stop the fire, with its attendant famine and pestilence. This was done by rain which fell from heaven, and mankind thanked the goddess by boiling milk in new pots. Thus, fire was opposed by water, and famine (depletion of fertility) was corrected in a symbolic manner by milk (fertility), also a prime cooling substance.

The contemporary rituals for Pattini are performed annually, or in times of drought and pestilence. The annual rituals among the Sinhalese and Tamils of the east coast of Sri Lanka generally occur around May. For the rest of the year the temple doors are closed. According to local belief, when the doors are opened there is an immediate increase in temperature. Human beings must be careful during this time to avoid eating heaty foods and to abstain from polluting activities. After about a week, the priests begin to sing the sacred texts which recount the myths of Pattini. This part of the ceremony among Tamil Hindus is known as *kulatti*, which literally means "cooling." By recounting the history of how the goddess' anger was cooled, the community is spared from drought, and people's bodies are cooled so that the pestilence caused by the excessive bile is controlled.

At the end of rituals for Pattini, people in all parts of Sri Lanka eat the foods consecrated to the goddess. The most important of these cooling foods are rice cooked in milk, turmeric water, and water in margosa leaves. Also, communicants drink sacred water in which the anklet, the primary symbol of the goddess, has been dipped. In Panama, on the east coast, villagers go in procession from the temple to the sea. After an offering of cool foods (*maḍai*) to the goddess, they jump into the water to cool themselves.

The attempt to control the elements of the universe is best seen in the water-cutting (*diya-kāpīma*) and fire-walking (*gini-pāgīna*) rituals performed every year in the major ritual centers of Sri Lanka. Several, sometimes contradictory, myths explain the origins of these rituals, but I will not examine this problem here. My purpose is to interpret the rituals from the metamedical point of view. In the fire-walking rituals the priest, and sometimes others in the audience who have purified themselves, walk barefooted across a 5-by-10-foot area (or larger or smaller area) of live coals. The priest tramples the fire (the Sinhalese term *gini pāgīma* literally means "trampling down the fire" and extinguishes it. Through this ritual he acts on behalf of the community to magically control the element of fire. He literally conquers the fire, and symbolically brings a turbulent element in nature under human control. Before trampling the fire he holds a pot of water in his hand and mutters a charm called the *gini sisila mantra*, "the charm for cooling the fire." He then sprinkles some water on the fire. The fire is not ordinary fire, but before it is trampled its extraordinary virulent "heat" has been "cooled" by the charm.

The water-cutting ceremony is performed soon after the fire-walking ritual, or it may be performed as an independent rite. In this ritual the priest goes in procession to a special place at a river, stream, or well symbolic of a waterway. He cuts the water in two with a sword and collects some in a pot, which is deposited in a temple and kept there until the following year. The rituals are conducted in great secrecy, the waterway being generally screened off with a curtain of white cloth.

This ritual is an attempt to control the element of water. The idea of keeping the water in the temple is to magically ensure a constant supply for the community during the year. It would be inauspicious if the water level in the vessel were to change in any way.

THE FIVE *Bhūtās* IN SORCERY

It is easy to demonstrate that the concept of the five elements pervades other areas of the ritual life. That the idea appears in sorcery is also to be expected since the *Suśruta Saṃhita* and other classic medical texts consider demonology (*bhūta vidyā*) to be one of the eight specialties or branches of Āyurvedic therapy.

In one sorcery ritual that I am familiar with, a figure representing the enemy is engraved on an ash melon fruit, together with the figure of Mahasona, "the demon of the graveyard." Then five letters for vowel sounds (*pañca akṣara*) are drawn on the enemy figure. More than one enemy may be drawn on the fruit, but each is depicted as shown by Figure 1. The five vowels are drawn at

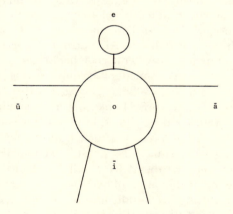

FIGURE 1. Sorcery image of enemy.

the five cardinal points, according to Sinhalese theory, as they are manifest in the body. They represent the five elements, the cardinal points of direction, and five planets (Table 1).

Two crucial agents that effect human life—the elements of the universe and the planets—are "roused" by the sorcery rite and attack the enemy from

TABLE 1

Correspondences of Five Vowels, Elements,
Directions, and Planets

Vowel	Element	Direction	Planet
ā	earth	east	Jupiter
ī	water	south	Venus
ū	fire	west	Mars
ē	air	north	Mercury
ō	ether, sky	meridian	Saturn

all directions. The elements in particular are upset by incantations, and destroy the body of the enemy. Two charms (*mantras*) are repeated 108 times, a conventional magical number that dates back as far as the *Atharva veda*. The charms activate or "make live" (*jīvan*) the ash melon.

One charm is known as the *rīri tīnduva*. *Rīri* means blood and refers to *Rīri Yakka*, the blood demon. *Tīnduva* is a crucial word connoting the consummation of any ritual act. This consummation is generally achieved by cutting some object—e.g., water-cutting. According to Āyurveda the five elements are converted into the seven *dhātus*, one of which is blood. The charm enlists the aid of the demon to destroy the enemy by casting a *diṣṭi* (look or gaze of a demon) on his blood. Since death may result, this demon is also known as *maru yakka*, death demon, and the five vowels are known as the *maru aksara*, death vowels. The *rīri tīnduva* is followed by another charm, the purpose of which is known as *maru ugullanava* or *maru avussanava*, to rouse (the demon of) death—i.e., to make him active in the body of the enemy and destroy his blood. This rite culminates with the ash melon being placed on the chest of the priest and cut by a sword-wielding assistant. Thus, a constellation of ideas from the medical tradition occur today in popular demonology.

When a layman goes to a professional sorcerer, he may be totally mystified by the esoteric letters drawn on the ash melon fruit. It is unlikely that he could construct the table of correspondences I have made, though this would be perfectly familiar to specialists. However, he probably could articulate the significance of the cool foods eaten during collective rituals, or of the cooling immersion at the close of these rituals. Although *bhūta vidyā*, the science of supernatural beings, was in antiquity a specialized subdiscipline of Āyurveda, it has become today the preserve of religious specialists. Contemporary Āyurvedic physicians in Sri Lanka do not usually engage in any form of supernatural curing. By contrast, religious specialists may prescribe Āyurvedic medicines along with their magico-religious curing techniques. The reasons will be apparent later.

I want to emphasize that the ideas in ritual curing belong to a specialized body of knowledge strongly influenced by Āyurveda. They are not popular ideas, any more than the technical aspects of Āyurveda are popular lore. Yet these ideas are consistent with the popular culture. For example, when a person goes to a famous sorcery shrine in Sinigama, on the West Coast of Sri Lanka, he is directed by specialists to grind seven types of spices on a flat stone. Most people will be aware that the spices are all "hot" foods and should cause an excess of heart in the body of their enemy, though they are not likely to connect the number seven with the seven *dhātus*, or body elements, of Āyurvedic medical tradition.

THE WIDER CONCEPT OF *Doṣa*

The most important concept which links the Āyurvedic tradition with the religious tradition is universally understood on the popular level. It is *doṣa*, which literally means troubles, and refers to the three humors (*tridoṣa*). In Sinhalese culture the term *doṣa* also refers to other "troubles" or misfortune that result from the actions of supernatural beings. The most common *doṣas* are:

preta doṣa	Troubles, generally sickness, caused by a mean ancestral spirit
yakṣa doṣa	Illness caused by demons
āsvaha doṣa and katavaha doṣa	Effects of the evil eye and evil mouth
deiyanne doṣa	*Doṣa* caused by the gods—e.g., punishment of wrongdoers by illness
hūniyan doṣa	Consequences of sorcery
graha doṣa	Misfortunes, including illness, as a result of inauspicious planetary influence
karma doṣa	Misfortunes due to a person's bad *karma*

None of these concepts are mutually contradictory; rather, a more limited concept is often contained within a larger one. The limited concepts generally pertain to disease, and the larger ones to a wider class of misfortunes. Thus, my illness may be due to *preta doṣa* (i.e., intrusion of a mean spirit). However, the *preta* may have been put into my body by the action of a sorcerer, *hūniyan doṣa*. This in turn had a particularly strong effect because of my astrologically bad times, *graha doṣa*, and this is surely due to my bad *karma* from a previous birth, *karma doṣa*. Illness may be due to naturalistic causes such as an upset humor from spoiled, inappropriate, or unbalanced foods. It may be caused by supernatural *doṣas*, or by a combination of both. And when both natural and supernatural causes are at work, both types of curing are in order.

Āyurvedic and supernatural theories of illness are ideologically linked by a formula distinguishing the external and internal causes for any particular disease. The external causes are such things as the consumption of bad food, while the internal causes are always upset *doṣas* or *dhātus*. Supernatural agents belong to the category of external causes. If they attack people, they upset the humors to produce sickness. The *doṣas* caused by supernatural beings thus excite the balance of three humors (*tridoṣa*) in the healthy person. Hence, in exorcistic rituals specialists not only expel the demon, but often prescribe Āyurvedic medications to restore the homeostatic condition of the humors.

CULTURAL PREOCCUPATION WITH *Dhātu* LOSS: *Prameha* DISEASE

I will now describe the way that Āyurvedic conceptions create diseases that could hardly exist in a different belief system, and a preoccupation or concern with diseases totally out of proportion to their "true" nature. I call these *cultural diseases* because they are created, at least partly, by the cultural definition of the situation. I will analyze two such diseases: phlegm (*sema*) diseases, which are related to the cultural preoccupation with the head; and a class of diseases dealing with *dhātu* loss, particularly the loss of semen. All physicians we interviewed were explicit that females secreted semen. This view may stem from Sanskritic tradition, for *Suśruta* was of the opinion that a sexual union between two women might cause conception if their semen somehow united in the womb of one of them (*Suśruta*, vol. II, 1963:132). Much of the information comes from three physicians in the suburbs of Kandy who acquired their knowledge through hereditary family traditions of Āyurveda, and have received no training in any of Sri Lanka's schools of Āyurvedic medicine. I shall call them physicians A, B, and C.

According to Physician A, *prameha* diseases arise from "urine trouble." They are not exclusively *vāta roga* (wind disease), though the term *vāta prameha* is used. There are twenty types of *prameha*; and they may, if untreated, develop into *vāta prameha* a symptom of which is swelling in the joints. They are caused by emission of semen (*śukra dhātu*) in the urine, by frequent night emissions, or when a "flour-like substance" of damaged semen (*piṭi*) is discharged with urine. The discharge of *piṭi* may diminish after a time, but the joints will then swell gradually.

Physician A says that the common causes of *prameha* are: (a) consumption of noxious substances like *gāñja* (*cannabis sativa*) and alcohol; (b) sexual excess; (c) congenital heaty body constitution; (d) excessive consumption of heaty foods.

The common symptoms of *prameha*, according to Physician A, are the passing of semen or of *piṭi* in the urine, and the discharge of oily matter (*tel kāran*) in the urine. The swelling of the joints is a later stage of the disease. The symptoms are similar in men and women, except that the semen leaves the vagina in the form of a white discharge (Sinhalese, *suda yāma; svetappradaraya*). Physician A claims that about 90 percent of the female patients who come to him with *prameha roga* have this symptom.

To cure *prameha roga*, Physician A prescribes cooling medicines and foods and advises patients, particularly men, to be on "good behavior." Physician A claims that university students come to him with *prameha* due to nocturnal emissions and deteriorated semen. He gives them medicines to calm or cool (*nivenna*) the body, and elixir (*rasāyana*) to increase their vitality by fostering the semen. He also recommends eating a paste (*kalka*) every morning and noon with cow's milk, and tonics (*arista*) after lunch and dinner.

Physician A described a case of *prameha roga* in a 23-year-old unmarried woman. The heat in her body was very great, causing "the *dhātu* to get heated and dissolve" (*unakarala yanava*). The *dhātu* was continuously secreted in the patient's vagina as white discharge. The discharge was not exclusively semen (*śukra dhātu*); although it resembled semen, it contained other *dhātus* as well. She also had *danava* (burning sensations). *Danava* is a popular term in Sinhalese discussions of symptomatology, and this patient suffered from burning sensations in her hands and feet, head, stomach, and chest, and in her eyes. When she slept at night, it was as if fire emanated from these body parts. Although this excessive heat is congenital in many patients, in this case it was due to eating harsh (*katuka*), heaty foods like tuna, prawns, and breadfruit, and to avoiding cooling foods like milk, oranges, and sago.

Physician I recommended cool medications, as follows: (a) *kasāya*, or decoction, to be drunk every morning, composed of *iramusu* (*hemidesmus indicus*), lotus stems, *sāvandarā* (*andropegon muricatus*), white and red sandalwood, and licorice; (b) various *kända* (*cunjee*) made of herbs like *pol palā* (*aeurua javanica*); (c) tonic to increase the semen; and (d) daily head bathing. He recommended that the patient refrain completely from eating heaty foods and spices like mustard, vinegar, meat, and salted fish. She was permitted relatively cool fish like fresh *tara* (*scombero motus*) and *parā* (*caranx*), and she was to consume cool foods like barley water, sago, young coconut, and red coconut water and milk (see Appendix I for a discussion of hot and cold foods).

After following this regime for three weeks the patient was completely cured.

Physician B claimed a special knowledge of *vāta prameha roga* (*prameha* caused by wind), which is the specialty of his family medical tradition. He said there are two types of *vāta prameha*: *prameha* of the young, which usually occurs before age 16; and true *prameha*, which develops in adults. The symptoms of *prameha* are: (a) swelling of joints; (b) crippled joints (*kora*); (c) tightening of nerves (*nahara*), so that the patient is pained, for example, in the knee, which subsequently becomes atrophied, a sure sign of *prameha*; (d) the semen (*śukra dhātu*) deteriorates, becoming thin (*hīta venava*); (e) backaches; (f) the kidneys (*vakugadu*) slowly dissolve; (g) tearing from the eyes.

Physician B was absolutely certain that "bad living" is the most common cause of *prameha* in adult men and women. This included illicit sexual relations, too frequent or prolonged sex, sexual fantasies, and the consumption of alcohol, *gāñja*, or opium. *Prameha* may also be hereditary, with the sins of the parents visited on the children.

The doctor claimed that patients between 10 and 16 years old were brought to him with swollen joints, most commonly the ankles. He also said that girls before first menses often discharge a white substance from their genitals. Though Western doctors do not see this as a disease, it is a disease according to his family tradition. Soon after menarche, women may discharge semen which has the consistency of *cunjee* (*kända*). This is known as *soma roga*, and is a type of *prameha*; it is also known as *karma roga*. This form of the disease can also arise from sexual shock or excitement. The symptom of the disease is that semen, or flakes of deteriorated semen (*piṭi*), are passed in the urine, or there may simply be excess urine, or the "white discharge" of women. At this stage the disease is not serious, but when the joints later swell it becomes a serious matter.

Physician B described a case of *vāta prameha roga* in a 21-year-old unmarried man. His symptoms were: (a) nocturnal emissions; (b) swollen joints, particularly the ankles; (c) palpitations (*hati*); (d) giddiness (*klānta gatiya*); and (e) backache.

Because this young man did not lead a bad life, his disease was caused by diet. He was an unskilled wage laborer who could not afford "vitamin" foods. Although his diet could not be greatly modified, the doctor prescribed a prepared tonic, *abhaya ariṣṭa*,[2] and barley water. The patient was asked to take the tonic eight times daily and to bathe daily to calm the heat (*uṣṇa nivenna*).

Physician C disagreed with Physician B that *prameha* is exclusively a *vāta* (wind) disease. He said that there were twenty types of *prameha* which fall into four broad classes:

2 According to Gabriel Gunawardene (1917:397–398), *abaya ariṣṭa* is made in the following manner:

198 oz. *terminalia chebala* (*aralu*)
99 oz. dried grapes
20 oz. *enbilia ribes* (*valangasal*)
20 oz. dried flowers of *bassia latifolia* (*mi pup*) cut into small pieces
2048 oz. of water

Boil all the ingredients over a low fire until one-fourth of its contents remain. Strain decoction, and then add the following ingredients:

198 oz. cane jaggery (treacle, *ukhakuru*)
4 oz. root of *tribulus terrestris* (*gotukola mul*)
4 oz. root of *impomoea turpethum* (*tirassa valu mul*)
4 oz. seeds of *coriandrum sativum* (*kotaimburu*)
4 oz. flowers of *woodfordia floribunda* (*malita mal*)
4 oz. tubers of *citrullus colocynthis* (*komadu ala*)
4 oz. bark of *piper chaba* (*siviya*)
4 oz. seeds of *peucedanum graveolens* (*satakuppa*)
4 oz. dried roots of *zingiber officianale* (*siddinguru*)
4 oz. roots of *baliospermum montanum* (*datta mul*)
4 oz. gum of *bombax malabaricum* (*katu imbul maliyan*)

Mix these ingredients together and pour the whole decoction into an earthen vessel and let it stand for one mouth. The mouth of the vessel must be covered and it should be airtight.
Dose: one ounce twice daily.

1. *Vātapradhāna*, where the chief agent of the disease is *vāta* (the *doṣa*, wind).
2. *Pittapradhāna*, where *pitta* is the chief agent (the *doṣa*, bile).
3. *Apapradhāna*, where *kapha* or *sema* is the chief agent (the *doṣa*, phlegm).
4. *Raktapradhāna*, where blood is the chief cause of the disease.

The first three are the three humors of Āyurvedic theory, but it is likely that the Galenic theory of four humors spread to South Asia with the Yunānī medicine of Islamic tradition, so that Āyurvedic practitioners sometimes classify diseases in a manner that resembles Galenic theory. While Physician C prescribes therapies according to this etiology, he believes that he must find out which of the three *doṣa* is predominant in each case, and then determine how this excited *doṣa* affects the blood. The blood is affected in all *prameha* cases, and through the blood the other *dhātu*. These are the internal causes of the disease. The external causes are: (a) sexual misbehavior; (b) alcohol; (c) *gāñja* (*cannabis*) and opium; (d) the wrongs (*vāradi*) in the body (*sarīra*) of the parents.

Physician C, like Physician B, argued that it is unlikely that children under 12 could have *prameha* caused by bad living. The belief that children are incapable of sexuality is widespread among educated Sinhalese. Physician C presumed that when children suffered from the disease it was caused by the bad living of their parents.[3] The symptoms are the same for both children and grown-ups. Physician C inverted the two stages mentioned by the other two doctors, and said that the first stage of the disease was the swelling of the joints. Acute pains may follow, if the wind humor has been excited or is the major cause of the disease. The second stage of the disease is when sugar, semen, or deteriorated semen passes out with the urine.

Physician C said that *prameha* was the most common ailment among the patients who attended his clinic. And he went on to say that one ancient sage expressed the view that women cannot get *prameha* but today evidence to the contrary is clear. In fact, nowadays *prameha* is more common in women than in men. The nerves become knotted and hurt badly; the patient limps, and bends her hands and knees with difficulty. After this stage a white discharge occurs in the urine, the vaginal path (*yoni mārgaya*) is wet with semen, and deteriorated semen (*piti*) passes out with the urine. If neglected, irregular menses may result in *prameha roga* in young women; and about half of the female *prameha* patients also suffer from hemorrhoids.

Physician C claimed that over 90 percent of the schoolgirls who came to him with *prameha* had the symptom of wetness in the vagina, and that he has treated patients who range from 15 to 40 years of age for this illness. The symptom is not mentioned when the patient initially describes her illness. Patients usually complain that they are weak, their bodies are thin (*kettu*), and when they work they quickly become fatigued (*hatiya*). Only when

3 There is a widespread belief among "educated" Sinhalese that the young are incapable of sexuality, a belief nowadays extended toward social inferiors.

questioned do they admit to wetness in the vaginal tract. Sometimes they confess that they have had the disease for several months, or even for years. They may have consulted Western doctors who told them that "this is no disease." But Physician C maintains that according to Āyurveda it is clearly a disease, and that his remedies cool the inside of the womb, the kidneys, and the urinary tract. If these medicines have no effect, he will try a drastic medication containing opium, which he says will "dry up the disease."

COMMENT

It is necessary to distinguish between the indigenous Āyurvedic tradition represented by these three doctors and the classical Sanskrit tradition, for they diverge from each other. Another Āyurvedic physician in Kandy, who was trained in Calcutta, asserted that the Sinhalese Āyurvedic tradition was wrong in its interpretation of *prameha*. His version of the subject was based directly upon the classic text, *Susruta Samhita*

According to *Suśruta*, the external causes of the disease are (a) idle, sedentary habits, which include sleeping during the day; and (b) the excessive consumption of sweet liquids and of fat-producing foods.

The bodily principles of Vayu, Pittam, and Kapham of such a person get mixed with improperly formed chyle of the organism. Thus deranged, they carry down the urinary ducts the deranged fat, etc., of the body and find lodgement at the mouth (neck) of the bladder, whence they are emitted through the urethra, causing disease known by the (generic) name of prameha. (Susruta, vol. II, 1963:43)

The premonitary symptoms are:

burning sensation in the palms of the hand and the soles of the feet, heaviness of the body, coldness and slimyness of the skin and limbs, sweetness, lassitude, thirst, a bad-smelling breath, a shortness of breath, etc. (Susruta, vol. II, 1963:43)

Prameha diseases, if neglected, may also cause abscesses and sores. The internal causes of the disease category are derangements of the three *dosas*. Ten forms of the disease are caused by the derangement of phlegm (*kapha*), six by bile (*pitta*), and four by wind (*vāyu*). Thus, there are 20 *prameha* diseases. A deranged humor may derange other humors and the *dhātus*, particularly blood, fat, and marrow. The discharge of semen in the urine is characteristic of one of the ten forms of *prameha* caused by phlegm, and is relatively insignificant in *Susruta's* discussion of these maladies. The *pramehas* caused by wind (*vāta*) are incurable. Ultimately, all types of *prameha*, if neglected, lead to diabetes, which is incurable.

The divergences between the classical text and the Sinhalese conceptions of *prameha* represented by Physicians A, B, and C are:

1. The Sinhalese physicians emphasize bad living, interpreted primarily as sexual promiscuity or indulgence, as a major cause of illness. The Sanskrit text does not have this emphasis.

2. The loss of semen (*śukra dhātu*) is of major importance to the Sinhalese physicians, but not in the Sanskrit text.

3. The Sinhalese physicians correlate the swelling and crippling of the joints with the discharge of semen, but this correlation does not exist in the *Suśruta Samhita* There the swelling of the joints is an entirely different category of symptoms, and one unrelated to the problem of night emissions, sexual excess, and secretions from the vagina. These latter symptoms the text identifies with other diseases (see *Suśruta*, vol. II, 1963:122–133 for a discussion of these illnesses).

By Western medical criteria, diverse maladies seem to be grouped together under the Āyurvedic term *prameha*. Among these illnesses would be kidney diseases and diabetes. Although our three Āyurvedic physicians claimed that many patients come to them with associated symptoms of swelling in the joints and the discharge of semen in the urine, these symptoms are not correlated in Western medicine, except in gonorrhea, where a white discharge may be associated with arthritis. Gonorrhea is rare in Sri Lanka, and two physicians (A and C) claimed that they referred "social diseases" to Western doctors. A likely hypothesis is that the reported swellings are due to rheumatic fever, which is common in Sri Lanka. The peak occurrence of rheumatic fever occurs in children around the age of 9. My impression is that the swelling associated with rheumatic fever is diagnosed as *prameha* among children, while the discharge of semen is the common symptom of adults. Be that as it may, I will now speculate on why these two classes of symptoms came to be associated in the thinking of Āyurvedic physicians, and the reasons for the massive cultural preoccupation with the loss of *dhātu*.

All three Āyurvedic physicians examine the urine of the patients only if they consider the case to be serious, or if they doubt the patient's report of *dhātu* discharge. The urine may be examined immediately; or for greater accuracy, the doctor may put some medicinal powders (*kuḍu*) in it and leave it for two hours, or overnight. He may then see oily matter (*tel kāran*) on top, and deteriorated semen (*piṭi*) which has settled to the bottom of the container. Semen is seen floating in between like fluffs of cotton or a cloud. Physicians A or C may also refer patients to a Western hospital or clinic for a urine test. This is done when a patient is suspected of passing sugar in the urine, and both doctors interpret these modern tests themselves.

How can we translate these ideas into Western medical idiom? Except for fat globules and possibly sugar, data that are viewed as relatively innocuous by Western medicine are considered pathological by the three Āyurvedic physicians. The chief interest of the Ayurvedic physicians is in the "flour-like substance" (*piṭi*), which may be phosphate deposits, and red and white cells. These deposits are considered pathological. Similarly, the white discharge in females, which may be secretions due to vaginitis or to hormonal changes in pregnancy or puberty, are interpreted as the pathological emission of *dhātu*, though not exclusively semen. The reported wetness in the vagina may be the lubrication caused by masturbation or sexual fantasies, or simply a normal physiological condition of moistness, but it is generally interpreted as pathological semen loss.

My description of *prameha* illustrates how the cultural definition of physiology and pathology creates a class of patients, some of whom might not be classed as ill according to a contemporary scientific definition of the situation. The Āyurvedic idea that the body is composed of *dhātus*, of which the most important are blood and semen, is practically universal among the Sinhalese. Semen is more important than blood, and the popular belief is that one drop of semen equals sixty drops of blood. The idea of semen loss causes a great deal of anxiety. It is likely that the anxiety provoked by this cultural definition of the situation may cause weakness, poor appetite, and weight loss, or aggravate these conditions when they have other causes.

Anxiety regarding semen loss is complicated by sexual anxieties and guilt feelings generated in a culture in which the expression of sexual and aggressive drives are radically circumscribed from very early childhood. In Sri Lanka, as in many other cultures, men and women have very little or no premarital access to each other. In this situation, nocturnal emissions and masturbation, as well as homosexuality, are a common outlet for the sex drive. Guilt and anxiety regarding sex are expressed by fear of semen loss. The patient says, in effect, "I am being punished for evil sexual thoughts and actions by the loss of body vitality and strength." Preoccupation with urine then occurs, and changes in its color, or the presence of deposits, are readily viewed as blood and semen. Also, semen deteriorates, and the idea is widespread that its deterioration causes impotence. (I am currently writing a monograph in which I show that "impotence anxiety" is manifest in rituals where the male genitalia are represented in exaggerated fashion.)

Thus, visits to Āyurvedic physicians for *prameha* are "overdetermined" by sexual guilt and impotence anxiety. The medications for cooling the excited humors and restoring virility are attempts to cope with these anxieties. Carstairs has a parallel discussion of this phenomenon among high-caste men in a Rajasthan community (Carstairs, 1961:83–88).

The recent massive increase in educational opportunities in Sri Lanka has swelled the ranks of the middle class, where sexual puritanism is most pronounced. Furthermore, unemployment has increased the age of marriage, which in turn increases the number of men and women with very limited means of resolving their sexual needs. The intuitive view of Physician C that there has recently been a large increase in female patients with white discharge and wetness of the vagina may be correct. I imagine a similar increase has occurred in men suffering from semen loss. The largest number of Āyurvedic advertisements in the Sinhalese papers deal with *prameha*. One Sinhalese newspaper has a weekly column entitled *veda-gedera*, the Āyurvedic Physician's Clinic. An examination of this column over eight consecutive weeks showed that 40 percent of the persons who solicited aid were worried

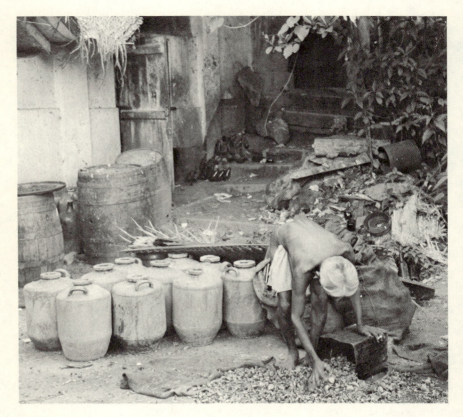

PLATE 1. The preparation of medicinal wines at the Gampaha Siddhayurveda College in Yakkala, Sri Lanka.

about weakness resulting from *dhātu* loss.

Certain food habits and pathological behavior are related to this concern about semen.

1. Many people select foods they believe will vitalize their semen. The *dūrian* fruit, pork fat, and tortoise meat are clear examples; indeed, the tortoise is threatened with extinction due to its imagined semen-fostering and aphrodisiacal virtues.

2. Many young unmarried men, particularly students in the university dormitories, eat raw eggs in the morning to enhance strength and vitality. I interpret this custom, also found in the West, as an unconscious attempt to compensate for loss of vitality due to night emissions, masturbation, or an imagined discharge of semen in the urine. In Sri Lanka the term for egg is *biju*, which is also used for seed, semen, and penis.

3. On the pathological level, I have interviewed several young men who claimed to drink their own semen, which they collected in their cupped palm

after masturbation. Such habits, though made understandable by the preceding discussion, are probably rare, since semen, like other bodily exuviae, is highly polluting. While the practice of drinking semen is probably rare, the fantasy may be more common.[4]

I believe that the total set of symptoms of *prameha* are brought together in a projective system which expresses and rationalizes sexual anxieties and feelings of guilt and inadequacy. My interpretation is analogous to Kardiner's interpretation of the nineteenth-century European medical view that "masturbation causes insanity." Kardiner has shown that the learned treatises and "scientific" accounts written about this "illness" were projections of sexual anxieties and guilt feelings in Victorian society. They also rationalized these anxieties in "scientific" terms (Kardiner 1946:32). The modern concept of *prameha* correlates swollen joints and *dhātu* loss on the assumption that punishment is required for the loss of semen, which is usually caused by bad living; and punishment in this case is swollen joints, crippled limbs, and aches and pains.

CULTURAL PREOCCUPATION WITH THE HEAD

Indian philosophical, medical, and astrological thought is greatly concerned with the head, and this concern is common to the South and Southeast Asian societies which have been influenced by Indian ideas. In Sinhalese culture the preoccupation begins to be learned when the mother massages the infant's head to mold its shape. Thereafter the head is more cared for than any other part of the body. Coconut oil is rubbed on the head to keep it healthy by persons of all ages. A portion of oil is placed in the cupped palm and applied all at once to the vertex of the head, then tapped with the palm so that it will permeate the skull.

The head must be protected from heat, and particularly from cold. The conception of cold is based on Āyurvedic theory, so that special care should be taken to protect the head from dew (*pinna*) and drizzle or rain (*poda, vässa*). Mothers of all social classes and educational backgrounds worry if their children are exposed to even the most meager drizzle. The concern is so great that adults may often be seen covering their heads in the rain with an ineffectual piece of cloth rather than leave it totally unprotected. To walk in the rain with the head unprotected is unthinkable; yet wet feet are of no cultural concern. Distinctions in types of bathing should also be seen in this context. For example, a basic distinction is drawn between a head bath (*hisa näma*) and a body bath (*änga näma*). A head bath should not be taken in the evening, or if a person has phlegm (*sema*) diseases. Cold water is ex-

4 Note *Susruta*'s comments on drinking semen: "A child born of scanty paternal sperm becomes an *Asekya* and feels no sexual desire (erection) without previously (sucking the genitals and) drinking the semen of another man" (vol. II, 1963:131). "The semen-carrying ducts of an *Asekya*, etc., are expanded by the drinking of the semen as above described, which helps the erection of his reproductive organ" (vol. II, 1963:132).

cessively "cold" and may aggravate the condition of the patient, whereas a a warm bath is only moderately "cold."

The cultural preoccupation with the head, and the Āyurvedic concept that to neglect the head may cause phlegm diseases, make people especially vulnerable to precisely the diseases specified. This self-fulfilling prophecy binds together in a single complex the cathexis of the head, medical theory, and environmental problems such as seasonal excesses of tropical humidity and heat.

TREATMENT AND DIAGNOSIS OF *Sema* (PHLEGM) DISEASES

The following examples of diagnosis and treatment of phlegm diseases are from Physician A. Though a general practitioner, he claimed special skills in phlegm diseases (*sema roga*), *pīnas rōga* (a special variety of *sema rōga*), and wind diseases (*vāta rōga*). According to him, 20 diseases arise from the excess or anger of phlegm. The external factors of this condition include staying up late at night; wetting the head by drizzle, rain, or dew; taking cold foods at the wrong time—e.g., when a patient is about to catch the common cold; and exposure to the fur of animals or the hairs of insects.

The simplest and commonest type of phlegm disease is the common cold. When one is about to catch a cold, one should not take cool foods like water of the young coconut. Foods that are neither too hot nor too cold (*sama-śītoṣṇa*—equally hot and cold) should be taken. The common cold is a source of considerable concern, and is thought to illustrate very concretely an excess of phlegm. It leads to more serious conditions, and may ultimately cause *unasannipāta*, a fever caused by all three humors, or to *pīnas* diseases. *Pīnas roga* is a cultural disease par excellence. Local newspapers are full of advertisements for this condition, and such patients form a considerable percentage of those who visit Āyurvedic physicians. It includes diseases like catarrh, sinus, tonsilitis, hay fever, and asthma. According to Physician A there are 18 types of *pīnas*. The most important are: (a) *sema pīnas*, where phlegm comes out in its own form; (b) *gal pīnas*, where the phlegm has hardened (*gal*, stone); (c) *lē pīnas*, where blood comes out with the phlegm; (d) *diya pīnas*, where the phlegm appears in watery form (*diya*, liquid); and (e) *laya pīnas*, where the phlegm has descended into the chest and causes conditions like asthma.

Although *pīnas* is always caused by phlegm, the external cause may even be something like a head injury. And, as usual, the remedy is to calm the aroused humor. It is necessary to avoid cool foods like milk and oranges. Milk especially has phlegm-rousing characteristics. Hot foods or medications should also be avoided, since the heat may dry up the phlegm to produce a more complicated condition. And of course the patient should avoid phlegm-producing behavior such as keeping late hours or wetting the head.

Physician A held a view frequently expressed in Sri Lanka, that Western medicine does not cure the *pīnas* but only dries the phlegm that causes the disease. The best foods to overcome the malady are those that are equitably hot and cold. Medications aid the patient to expel phlegm through the mouth and nose. For this purpose oil should be applied on the head, and Physician A gives smoke wicks (*dum pandu*), which are soaked in medicine and burned for the patient to inhale the fumes. Medicine may also be rubbed on the throat, and powders (*pīnas kudu*) inhaled to help expel phlegm.

Pīnas is a major disease preoccupation of the Sinhalese. The view that phlegm must be gotten out of the system is expressed by popular customs. For example, people commonly expel mucus from the nose in a public manner. Clearing the throat loudly (*kāranava*) is a well-established habit, and noises that usually emerge from Sinhalese bathrooms in the morning are made by people clearing the throat. This may be done by placing two fingers on the back of the tongue and vigorously rubbing it, causing retching, which often induces salivation and regurgitation, or vomiting.

STATISTICAL DATA

Insofar as cultural diseases are based upon conceptions of the body and the causes of illness which are coded into Sinhalese and Tamil religion, magical rites, and everyday manners, they evade the categories of Western medical science, and its physicians are not likely to cope with these diseases in an effective manner. Yet it is probably true that when practitioners of Āyurvedic and of Western medicine are in competition, the scientifically superior and pragmatically more effective system of Western medicine will gradually erode Āyurveda (see Appendix II). The slowest elements to erode will probably be the cultural diseases. Many patients who visit Āyurvedic physicians and clinics are afflicted by these diseases. It is not possible at this stage to make a precise statement about the numbers involved, though this information could be gotten from the records kept by all registered Āyurvedic physicians. In June 1971 about 87 patients, or 35 percent of all the patients who came to Physician A's clinic, suffered from *pīnas* or *semapratiśyāva*. Physician B treated 132, or 12 percent of his patients, for *dhātu* loss. Obviously, some kind of specialization goes on among Āyurvedic general practitioners.

Are there other diseases for which people seek Āyurvedic treatment in unusual number? I administered a questionnaire in Sinhalese to 58 final-year students in the College of Āyurveda at Colombo. The students were asked to list those diseases which they believed could most effectively be treated by Āyurveda. I have summarized below the responses of 54 students who answered this question by naming 62 diseases.

Diseases		*Responses*
37 received	less than	5
14 received		5–10
6 received		10–20
5 received	over	20

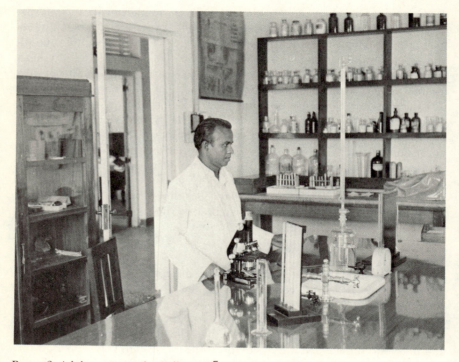

PLATE 2. A laboratory at the College of Āyurveda in Colombo, Sri Lanka.

TABLE 2

Five Diseases Which Final-Year Students in the College of Āyurveda
Believe Could Most Effectively Be Treated by Āyurvedic Medicine

Name of Disease	Western Terms	Agreement: number of responses	Percentage of possible total responses (n = 54)
āmavāta	rheumatism, arthritis	44	81.5
kuṣṭa	rashes, skin diseases, eczema	39	72.2
pakṣagāta	paralysis of limbs; loss of ability to use limbs	32	59.2
vātarakta	neuralgia, neuritis, swelling and cracking of skin below knee, varicose veins	24	44.4
arsaṣ	hemorrhoids	22	40.7

Thus, while 62 diseases were listed, the students showed a fair consensus about five diseases as ones for which Āyurvedic medicine is most effective. These diseases are listed in Table 2.

We also asked which diseases could most effectively be cured by Western medicine. The first four diseases in Table 2 were not mentioned in the lists of any students responding to this question. However, four students mentioned hemorrhoids (*arsaṣ*) as a disease that could effectively be treated with Western medicine.

Since Āyurvedic students indicated that their system of treatment is especially effective for five diseases, defined in Āyurvedic terms, we may ask if this view has any objective validity. In order to verify this problem, we looked at records for patients admitted to the hospital of the Āyurvedic college in Colombo for a three-month period. This is the largest Āyurvedic hospital in Sri Lanka. Table 3 shows that 163 patients, or 61 percent of all the patients admitted to the hospital, were diagnosed as having one of six diseases. Table 4 gives the number of admissions for each of these diseases.

A comparison of Tables 2 and 4 indicates that the diseases which the students believe to be most effectively treated by Āyurveda are ones that constitute the majority of cases in their teaching hospital. The only disease on the hospital list that is not in the student list is *nāḍi gatavāta*, a subcategory of *vātarakta*, which is on the student list.

It looks as if the judgments of students regarding the efficacy of Āyurvedic treatment are based on their experience in the wards. Interviews with hospital authorities convinced me that the hospital has specialized in treating the illnesses in Table 4, and that its doctors refer the cases they cannot handle to hospitals for Western medicine. This practice of referring patients to Western medical facilities may encourage the public to recognize a division of labor between the two systems of medicine, so that patients themselves selectively resort to the Āyurvedic hospital for certain maladies.

Āyurvedic physicians in private practice also commonly recommend that their patients consult doctors of Western medicine. All of the practitioners we interviewed said that they refer patients to Western doctors, and sometimes consult Western doctors themselves when they or members of their families are ill. Since they are prominent members of their communities, their example would help produce a division of labor between the two systems.

Four of the diseases in Table 4 are caused by excesses of wind (*vāta*) and involve pain or incapacity of the limbs or joints. They are chronic illnesses, and their Western equivalents are identifiable. Āyurvedic treatment requires various types of medication, but massaging with medicinal oils is always used for these diseases. The treatment itself is probably effective and, in any case, gives psychological relief. Western medicine has no cure for these conditions, and the way that it is practiced in Sri Lanka does not provide the psychological support that Āyurvedic medication gives. The same thing may be said of eczema (*kuṣṭa*), which involves a strong psychological component. And finally, people with hemorrhoids resort to Āyurveda because it claims to cure the condition without surgery.

TABLE 3
Summary of 275 Cases Admitted to the Government
Āyurvedic Hospital, Colombo
Feb. 1 to April 28, 1971

	Diseases	*Patients*
Diseases only 1 patient was diagnosed as having	36	36
Diseases more than 1 but less than 5 patients were diagnosed as having	12	33
Diseases 5 to 10 patients were diagnosed as having	5	34
Diseases 10 or more patients were diagnosed as having	6	163
No information	?	9
Total	59	275

TABLE 4
Six Major Diseases Treated in the Government
Āyurvedic Hospital, Colombo
Feb. 1 to April 28, 1971

Name of disease	*Western terms*	*Number of cases*	*Percentage of total (n = 266)*
pakṣagāta	paralysis of limbs	52	19.5
āmavāta	rheumatism, arthritis	40	15.0
kuṣṭa	eczema, skin diseases	25	9.4
vātarakta	neuralgia-neuritis	20	7.5
nāḍi gatavāta	neglected neuralgia, causing swelling and pain in nerves	16	6.0
arsas	hemorrhoids	10	3.8
Total		163	61.2

Many patients at the hospital were old, incurable, or chronically ill people who probably sought Āyurvedic treatment as a last resort. It was easy for me to get information on age and chronicity of illness from the hospital register of admissions. In scrutinizing the 275 admissions for a three-month period in 1971, I found that 62.9 percent were listed as chronic and 26.3 percent as acute. Despite the gross underenumeration which I believe occurs for the chronic category, this is a very large proportion. The average age of the patients was 51.6 years.

I also asked how Western medical practitioners viewed the efficacy of Āyurvedic medicine. I sent a questionnaire to 38 general practitioners who belonged to the Kandy Society of Medicine—excluding from the survey all government and university doctors—and 24 doctors replied. One question asked whether respondents considered Āyurvedic treatment efficacious for some maladies to which 13 doctors answered yes and 11 answered no. I asked affirmative respondents to list the maladies for which they thought Āyurvedic treatment was effective; and 12 doctors mentioned 36 diseases in all, while the thirteenth doctor stated that Āyurveda had only a placebo effect (several physicians stated that their views should not be construed to mean that Western treatment was ineffectual). Table 5 translates the categories these doctors used into indigenous terms, wherever feasible.

TABLE 5

Types of Diseases for Which 13 Western-Trained Doctors in Kandy, Sri Lanka, Thought Āyurvedic Treatment Could Be Effective

Malady	*Number of times mentioned*
sema diseases	11
(hay fever, asthma, colds, headaches, catarrh)	
āmavāta and *vātarakta*	8
(muscular pains, arthritis, swelling and pain in the joints)	
fractures	4
(massage with oils after the fracture has set—physiotherapy)	
kuṣṭa	2
(skin diseases)	

NOTE: Diarrhea and hypertension were each mentioned twice.
Urinary calculi, drastic purgation, diabetes, worm infestation, early nephritis, and hemiplegia were each mentioned one time.

When asked whether they referred patients to Āyurvedic physicians, all Western practitioners answered no. The question was badly phrased, since formal referral to Āyurvedic physicians is against the ethics of the profession.

However, three doctors wrote that they "advised" their patients to seek Āyurvedic treatment for phlegm diseases when Western medicine had failed, and for massage with medicinal oils.

That Āyurveda is popular for particular maladies was confirmed by examining the case records of six free Āyurvedic clinics maintained by the Kandy Municipal Council. The total number of patient visits was 112,693, and the total number of diagnostic categories was 94. Each of 71 categories had under 1 percent of the total patient visits. These cases altogether constituted only 13.14 percent of the total, while 86.86 percent of the cases were diagnosed as having one of 23 illnesses. Over 63 percent of the cases fell into 10 categories, which I judged to be the popular illnesses for Āyurvedic therapy. They are listed in Table 6.

TABLE 6

Ten Most Popular Categories of Illness
Used to Diagnose Over 63% of 112,693 Patient Visits in 1970
To Six Free Āyurvedic Clinics in Kandy, Sri Lanka

Name of disease	Western term	Number of visits	Percentage of total
krimi rōga	worm infestation	10,709	9.50
kusṭa	eczema, skin diseases	9,260	8.22
vāta vyādi	"wind-caused" diseases;		
	aches and pains	9,249	8.21
pratisyāva	cold	8,458	7.51
vātarakta	neuralgia-neuritis	7,732	6.86
jvara	fevers	6,365	5.65
pradara, śvetappradara	discharge from vagina	5,578	4.95
ajīrna	indigestion	5,163	4.58
āmavāta	rheumatism, pains in joints	5,123	4.55
pīnas	catarrh	4,312	3.83
Total		71,949	63.86

With the exception of worm infestations, fevers, and indigestion, the kinds of diseases we have discussed in the preceding pages are also included in Table 6. An explanation is required regarding *vāta vyādi* and *pradara*. *Vāta vyādi* simply means wind diseases, those not covered by the conventional terms for neuritis-neuralgia and rheumatism. The chief physician of the Municipal Council said that most of these patients have "aches and pains," or "trouble with their joints." *Pradara* includes white discharge and discharge of nonwhite secretions from the vagina. Some clinics treat these diseases separately; others ignore white discharge (*śvetappradara*), and list only *pradara*. We have combined the two categories because both are viewed as discharge of *dhātu*. This category does not include discharge of blood from the vagina, which is listed as *rakta pradara* (0.09 percent). *Pradara* does not include *prameha*, either; this was listed separately (3.01 percent; 3,386 visits). Male semen loss was most likely treated as a symptom of *prameha*.

Table 6 confirms our view that Āyurveda draws patients with the cultural diseases and chronic ailments we have described. *Pakṣagāta* (partial paralysis), which formed an important category in the Āyurvedic hospital, accounted for only 0.20 percent of the free-clinic cases because the clinics did not treat these cases.

CONCLUDING REMARKS

This essay has had two major topics: (1) the metamedical extension of Āyurvedic ideas in Sinhalese culture, and (2) the description of cultural diseases. I have also suggested that Āyurveda is often a last resort for patients with chronic illnesses, and that the overall medical system is structured by a division of labor between Āyurveda and Western medicine. Although I believe that Āyurveda is effective for many types of diseases, I have not discussed its therapeutic efficacy because this problem is outside of my competence.

I am not entirely satisfied with my treatment of phlegm (*sema*) diseases as cultural diseases, since I cannot specify the effect of the cultural preoccupation with the head on the etiology of these illnesses. I can only suggest that *sema* illnesses may be in part caused or aggravated by the cultural preoccupation with the head. On the other hand, illnesses attributed to *dhātu* loss are clearly related to indigenous theories of body functioning which have no scientific validity. All cultures, including popular cultures in Western society, have modes for conceiving body processes that are objectively false. These processes are subjectively real to individuals, however, and symptoms related to these "false" conceptions may reasonably be viewed as products of true illnesses—i.e., as genuine maladies generated by physiological reactions to false concepts and the behavior based upon them. From the point of view of Western medical science, symptoms belonging to different categories of illness may be conceived of as representing a single illness. It is clearly misleading to say that a cultural disease like *dhātu* loss is not an illness, as Western medical practitioners do. Such statements are nonsense to the patient, who perceives and feels himself afflicted. These statements would make sense only when comprehensive cultural changes lead to a redefinition of the situation.

Finally, an analysis of metamedical concepts should be possible for any medical tradition. The concepts of Chinese medicine would clearly lend themselves to the kind of analysis I have made of Āyurvedic concepts in Sri Lanka. Further research will, I am sure, indicate the value of studying the Western medical tradition in this manner. It is misleading to characterize this tradition as "scientific," and to assume that it therefore lacks metamedical dimensions. Science itself has a meta-dimension, and science is only part of the Western medical tradition. Analyses of the metamedical dimensions of Asian and Western medicine will open a fruitful and relatively unknown area of comparative research.

APPENDIX I

Hot and Cold Foods

The classification of food into hot and cold categories is known and used by Sinhalese people at all levels of education, and at every degree of social-class differentiation. The analyses of food and dietary habits are extremely complicated in Āyurveda. Foods are prescribed on the basis of at least two principles: (a) the relative presence of the five *bhūtas*, and (b) the capacity to foster and build the seven *dhātus*.

A food may be bad under some conditions because it is excessively hot, but under other conditions it may be good because it builds up the *dhātu* of blood. In Āyurvedic prescriptions the binary distinction into hot and cold is complicated by consideration for other properties. In the popular culture, however, the major distinction is a binary one between hot and cold foods. Sometimes people postulate a category in which these two elements are balanced (*sama*), and foods may also be differentiated by their capacity to produce or reduce wind. Wind-producing foods may be hot, cold, or *sama*.

The impact of Āyurvedic ideology on the culture is probably strongest in the area of food habits and dietary prescriptions. In this research, 24 physicians of Western medicine in Kandy were asked whether they gave advice to their patients regarding hot and cold foods; while 14 replied that they did not give such advice, 8 said they did, and 2 advised patients to eat the foods that agreed with them. Several doctors tried to interpret the hot/cold theory in scientific terms by saying that hot foods contain excessive uric acid, or that the distinction corresponded to high and low caloric content. Several said they did not believe in the theory personally, but tried to meet the prejudices of their patients in a reasonable manner. I am convinced that at least 5 of these doctors had some kind of personal belief in the validity of prescribing foods by using the humoral concept of hot and cold properties. One doctor who did not give advice to his patients regarding these dietary habits practiced them at home. Another said, "About 95 percent of my patients believe in this. They have been indoctrinated in these beliefs by the older generation, and I think that if I try to explain the fallacies in these beliefs, I might lose my practice! However I tell them this: 'If there is any food which disagrees with you, please avoid it. I cannot lay down a rule and say this is good and this is not good, because various people are sensitive to various types of food.'"

One doctor who said that "Āyurveda is a waste of time and money" had this to say about hot/cold foods: "We advise cooling foods for people who are nervous and excitable and for mental cases; cooling foods are milk, spinach, ladies' fingers (i.e., okra), tomatoes. Heaty foods for rheumatic patients. For asthma patients: breadfruit, meat, and fish."

APPENDIX II

The Idiom of Expression and Communication of Illness

Scientific effectiveness is not the only criterion for consulting a medical practitioner, for patients want to feel they have effectively communicated their problems to the doctor. A major problem of Western medicine in Sri Lanka is that patients, particularly among the peasants, and doctors talk in mutually incomprehensible idioms. This is not true for the Āyurvedic physician and his patient. The language by which the patient describes symptoms is perfectly comprehensible to the Āyurvedic doctor, since it is derived from Āyurveda. Thus, patients establish communication and rapport with Āyurvedic physicians that are sadly lacking in interactions with Western doctors. For many peasants, Western medicine is effective but nonrational, whereas Āyurvedic prescriptions flow logically from a shared body of assumptions.

Consider the following typical statements by patients suffering from *dhātu* loss: "Blood is heated and passes out" (*lē unu karala yanava*); "the *dhātus* get heated and pass out" (*dhātu unu karala yanava*). Similarly, a patient may say that a serious headache is because "wind has struck the top" *vāte inhalata gahala*—i.e., an excess of wind produced in the region of the stomach has moved toward the region of the head). These statements are nonsense to a Western doctor, but not to an Āyurvedic physician.

Indeed, the good opinion Sinhalese have of Western medicine does not imply acceptance of its theories. Educated persons may simultaneously adhere to the germ theory of disease and to Āyurvedic humoral theory. Attempts are sometimes made to reconcile the two theories. Articles on this subject have been written in *Ayurveda* and *Ayurveda Pradeepika*, the scholarly journals of the profession. I quote below the statements of Āyurvedic College students who said they could reconcile the germ theory and the *tridoṣa* theory.

1. *Germs upset the three humors, which then cause illness*:
   a. "In Āyurveda it is shown that bacteria upset the three humors, and subsequently diseases arise."
   b. "Sometimes bacteria enter the human body but get destroyed. This occurs when germs fail to break the equilibrium of the *tridoṣas*."
2. *Humoral equilibrium provides immunity to germs*:
   a. "The state of equilibrium is similar to antibodies. Diseases cannot be caused if the *tridoṣas* are in a state of balance."
   b. "It is possible to state that immunity is simply the equilibrium of the three humors."

    c. "It is difficult for germs to attack the body when the *tridoṣa* are properly balanced."

3. *The germ theory and the humoral theory are independent, equally valid theories of disease causation*:

    a. "If one of the three *doṣas* are aroused, the other two humors are also affected. Disease cannot arise if the three humors are in good order. When a germ enters the body a similar thing happens; a certain section of the body becomes weak or damaged. . . ."

    b. "*Tridoṣa* frequently get upset owing to changes in climate or food; germs also cause illness. I don't say that diseases are caused only by *tridoṣa*; . . . *tridoṣa* and germs are two different things."

Literature Cited

Carstairs, G. Morris
    1961 *The Twice Born: A Study of a Community of High Caste Hindus*. Bloomington: Indiana University Press.
Das Gupta, S. N.
    1932 *A History of Indian Philosophy*, Vol. II. Cambridge: Cambridge University Press.
Filliozat, J.
    1964 *The Classical Doctrine of Indian Medicine*, trans. from the French by Dev Raj Chanana. Delhi: Munshiram Manoharlal.
Gunawardene, Gabriel
    1917 *Medicinal Plants of Ceylon*. Colombo.
Kardiner, Abram
    1946 *The Psychological Frontiers of Society*. New York: Columbia University Press.
Susruta
    1963 *Susruta Samhita*, Vol. II, ed. and trans. K. L. Bhisagratne. Chowkhamba Sanskrit Series Office, Varanasi I.

The Social Organization of Indigenous
and Modern Medical Practices
in Southwest Sumatra

M. A. JASPAN

THE REJANG FOLK DOCTOR

Among the Rejang of Sumatra, and in Southeast Asia generally, traditional theories of pathology relate to four main categories: (a) the action of natural elements, particularly water and wind; (b) deistic or ancestral retribution; (c) sorcery and witchcraft; and (d) poisoning.[1] These ideas are considered when the folk doctor examines a patient, and almost always constitute a core part of both the patient's own account or explanation of his illness and the doctor's case history, diagnosis, and therapeutic program. In the absence of modern epidemiology, the Rejang doctor is left with metaphysical interpretations, such as retribution for evil, in the sense of anti-social actions or thoughts, serious breaches of custom, or the neglect of ancestors, kinsmen, or living dependents who are in need.

Pathogenesis and therapy are centrally related to a conception of balance and imbalance that Henry Sigerist referred to as a "Plus" or a "Minus," a "Too-much" or a "Not-enough." He wrote: "A person is ill either because his organism contains something it does not require, or does not belong to it, or because something necessary to it has been removed" (1951:128). Thus, the folk doctor tries to extirpate or exorcise injurious intrusions into the body, or to recover and replace what has been lost.

The Rejang, who live in the highlands of southwest Sumatra, have a population of almost a quarter million people. From 1961 to 1963 I conducted nearly two years of field research among them (Jaspan 1964), and for approximately a year of this time I chose to be apprenticed to Man Aher, a man in his seventies who was regarded as the greatest Rejang folk doctor, historian, and bard. (The phenomenon of the versatile doctor who was also an accomplished natural historian or man of letters was common in Europe

---

1 I have described these ideas in another paper (Jaspan 1969), which used material from Burkhill's classic study of Malay village medicine (Burkhill 1930) and my own anthropological field work in several parts of Indonesia and mainland Southeast Asia. The present essay complements my 1969 paper, which went on to describe the public nature of diagnosis and treatment; the close link traditional medicine apprehends between natural environment, interpersonal relationships, and ill health; Southeast Asian concepts of basic metabolism, and the effects of modifying it; the specialized fields of indigenous medicine, mental illness, personal hygiene, pastoral care, and patient management; and, finally, the connection between medical theory and medical training.

until the nineteenth century.) It was the custom for a Rejang doctor to train one of his own sons or nephews in his art of medicine, if he had the right personality and a sense of dedication or calling, but the pressures of war, revolution, and rebellion had turned young men's inclinations elsewhere. Until I arrived in 1961, both Man Aher and others thought that much of his knowledge would die forever, with him.

One of the most significant holistic attributes of Man Aher's system of medicine was its "transparency." The Rejang folk doctor did not regard his knowledge and techniques as professional secrets, nor was there an aura of professional taboo separating doctor from layman, or medicine from all else. This does not mean that he did not have substantial professional equipment in the sense of training, experience, techniques, pharmacopoeia, and religious actions. His principal fear was not imparting or losing these to competitors or laymen, but that economic and modernizing pressures had deprived him of medical trainees or apprentices, and his knowledge and skills might therefore not be transmitted as an integral corpus of professional learning.

In retrospect I am astonished that a bond of rapport and understanding should have been struck between Man Aher and myself from the first day I came to his village, Topos. Some others regarded me with suspicion, though in most cases it gradually gave way to cooperation, except for a few who held out and kept their distance. Topos village is the most isolated in Rejang country, and is still largely dependent on subsistence hill rice farming in swidden clearings in the jungle. But villagers had heard I would be coming that day, and Man Aher was at the entrance of the village dressed in ceremonial costume to greet me. Beside him were four nubile girls, also in festive costume, to honor ancient custom by bearing a tray of betel perquisites symbolizing respect, friendship, and readiness to accept a stranger of good will into their community (Jaspan 1968). The folk doctor then stepped forward from the inquisitive crowd and issued a long speech of which I understood hardly a word. A few weeks later I asked him what it meant, and he agreed to repeat it; but I preferred first to record it on tape, and then go through it laboriously with him, line by line, while I transcribed both the original text and an English translation. This, incidentally, was a technique I later used in order to register and express the meaning of many medico-religious incantations.

The full text of Man Aher's honorific speech is not relevant to this paper. What struck me greatly in it, however, was his description of the Rejang heartland in Lebong, not in terms of its area, population, or government, but in a succinct quatrain of ten Rejang words as

Tanea ubeut,	A land of medicine,
Tanea guau;	A land of learning;
Tanea ubeut kaeun	Of medicine that brings recovery
Tanea guau patjo'	Of learning that brings insight.

I naturally asked Man Aher why the Topos region in Lebong was considered more important for its medicine and learning than anything else. To this he replied: "It has always been so. I inherited this from my father and my medical teachers, and they from theirs." He added that in the cool mountain heights where the water in the fast-flowing streams is clean and pure, and many forests have never been touched by man's adze, there are plentiful herbal medicines, a healthy climate, and what might best be called a psychic and physical purity which the Rejang associate with the source of a river, rather than is mouth. For the Rejang, Lebong is also a sacrosanct place of origin where their ancestors first entered the country, and are thought to be buried in the mists of the mountain peaks. This notion of physical purity in the highland peaks, jungle, and streams extends to the people—all Rejang regard the people of Topos as the most robust, incorruptible, and morally tough-fibered of all Rejang. But a folk doctor such as Man Aher is expected to have even higher qualities of character than those of other Topos villagers.

My apprenticeship in traditional Sumatran medicine consisted of accompanying Man Aher on his calls to patients and assisting in the preparation and administration of drugs, in the propitiation of ancestors to heal their living descendents or to exorcise nefarious spirits, and in procedures relating to preventive epidemiology. This was not however my sole task as an anthropological field worker: I was simultaneously studying Rejang ethnohistory, social organization, law and economic life, and their literature and arts. But as Man Aher turned out to be a sound informant on several of these other fields as well as medicine, my association with him grew even closer. As a "national bard" (in a figurative sense, for the Rejang have no such established category), an acknowledged expert on customary law, and an accomplished rice farmer and hunter, there was scarcely any part of my inquiry where his assistance was not sought and valued.

Yet despite all his versatile knowledge, Man Aher was illiterate—something he much regretted, for there had been no opportunity for schooling when he was a boy and a young man. He encouraged his children, grandchildren, and great-grandchildren to attend school and go on to the university whenever possible. He had deeply progressive views on most matters, though not a facile penchant for modernity and change for its own sake. He believed that man still has much to learn; but conversely, many generations of accumulated human learning must not be lightly discarded.

While believing in the merits of traditional Sumatran medicine, he was not opposed to modern medicine. On the contrary, he welcomed it and hoped it would assist him in his lifelong efforts to heal his own people. Thus far, modern medicine had made little more than occasional forays into the village, seldom lasting more than a few hours. Contact with doctors and hospitals, when villagers went to a town, tended likewise to be brief, spasmodic, and rather impersonal. Although Man Aher often asked his patients about the nature of their treatment by "Western" doctors, his interest in modern medicine did not diminish his belief in the professional legitimacy, propriety, and efficacy of his own corpus of medical theory and practice. He saw the two as complementary: if used *together* in treating a patient, they might significantly reduce the gap between knowledge, on the one hand, and ignorance or uncertainty on the other.

Man Aher particularly stressed the therapeutic success of Rejang medicine in two fields that lie outside surgical technology: metabolic ailments and mental illness. With regard to internal medicine, he had a substantial body of empirically derived knowledge of the therapeutic properties of forest plants and their prescriptive effect when administered for indigestion, diarrhea, constipation, and diuresis. With regard to mental illness, he believed that mental health or ill health are a function of an individual's reciprocal acceptance by kin, neighbors, and the village community generally. Experience inclined him to relate illness in which manifest somatic abnormality or malfunctioning were absent to a psycho-social disturbance or dysfunction in the social-relations continuum linking the patient to his or her nuclear family, kinsmen, and neighbors—although he would not of course state this in these terms. But in addition to such interpretations, and the theistic rites he conducted to cool aggression and restore psychic equanimity, he nonetheless used his knowledge of herbal drugs for relieving his patients' anxiety states and hypertension.

It is neither possible nor appropriate to describe here the full extent of a Rejang doctor's medical skills, techniques, pharmacopeia, and practice of both therapeutic and preventive medicine. But unless some examples are given, the premature and false conclusion may be reached that all I am doing is to wrap a load of primitive, superstitious mumbo-jumbo into a seemingly scientific package. I do not deny that there is both humbug and quackery in the methods of shamans, herbalists, and other traditional practitioners in much of the Third World—as there was in our own pre-20th century society and, if we are to be truthful, which is still with us in a number of unillumined corners of modern medical practice. To return to Man Aher, however, I think three prime factors mark him off from a great many shamans, witch doctors, or medicine men of tropical Africa and Asia. These are, firstly, his deep concern for empirical scholarship; secondly, a kind of Hippocratic code of ethics which forbade him any personal gain from the practice of medicine; and thirdly, his genuine success as a family and community doctor.

SUMATRAN PRACTITIONERS

The generic term for doctor among he Rejang is *dukuen*, etymologically akin to the Javanese *dukun*. There is, however, an older word, *piawang*, akin to the Malay *pawang*; but the Rejang have tended to narrow the meaning of this term to denote either a specialist in gynecology or a midwife. *Piawang* is used more frequently than *dukuen tjupi*, a baby doctor. *Bidan*, the Malay and Indonesian term for midwife, is seldom used by village Rejang. Thus the generic *dukun*, without further qualification, is understood to be a specialist in medicine irrespective of whether his patients are women only, or children, or any other category.

Such specialists might be regarded as equivalent to general practitioners in Western societies. Among the Rejang they are more often men than women. Their functions are to diagnose and heal the sick, to advise and direct measures for the prevention of epidemics and noncontagious diseases, and to preside over the psycho-moral well-being of the community. This does not mean that every village has its own doctor, or that a doctor's clientele consists only of his own villagers, or that his villagers have no choice in selecting a doctor. There was indeed one other doctor in Man Aher's village, whose practice took in about a fifth of the village population. But Man Aher had almost as many patients from other villages, some more than 150 miles distant. There is thus no form of administrative structuring of relationships between patients and doctors in the traditional system.

Doctors who have from the start specialized in one field of medicine or who have moved from general practice into either a medical specialization or a related nonmedical field retain the title *dukuen*, but this is qualified by the specialization. Thus there is, for example, *dukuen tjido'*, a thoracic specialist dealing with cases of asthma, chronic coughing, and what is probably pulmonary tuberculosis.

There is, however, one relatively large category of seriously ill persons whose symptoms do not yield to the treatment of either Rejang or "Western" doctors. The Rejang consider such patients to have been poisoned, not perhaps by atmospheric fumes or yet undiscovered viruses, as sometimes predicated in Western medicine, but by the administration of toxic substances by personal enemies, or through sorcery. Rejang general practitioners are often reluctant to treat patients who are convinced they have been poisoned. They are skeptical of both the theory and the clinical methods of the poison extractors (*dukuen atjuen*), though the level of professional tolerance varies from one doctor to another, perhaps as Western doctors vary in their attitudes to osteopaths.

In this sense, however, the use of the term *dukuen* is more akin to *tukang*, or specialist, and the poison extractor is a technician specializing in this sole pursuit, just as a blacksmith is considered a technician specializing in yet another craft or skill. In this more general sense, the term *dukuen* also occurs in the designation *dukun jerat*, for "hunting specialist," a man whose advice is sought on when to go out hunting, where to hunt, and what methods to use. Apart from giving excellent advice based on long experience, most *dukun jerat*—like most medical *dukun, mutatis mutandis*—believe in strengthening the chances of success in a hunt by first propitiating the names of famous hunters of yore, or the particular tutelary spirits of that part of the forest to be traversed.

This interdependence of empiricism and supernatural resort is not confined
to the hunting specialist, but is indeed central to the theory and practice of
Sumatran folk doctors. To condemn this as unscientific, primitive, or just
scornworthy would, in my view, be arrogant, pontifical humbug on our part.
It would also imply an assumption in Western medicine that all disease
or ill health is susceptible of successful treatment solely by our present knowledge and practice of medicine. Fortunately, however, few would make such
claims; indeed, the most advanced schools of medicine are only too aware
of the many lacunae in medical knowledge and ability to successfully treat
a variety of diseases. Furthermore, do we not have hospitals or special wards
for the chronic ill and for incurable diseases? And are there not vast numbers
of mentally ill condemned to spend years in mental hospitals where the
efficacy of treatment is often not particularly impressive and where, despite
all our scientific knowledge, so much still depends on an intuitive approach
to patients?

OCCUPATIONAL PROFESSIONALIZATION

In no case is the Rejang doctor a full-time professional worker who depends
for his livelihood on his practice of medicine. Like everyone else in the village
community, he is primarily a rice farmer; but his medical training and skill
give him a high social status, and he is a respected member of the executive
committee, so to speak, of traditional village government. Most of his consultations, especially during busy farm work seasons, take place at patients houses
either in the evenings or in the mornings before about 8:30. He does not keep
a surgery or consulting room, but sees patients mainly in their own homes.
Sometimes a casualty patient is brought from the scene of an accident direct
to his house.

In some cases he keeps a small medicine chest (*ganiet*) of *materia medica*
that can be stored dry. However, most of his prescriptions are dispensed
from freshly gathered and prepared herbal ingredients. Man Aher would
see a patient in the morning, and later when he went through the forest
trails to his swidden farm would tarry awhile here and there to seek the leaves,
stems, or roots he required. These would be taken either from one or two
trees or from several different trees or shrubs, and not necessarily all from
the same part of the secondary forest or jungle. After collecting what he
needed, he continued with his routine farm work, unless the patient's condition was critical and required an immediate administration of his drugs.

MEDICAL EXAMINATION

What is the nature of a Rejang doctor's examination of a patient? By
what criteria does he select a therapeutic program? How does he prescribe
and make up a drug, and how does he supervise or ensure the efficacy of his
treatment?

The Rejang do not have the habit of seeing a doctor at regular intervals for a periodic examination or checkup irrespective of their feeling ill or well. They nonetheless recognize a need for ongoing attention to the individual's and the community's health requirements, through both preventive medicine and promotive health activity—to which I shall return later.

A doctor becomes aware of a case when he is summoned by the patient's kinsmen. The visit consists of examination, preliminary treatment, and advice to the patient and his or her kinsmen, and is followed by drug preparation and subsequent visits. Generally speaking, a patient has to be quite ill to warrant calling a doctor. For transient abdominal discomforts or headaches, alimentary ailments such as mild indigestion, diarrhea, constipation, etc., most people have or can borrow home remedies, or may seek advice from close kinsmen or neighbors. Summoning the doctor is not, however, inhibited through a fear of having to pay high fees—a Rejang doctor does not accept money as payment for his services, and the standard gift of a small basket of rice, a coconut, and a chicken is only payable if the treatment of the patient has been successful. I have, furthermore, never heard of a Rejang doctor reproving a patient for having summoned him inopportunely, needlessly, or at an uncomfortable hour of the night or the weekend.

The doctor responds to a summons by going to the house of the sick person as soon as possible. There he conducts his examination of the patient in a room crowded with solicitous kinsmen and friends. Both Rejang doctors and the lay public believe that a seriously ill patient requires his kith and kin near him because they give him moral support, material succor, and tangible proof that he is loved and wanted. It is also thought necessary, in the perilous twilight state of body and mind weakened by disease and within sight of death, to guard the patient's soul lest it stray or be enticed from its body. Thus the atmosphere of silence and subdued speech associated with illness, and especially grave illness, in Western society, is quite alien to Rejang, and indeed to most Southeast Asian societies.

On arrival at the patient's mat-side, one or more close relatives describe to the doctor how in their view the patient's present illness originated and developed; they also venture their own diagnosis and suggestions for treatment. The doctor listens to all this with patience and empathy. He is certainly not intolerant of lay opinion; nor does he consider it irrelevant. Perhaps this is because their professional–secular dichotomy is not as finite as in Western society; they would certainly not wish it to be so. This absence of professionalization applies to other areas of Rejang life, such as religion, where there is no division between professional priests and a residual laity. The priests, like the doctors, are primarily farmers: when public services make heavy inroads into their private economic time, they are recompensed in kind, in the manner already noted.

After a case history has been obtained, orally and in the company of many, the doctor examines the patient—who generally remains lying on the mat—

by palpation. He then makes an ausculatory check, placing his ear above
the patient's heart, and manually examines the viscera of the lower abdomen.
Experience has taught him the importance of an enlarged spleen, particularly
where there is a fever, marked lassitude, loss of appetite, and profuse perspiration. While examining the patient, he asks the patient's spouse, parents,
or adult children about the nature and frequency of the patient's bowel
movements, body temperature, perspiration, and appetite. Except in malaria,
sweating is regarded as a positive index, something that is likely to reduce
the fever and in a sense counteract and destroy pathogenic viruses. If there
is an absence of perspiration, the doctor prescribes a sudatory infusion to be
taken until perspiration is both free and regular. The onset of perspiration
is usually taken as an indication that the febrile crisis has been reached and
passed.

DIAGNOSIS AND TREATMENT

When an examination has been completed the doctor is usually offered
sweetened black coffee or tea—sugar is a luxury—with a handful of bananas
or rice-flour biscuits. He discusses his diagnosis and proposed treatment,
going over or elaborating points already made. These are not kept secret,
and it is never considered improper or undesirable that the patient or his
kinsmen should hear and know the diagnosis, or the proposed therapy
and prognosis. The conspiracy of professionalism, so widespread in Western
society, is largely absent in the behavior and medical ethic of Rejang doctors.
Before leaving, the doctor gives general directions for the management of
the illness and its proposed treatment. In most cases the patient is to be kept
indoors, warm and confined to his or her mat. A sick-mat diet must be soft
and easily digested: rice, in particular, must be prepared as a gruel. Meat
and fish are usually avoided, though boiled chicken and the broth in which
it is cooked are often prescribed.

The patient is strictly forbidden from going to the river—where bathing
and defecation normally take place—as this is often a walk of several hundred
yards down a steep descent and then up again. This is partly because of
exposure to chill winds and cold water, but also because of the belief that a
river plays a predominant part in the introduction and spread of infection
and contagion.

After leaving the patient, the doctor seeks certain herbs, as already indicated. When he returns to the village in the late afternoon he shreds the roots,
leaves, or bark, as necessary, and boils them. Thereafter he strains the potion
and pours it into a bamboo cylinder, calabash, glass bottle, or any other
convenient container. This is brought to the home of the patient, and instructions are left about when and how often the medicine is to be taken, and the
dosage. If the patient reports feeling cold or stiff, or has muscular pain,
the doctor often advises massage—at which the Rejang are highly skilled—

but may initiate it himself until arrangements are made to have a masseur (again an ordinary farmer-villager) attend.

I mentioned the doctor's concern about pathogenic viruses, and this may have appeared strange and perhaps out of character with a non-Western or pre-modern system of native healing. Nevertheless, the concept of viruses is well understood in Rejang medicine: indeed, their language has a specific word for virus, *kuman*. They have no doubt—possibly as a result of thorough health education by the Dutch—that certain diseases such as cholera, influenza, and smallpox are virus-borne. They also believe that many of these diseases were introduced to Sumatra and their own interior highlands by virus-bearers from elsewhere. Until recently, most persons entering Sumatra came by sea, and travel to the interior was by river. Because of this, pathogenic virus infections and contagions were believed to come from the sea and rivers. While the sea is far away, however, the rivers—whose surfaces are generally windy in the Rejang highlands—are thought to be the sort of place where chills, sore throats, coughs, and influenza are unsuspectingly picked up. This ties in with a sizable body of Rejang magico-religious belief about spirits and devils inhabiting riverbanks and seacoasts.

Apart from febrifuges, drugs to reduce or ease splenetic enlargement, and other specific drugs, a doctor often advises the application of poultices and semi-dry compresses or poultice plasters. These are generically described as *tapea*. The compress usually consists of a number of herbs ground together, sometimes mixed with boiled rice, and wrapped in leaves. These are then affixed to such parts of the body as the forehead, neck, abdomen, arms, or legs. Forehead compresses are most common for migraine and other severe headache; abdominal compresses are used for cases of internal swelling, hemorrhage, or other felt but indiagnosed pain.

PATHOLOGY AND DIAGNOSIS: PRINCIPAL PATHOGENIC CAUSES

Man Aher's first step in any diagnosis was to determine whether the ailment or disease belonged to the hot or cold variety. The theory underlying such dichotomization contains both metaphysical and somatic elements. Once decided, however, the therapeutic regime accords with one of the two major types. "Hot" illness requires febrifuges such as quinine (which is also used as an analgesic and anti-depressant) and cooling drugs. "Cold" ailments, on the other hand, require heat and sudatory treatment.

A further method of categorizing maladies is based on four principal pathogenic sources: wind, spirits, poison, and worms.

If a patient has a severe chill, with thin nasal mucus and a painful head and joints, he is diagnosed as "entered by wind" (*masuk angien*), a concept that includes catching a chill or draught, or getting a cramp or a stiff neck. All such ailments require heat treatment, and the patient is instructed to stay indoors near a fire and to take hot drinks and sudatory drugs. The absence of sweat in a patient "entered by wind" is regarded as a negative, and sometimes dangerous, symptom. The sudatory dosage may be increased, and the patient brought nearer to the fire. When *météng* or free perspiration begins, there is general relief, and a belief that the malady will take a natural course leading to recovery in a few days.

The evidence for worms is their visual sight in stools or an anal itch, in the case of threadworms; but tapeworm is not always easily sighted, especially since defecation takes place in fast-flowing rivers and streams. Man Aher used the herb *teriba* (*Rhinacanthus communis*) in treating ringworm and ascarides. Extremely bitter drugs, such as quinine and similar preparations from bitter tree bark or roots, are also used to flush worms out of the alimentary tract.

The second principal pathogenic category after wind is that of spirits. I think this is an area where the empirical competence of Rejang medicine no longer operates, and the doctor virtually says: "I have examined the patient, diagnosed such-and-such symptoms, and treated him accordingly, but without success. There are probably more powerful influences at work." The patient's kinsmen conclude from this that they must now turn to either expelling some harmful spirit or poisonous substance from his body. In other cases, the doctor's examination may have shown no recognizable or identifiable symptom, yet the patient is manifestly ill or is wasting away. Here again the doctor suggests the possible interference of nefarious spirits or poisoning. The procedure for exorcising such spirits necessitates a *kedurai* rite in which certain ceremonial foods are offered to the patient's ancestral spirits, who are exhorted to assist their ill and suffering descendant by evicting the troublesome demon or devil. In some cases the doctor, now in a role of devil-exorciser, directly confronts the devil assumed responsible, saying: "We offer you food to satisfy your hunger. Take it and eat it, but do not eat this child." The ritual food offering at such *kedurai* rites consists of rice boiled in saffron, parched rice, coconut oil, and a grilled leg or wing of chicken.

Here again this mixture in Man Aher of diagnostician and healer, using extensive empirical knowledge, on the one hand, and of shaman/magician on the other, may only confirm the view of some Western medics that all non-Western medicine is in the last resort witchcraft or sham. But we need only recall that many distinguished Western doctors do not consider they are betraying their scientific training and professional standards if to their professionally-based efforts to effect recovery they add a prayer to God. And religion apart, I am by no means sure that the imbibing of tonics and mineral waters, or resort to secular or religious spas, are not epistemological equivalents of the non-empirical, irrational, and supernatural elements in the Rejang practice of medicine.

In my experience of Man Aher's practice, his greatest and most frequent successes were in treating such conditions as diarrhea, constipation, colic, stomach cramp, headache, and bone fractures—and most of all, malaise, anxiety, or depression due to psychological causes. On the other hand, not having any substantial knowledge or experience of parasitology or surgery, he could not go further than to diagnose and alleviate such diseases as tuberculosis, hepatitis, and bacillary intestinal infection. Nor did he have the knowledge or skill to perform surgery in cases of appendicitis and tonsillitis, or where caesarian section would have saved a mother and her baby. Rejang medicine stops where its incipient knowledge of parasitology, antibiotic pharmacopeia, and surgery ends, since from there it gives over to extra-medical ideas, beliefs, and practices. In these areas the Rejang doctor recognizes the greater competence of Western medicine, and he is quick to advise a patient to go to a Western-trained doctor (until recently, mostly European or Chinese) for antibiotics and surgery.

TAXONOMIES OF ANATOMY, PATHOLOGY,
AND MATERIA MEDICA

My field notes make possible the compilation of an extensive list of Rejang medical terms for anatomy and physiology, for abnormal and pathological body conditions, and for methods of treatment, and of their pharmacopeia. I shall here give only a few examples of such terms.

In anatomy, there are special terms for almost all the bones of the body, the main arteries and veins, the viscera and external characteristics. There are separate names for each finger and toe (not just big, little, middle, second, and fourth); for an unmarried woman's breasts and those of an old woman; for a skin in healthy condition and a dull skin; etc. In pharmacopeia the Redjang have several antidotes for snake poisoning such as *batu geliga* and *baleut mleu*. *Daun tidur-tiduran* leaves provide a sedative infusion for restless children; *putjeui glenyer* is made into a soporific or sedative potion for adults; *tjergayu* or *sergayu* is used both as a febrifuge and as what might be translated as a broad-spectrum prophylaxis against communicable diseases. Chest ailments are often treated with the herb *stanguen*, while congested lungs in babies and children are treated with an elixir made from *tjekur, Kaempferia galanga*. Ringworm and ascaris are initially treated with *teriba, Rhinacanthus communis*; but if that is not effective, more potent root potions are resorted to, some including a strychnine constituent. Strychnine beans are also used for respiratory stimulation and to stimulate cardiac action.

Man Aher's treatment consisted as much in advice to patients as in the prescription of drugs. Where a patient had overindulged in what he considered "hot" or "rich" foods, such as durian fruit, deer venison, or goat meat, he advised a light diet with rice gruel and weak tea. Where he diagnosed a stomach chill, this was often ascribed to eating acid foods or drinking palm toddy on an empty stomach. There are other drugs to treat burns and lesions, to relieve diuretic complaints and dysmenorrhoea, to induce abortion, to reduce inflammation, and so forth. Many of these drugs were of proven efficacy; but their composition and function, generally speaking, remain unknown to modern medicine.

POISONING

This is a syndrome that accounts for over half the cases of illness in the South Sumatran highlands. Sudden nausea, and a sense of being flushed or of weakness in the knees, are considered the first symptoms of poisoning, and the doctor's first step is to administer an herbal emetic. If this does not bring relief, antidotes to known poisons are attempted; but if these fail, it is thought that the poison is likely to be organic, in the sense of a culture bred by a poison specialist or sorcerer, and inadvertently ingested by the patient when invited to eat outside his home, particularly at a wayside restaurant. Man Aher declined to treat such confirmed poison cases; he was indeed cynical about the increasing number of poison extractors who claimed to remove visible specks of poison from a patient's abdomen or back through a process that might be described as psycho-magnetism. Indeed, he showed the same polite skepticism of the widespread public vogue for the poison specialist as he did for such locally sold Chinese patent medicines as Yee Tin Medical Oil, whose stated composition is

Dragon's Blood	3%	Oil of Artemesis	3.50%
Oil of Teaseed	10.50%	Leaf of Artemesis	5%

and which is prescribed for "all colds, coughs, diarrhea, vomiting, cholera, sunstroke, burns and scalds, and internal colic"!

PUBLIC HEALTH AND PREVENTIVE MEDICINE

Traditional

There is no system of separate public health officers or sanitary inspectors in Rejang villages. These functions are both understood and considered necessary by the village people, but there is no division between preventive and therapeutic health services. Once a year there is a "Cleansing the Village Ceremony"; this is both pragmatic and an occasion for feasting and entertainment. Man Aher presided over the public angle, visiting each house in turn to inspect its cesspool and yard. The cesspool, which collects kitchen and toilet waste from the scullery (which, like the house, is raised 8 to 14 feet on piles), must be covered with soil or river sand, and Man Aher insisted that each householder should have a heap or bucket of sand reserved for this purpose. He also ensured that each house had a barrel or bucket of water kept in case of fire. The courtyard around each house, in some cases reaching back to the bush or forest, had to be kept cleared of scrub, grass, and weeds, to discourage mosquitoes, ticks, midges, and carriers of dengue or glandular fever. Anyone failing to meet the required standard was reported to the Village Headman, who discussed the matter with his Council of Lineage Elders. This soon brought any backsliders to heel.

Other aspects of preventive medicine were an emphasis on sound diet and an avoidance of alcohol and of extremes of heat and cold, especially of iced water and of hot beverages at near-boiling temperatures. Bodily cleanliness is considered important, with everyone brought up from childhood to know that at least two baths a day—in the morning after rising, and in the late afternoon after work—are essential for good health. These examples by no means exhaust the numerous other instances I recorded of promotive health practices, beliefs, and injunctions.

Modern

Apart from the traditional medical services thus far described, rural South Sumatra is also served by a public health service, conceived on a Western model by the former Netherlands Colonial Government and for which the Government of Indonesia is now responsible. The state health service does not have its roots in either popular conceptions or traditions of medicine. Nor does it acknowledge or recognize the traditional theory and practice of medicine.

The South Sumatran public health service is administered by a provincial department of health. The department's head officer is appointed by the minister of health of the central government in Jakarta, but increasingly he is responsible to the provincial government as well. There is sometimes an area of ambiguity or overlapping in the degree of jurisdiction of the central and the provincial authorities.

Each regency or *kabupaten* in the province has a public health department (*Dinas Kesehatan Rakyat*), the head of which is a qualified (modern) medical practitioner (medical officer of health—M.O.H.). In view of the serious shortage of Western-trained doctors after World War II, the government had to recruit many of the doctors it needed from abroad, and later—in the 1960's—to draft graduates of the medical schools in Java to serve in the outer islands. The Rejang—Lebong Regency lies in the province of Bengkulu—until 1966 it was in the province of South Sumatra—and in this province the post of head of regency medical services could be filled for only two of the three regencies. And in both of these, the doctor chosen had also to serve as medical officer to the armed forces, normally a separate appointment in areas more generously supplied with medical personnel.

In theory the civil and military medical officer is fully occupied with the public health work, hospital supervision, outpatient clinics, and health administration of a regency with a population that lies between about 120,000 and 200,000. In practice, however, the salary offered by the state has not been sufficient to maintain a doctor in rural areas such as these. Consequently, the doctor is permitted to maintain a private practice after official office hours. As these are 7 A.M. until 2 P.M., the doctor has the greater part of the afternoon (i.e., after the almost ubiquitous siesta) and the evening in which to conduct his private practice.

The lack of trained modern practitioners places an enormous handicap on the efficacy of public health services, however well these are conceived and organized in Jakarta or the provincial capital. The result is an over-burdened doctor who has to fragment his energies between administration, hospital management, a house surgeonship, hospital surgery of all kinds (including obstetrics), and the maintenance of isolated district clinics; and parallel to this, another self-contained service comprising a military surgery and hospital. In practice, many of the duties of the M.O.H. have to be delegated to less qualified personnel, such as certificated health assistants (*mantri kesehatan*) and male of female nurses (*jururawat*).

No attempt is made to recruit the assistance of traditional doctors. On the contrary, modern medicine treats its traditional counterpart with contemp-tuous repudiation, and would undoubtedly resist any attempt at the profes-sionalization of traditional doctors within the framework of the state or any other modern medical system. This attitude is, however, assymetrical, for the folk doctors are willing to share their knowledge with modern doctors and to be trained in some aspects of modern medicine.

Between the folk doctors, who provide the mainstay of effective medical service in the countryside, and the one or two modern doctors in the province, a substantial volume of treatment is carried out by the government health assistants, once again mostly outside their office hours. These *mantri* have access to the most advanced drugs, either through purchase on the open market or by agreement with the medical officer under whom they serve. Not having full medical qualifications (they have usually completed a three or four-year medical course), their charges to patients are less than those of fully qualified doctors—in the approximate proportion of half to two-thirds. Should the *mantri* doubt his capacity to diagnose or treat any case, he may refer it to the doctor. This indeed epitomizes the professional relationship between the two, in most cases.

Whereas the medical officer of health usually serves only a two- or three-year tour of duty, sometimes renewed if no replacement can be found, the *mantri* tend to be local residents. At times, when the doctor is on leave or is summoned to the provincial capital for a conference or briefing, the *mantri* has to hold the fort and deal with everything normally handled by the M.O.H. He thus has the closest relations, both in an administrative and a private medical-consultant sense, with the civil, military, commercial, and intellectual elite groups of the regency. The *mantri* consider their professional status and salary-grade position in the hierarchy of medical personnel far from satis-factory. They tried to obtain better recognition in the 1950's and 1960's, and thought they might succeed because of the growing popular awareness of and need for modern medicine, and antibiotic drugs in particular. At that time the medical profession succeeded in holding back these demands, although in the socialistic Guided Democracy period of 1958–1965 the government was increasingly sympathetic to the *mantri* viewpoint. But their hopes are now waning, because of the vastly increased production of qualified doctors from Indonesia's nine medical schools, especially from Jakarta, Surabaya, and Jogjakarta.

Perhaps the greater tolerance of *mantri* toward the notions and practice of traditional medicine reflects their role-anxiety. This derives, firstly, from an incomplete medical training; secondly, from their having struck roots in a predominantly rural society where culture and belief have proved resilient to an international modernizing technology and culture's bulldozing of non-Western social structure and belief.

CONCLUSION

I have touched on only a few aspects of Rejang medicine. Perhaps more important than anything else in Man Aher's practice of medicine was the way in which he saw body and mind as indivisibly linked. A morbid somatic condition was not something entirely objective and outside the patient's consciousness, which could or could not be cured according to the precision of the diagnosis and the chemotherapy. For him, the conscious understanding and efforts of patient, relatives, and friends are a vital factor in the therapeutic process. This process furthermore included the doctor's own active and devoted concern for the patient. In following through many of his cases, I became aware how greatly this concentration of attention on a patient brought about relief or a cure, even without chemotherapeutic or surgical intervention. This giving of intensive support by the doctor contributed to the patient's sense of being deeply involved in his or her own therapy, in conjunction with many other people all working toward the same goal.

Such concentration of attention may be compared with the special care given to the fortunate few in Western society who are in private wards where the doctor tends to call more often, and to stay longer; where the nursing is more intimate and often more attentive; and where visitors may also stay longer. All this certainly assists treatment and recovery. But in Redjang country, this is the right and privilege of all. Perhaps that is why, as I mentioned at the beginning of this paper, its people call their country

> A land of medicine:
> Medicine that brings recovery;
> A land of learning:
> Learning that brings insight.

Literature Cited

Burkhill, I. H., and Mohamed Haniff
  1930 "Malay Village Medicine." *The Gardens' Bulletin, Straits Settlements* 6 (April).
Jaspan, M. A.
  1964 *From Patriliny to Matriliny: Structural Change Among the Redjang of Southwest Sumatra.* Canberra: Australian National University.
  1968 "Symbols at Work: Aspects of Kinetic and Mnemonic Representation in Redjang Ritual. *Bijdragen tot de Taal-Landen Volkenkunde,* 123 (4): 476–516.
  1969 *Traditional Medical Theory in Southeast Asia.* Hull, England: University of Hull Publications.
Sigerist, H. E.
  1951 and 1961 *A History of Medicine,* 2 vols. Oxford: Oxford University Press.

Chinese Traditional Etiology
and Methods of Cure in Hong Kong

MARJORIE TOPLEY

The position of Chinese medicine in Hong Kong and the problems of official recognition are complex. When in 1841 a certain Captain Elliott negotiated the preliminaries for a Sino-British treaty for the cession of Hong Kong island, one of his proclamations stated that the Chinese were "secured in the free exercise of their religious rites, ceremonies, and social interests. . . ." Many local inhabitants regard this statement as meaning that Chinese customs insofar as they are not harmful or contrary to natural justice should be protected: that no law which would interfere with their integrity should be applied to them. By and large this has also been the official attitude. But what is custom in the traditional medical profession? And what is or is not harmful in traditional methods of cure? As society changes, so does custom: new ways of training traditional doctors exist, as we will see, and many persons now practicing medicine have no medical training.[1]

It is difficult to say among contemporary practitioners who should be officially recognized as a traditional doctor, and sometimes even what constitutes a customary cure. Eventually such problems may have to be faced, but at present most of the controls which are exercised over traditional medicine have emerged as the indirect effect of pharmaceutical laws, food hygiene regulations, or other measures aiming to prevent hardships or dangers to the public. Thus, no traditional doctor is required to register, except as owner of a business, but no doctor without legally valid modern medical training may use certain listed poisons or treat any eye diseases.

1 The version of the paper for the Burg Wartenstein Symposium was based entirely on data collected in 1969. For this published version, the statistical information has been updated and augmented, and material from specialists in traditional medicine and other sources replaces or expands some of the sections. This new material was acquired late in 1971. The individual sources are indicated as they appear, but the overall source is a two-year project on which I am currently engaged at the Centre of Asian Studies which is specifically concerned with the operation of dual systems of medicine—modern and traditional—in the Colony. The study began in September 1971 and the data is, therefore, very preliminary. But since it will be some time before a report on the study can be written, it seemed worthwhile to include it here.

The inclusion of the new material does not shift the original emphasis of the paper, which is on differentiation within the traditional system itself, but enables more attention to be given to organization and structural features of the traditional system than was possible in the earlier paper.

Largely as a result of this situation, there is not only no official information readily available to the public on Chinese medicine, but little in government files, either, except as it arises through encounters with the law or in connection with the registration of medical associations. No specific research concerned with the sociology of Chinese medicine in Hong Kong had been undertaken before 1971.

A number of official sources indicate that modern medicine is a popular profession. The University of Hong Kong had a medical faculty with almost 700 students in 1971. Early in that year, more than 2,000 doctors were on the medical register (although some may not be active in the Colony), with more than 600 government medical officers. There were also more than 400 unregistrable doctors, mostly working in government services and exempted from registration, or in charity clinics themselves having exempted status. There were nearly 200 registered and government pharmacists. In addition, an unknown number of unregistrable doctors, occasionally without any qualifications from anywhere, practice illegally in the Colony under the guise of "Chinese practitioners" or "herbalists."

How popular does the traditional profession appear to be? "Schools" operate in Hong Kong as new kinds of institutions for training students of traditional medicine; located for the most part in small apartment buildings, their number is probably increasing. At least 16 associations of traditional doctors exist, 4 of which appear to be very active and alert to any new government measure that might have implications for traditional practice. Looking at the membership lists of such associations, I estimate that among them they have approximately 3,000 members. There may in fact be more, since this is the same estimate as was made several years ago by the present director of Medical and Health Services (Choa 1967:31). Some members do not keep strictly to Chinese medicine. A large number of "herbalists" with no medical training, some combining modern and Chinese medicine, join these associations. They are a concern to the government and also to a comparatively small elitist group of traditionally trained secular doctors.

At least 12 associations exist for selling or manufacturing Chinese medicines, 3 of which are for employees in medical shops. There is also an association for herb gatherers. In 1966 approximately 4,000 shops, stores, or other premises were in the business of selling or dealing with Chinese herbs and medicines. More than 2,000 were said to be herb shops that sold prescriptions to the public, employing more than 10,000 people. These figures may be exaggerated, since they come from a petition to the governor and a letter to the Secretary for Chinese Affairs by medical associations, to protest a proposed ordinance restricting the uses of poisons.[2]

2 The ordinance was passed. I am grateful to the Secretariat for Home Affairs for information about this petition and letter, and for much of the information later in this paper on problems between the government and medical associations about the operation of laws and ordinances. The Secretariat for Chinese Affairs was reorganized in early 1969 and became the present Secretariat for Home Affairs.

There appear to be nevertheless at least as many doctors and pharmacists in the traditional sector of the medical system as in the modern. It is too early to say with any assurance whether this is a function of direct and popular demand for traditional services, or conceals a demand for modern services which is not yet satisfied. In general, however, public health specialists in Hong Kong believe that Chinese laymen use traditional and modern medical services as complements rather than alternatives.

In 1966 Dr. G. H. Choa, who was then Senior Specialist, tried to find out what prompted patients to go to traditional practitioners. He asked his general-ward patients if they had consulted a traditional practitioner at any time in connection with their current illness, and if so, for what reason. He asked these questions of 100 male and 50 female patients, of whom 42 males and 19 females had consulted a Chinese doctor at some time for their illness—24 males and 4 females at the onset of illness, and 18 males and 15 females between modern treatments. As for the reason, 18 males and 4 females gave "faith," 4 males and 2 females gave "economy," 4 males "convenience," and 16 males and 13 females "no improvement" (Choa 1967:32).

Chinese medicines are often more expensive than the modern medicines that might be used for approximately equivalent complaints. While a modern doctor in private practice may earn on an average HK$10 to $15 per consultation (HK$6 = approximately US$1), usually including medication, a traditional doctor may charge an average of HK$5 for consultation and an extra HK$5 for prescription. Chinese medicine is one traditional profession which seems to be lucrative. Consulting a Chinese doctor is probably more convenient for the poor than joining the queues and crowded waiting rooms at government and government-subsidized clinics. But what about the layman's faith in Chinese medicine? Faith in what? This is one of the main questions I deal with in this paper.

In a study of child-rearing in 1969, I held four approximately 1½-hour depth interviews with 20 non-English-speaking mothers (19 were Cantonese and 1 was a Hakka married to a Cantonese) in the Cantonese dialect.[3] They lived in government high-rise housing estates in the urban district of Kowloon. Many of the questions I asked at each session related directly or indirectly to matters of health, particularly in children. I found that when their children were sick, the mothers sometimes took them to modern doctors. They also sometimes treated them themselves, on the basis of knowledge acquired from kinsmen and neighbors, usually elderly persons. Additionally, they sought advice from shops that sell Chinese medicines, and from traditional doctors. And they went to a range of other specialists for advice and treatment: diviners (horoscope readers); Taoist, Buddhist, and other priests;

3 This nine-month study was a part of a project on child development in Hong Kong which is being undertaken by the Pediatrics Department of the Faculty of Medicine, University of Hong Kong, with a grant from the Nuffield Foundation and other organizations.

women experts in ritual performances; and even spirit-mediums.

I subsequently discovered in follow-up interviews that these specialists sometimes combine medical (usually herbal) treatment with ritual treatments; that not all traditional doctors would assert that ritual treatment was without value, although none regarded ritual as their own province; and that some modern Chinese doctors would not say there was nothing in Chinese traditional medicine. One physician I interviewed used a combination of Chinese and modern medicine in his practice, and a few thought ritual, although not a true method of cure, might have value for certain kinds of patients.

The present analysis was prompted largely by these discoveries. The data obtained in 1969 have been augmented with information from additional specialists. Nevertheless, I do not generalize for the whole of Hong Kong. My study has been limited, and my informants mainly Cantonese. While the Cantonese are Hong Kong's major dialect group, dialect differences often go with other subcultural differences, and it is possible that some things I say, particularly about ritual practices, have no relevance to other groups. None of the conceptual and behavioral data is oriented to any specific social strata, however. The oldest mother interviewed in the child-rearing sample was 45, and most came from rural areas; 5 mothers had no formal education, 8 had incomplete and 3 had complete modern primary education, and 4 had incomplete secondary schooling. The husbands' monthly incomes ranged from HK$200 to $800. The traditional doctors I have interviewed recently came from educated middle-income families, and most of them were born in China. The herb-sellers and other related specialists were from poorer, less educated families, and most of them were also born in China.

THE DIFFERENTIATION OF CONCEPTS

Chinese medicine has not stood still over the centuries. Its progress appears to be marked by increasing abstraction in the handling of concepts and the sloughing off of religious ideas and ritual practices once associated with the physician's profession. How these and other changes came about is a matter currently occupying some specialists in the history of Chinese scientific development, as we can see from the work of Needham (cf. 1970), and in the papers by Otsuka and Porkert in this volume. Traditional medicine continues to change in China today, where dialectical materialism is being used to attempt a synthesis of the Chinese and modern systems. According to an article in *Red Flag* magazine, this is in accordance with the "law of the unity of opposites" which is "the basic law of the universe" (Hon 1970). In the present volume such matters are Dr. Croizier's special concern. The upshot of all this is, however, that much of what appears in the T'ang dynasty to have been part of the scholarly tradition in Chinese medicine now exists in parallel systems with their own specialists in Hong Kong. This is a matter which will concern us.

I have analyzed the traditional conceptions of two childhood diseases in an essay showing that disease concepts and therapy involved *rites de passage*, the ritual handling of transition and change (Topley 1970). While I looked at these diseases (measles and a syndrome called *haàk ts'an*[4]) as *internal* problems, I pointed out that metaphysical notions about *external* connections between the individual and the world around him were relevant to understanding ritual treatments. We shall now have to look briefly at a Chinese theory of internal and external balances in order to understand the kinds of specialists and cures in contemporary Hong Kong.

The cosmos is composed of ethers of heaven and earth, which are *yang*—having the attributes bright, light, and male—and *yin*, with the attributes dark, heavy, and female. It contains phenomena created by the dynamic action upon these ethers of Five Agents (*wu-hsing*): the elements water, fire, metal, earth, and wood. They mutually create and destroy each other: water puts out fire, fire burns wood, and so on. These attributes and elements are symbolic representations of aspects of nature, and have functioned widely within Chinese culture to think about complex sets of relationships between people, between mankind and the physical environment, and between man and chronological processes. Rather like numbers, they have been used to work out correlations among phenomena. This has sometimes led to the discovery of meaningful causal connections, and has involved a degree of rational experimentation (Lévi-Strauss 1962:9f. and 11f.). But they have also been used in a mystical manner. Again like numbers, they are used to describe the indescribable, or metaphorically, as one uses the sensations of hot and cold to describe colors to a class of blind children (Welch 1957:51f. and 59). They have been cloaked in allegory, and used in iconography.

According to this theory, an individual's physical and psychical character is determined by the movement of cosmic ingredients—the elements acting on the ethers, which have the additional attributes hot (*yang*) and cold (*yin*) with reference to the human constitution. In their natural state, the relationship among phenomena is one of balance or harmony. This is the so-called Will of Heaven; and when man is in harmony with things of the cosmos, he can be said to comply with Heaven's will. The approximate position is depicted in Figure 1.

Imbalances occur for a number of reasons. Some are inevitable. The cosmos is in flux, and relationships change with the years and the seasons. Human society is in flux as people are being born, marrying, and dying, and these

---

4 Nearly all technical and other terms and expressions used by informants or in the literature are romanized in Cantonese, following the system used by Meyer and Wempe (1947). The exceptions are the philosophical concepts *yin*, *yang*, and *wu-hsing*, and the "internal" and "external" classics *nei-ching* and *wai-ching*, which I leave in their more familiar mandarin form.

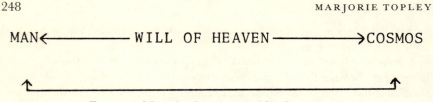

FIGURE 1. Man in harmony with the cosmos.

transitions create metaphysical instabilities. These instabilities in turn affect internal balance in the human body. Inevitable external instabilities are amoral, although to avoid imbalance as far as possible is a moral duty. Individuals with a particular combination of cosmically interacting elements should avoid unstable situations such as weddings and funerals, and the persons in these events who are undergoing transitions. One knows when to observe these avoidances by consulting the astrological tables in an almanac. Some people have cosmic balances that clash with those of people with whom they have a continuous relationship. In marriage, traditionally this state of affairs was avoided by comparing the horoscopes of the prospective bride and groom (Freedman 1967, 1970). But it can also happen with mother and child. One cannot choose the time of birth of one's children—yet. This results in both parties having difficulties in getting along, suffering constantly from sickness, and a mother feeling little or no affection for her child (*mŏ sam-ts'īng*) (ĩopley 1974).

Here, then, we have a "physiomorphism" of man and a "naturalization of human actions." Systems of action based on such concepts have been called *magic* (Levi-Strauss 1962:221). But a number of extremely subtle and complex relationships exist among the techniques which have developed in Chinese culture for handling problems of imbalance. For their examination I prefer to talk about the mystical and nonmystical applications of the cosmic theory.

Chinese medicine has come to focus on the *internal* problems of homeostasis, regarding the problems of *external* balance as the province of others. I propose to use the term *quasi-science* for the treatment of internal problems and the term *mystical science* for the treatment of external problems by rebalancing the individual with outer phenomena. Chinese medicine has largely given up the treatment of the external imbalances, but the body of knowledge on which treatment is based has continued as a separate and parallel—even, for some people, a complementary—system. Its specialists are diviners who deal with the horoscope, priests who perform transitional and rebalancing rites, old women of the family, and other women who are acquainted with the almanac and problems of working out the external causes of sickness. At one step removed is the geomancer, who sees that people erect buildings in a way that will not disturb the balance of nature (Freedman 1968).

Mystical science consists of literal and ritual rearrangements, and quasi-science of the literal, nonritual treatment of imbalance and disease. But quasi-science has its symbolic counterpart in acts which are directed to internal rearrangements, and which are not performed by doctors. These categories will be clear when I give examples of treatments and discuss their connections with each other. But I should first make several points about the terminology I am using.

I am aware of the hazards of developing an observer language from Western science for the analysis of non-Western systems. But I am also conscious of the analytical hazards of using participant language, and of the need to establish a universal-observer discourse as new comparative studies are undertaken.[5] The use of language developed within the terminological and conceptual framework of the system itself is dangerous, in my opinion, when the type of analysis for which the language is employed has not been attempted by users of that language. But whatever language one uses needs to be justified.

I used the terms *internal* and *external*, and so do the Chinese, but our meanings differ. According to Professor Needham, "internal" in Chinese medicine means "everything . . . rational, practical, concrete, . . . in a word, scientific." "External," or outside, means "everything . . . to do with gods and spirits, . . . everything . . . miraculous, . . . unearthly. . . ." He demonstrates this distinction from the titles of the Yellow Emperor's classics of medicine. The so-called Internal Classic (*nei-ching*) deals with disease taxonomy, classification of parts of the body, and the internal workings of the human being. Needham claims that the External Classic (*wai-ching*), now lost, must certainly have included "cures effected by charms, cantraps, and invocations." His assertion that the fact that this classic was lost at an early period emphasizes the secondary character of the magico-religious aspect of medicine in China seems doubtful to me (1970:271f.). But the point I would make is that, as it is used in China, external includes religion, as well as what I would call mystical science. In my usage they are not the same. Both quasi-science and mystical science are concerned with matter-of-fact relationships among phenomena, while religion is concerned with matter of principle.

But why do I use the terms quasi-*science* and mystical *science*? We know of course that Chinese medicine is not scientific in all senses of the term. It does not include a full understanding and use of the experimental method, or a full application of mathematical hypotheses to nature (Needham 1969: 15). But some experiment was certainly there, and structures of considerable sophistication were developed to categorize and analyze various aspects of the natural world. If "the whole aim of theoretical science is to carry to

5 On the question of "observer language" and problems of the comparability of cultural material, I am grateful for discussion with Professor W. T. Jones of the California Institute of Technology. He is not, however, responsible for the terms that I use, or for the form in which I express the problem.

the highest possible and conscious degree the perceptual reduction of chaos" (Simpson 1961:5), then China has had theoretical science.

I have to distinguish the literal and symbolic aspects of the internal approach. Some of the things that patients do to effect treatment are based on symbolic associations between cause and effect, and generally traditional doctors self-consciously disassociate themselves from such actions. However, the literal and symbolic approaches are not completely differentiated, and the efficacy of many medicants that doctors use is based on symbolic connection (cf. Anderson and Anderson 1968). For this reason I use the term *quasi*-science with reference to the internal approach in medicine. In employing the term *mystical* science I follow Freedman, who used it to refer to geomancy (1968). Geomancy deals with external imbalance and its correction, but the geomancer is not a priest, and geomancy is not a religion.

I turn now to a religious view of disease which contrasts with the amoral conceptions we have dealt with so far. This view involves the anthropomorphism of nature and the humanization of natural laws. It deals with problems of morality, and it complements the other systems. In Chinese thought, man's nature is part of a universal order, but culture teaches him how to comply with this order by preserving inner and outer harmony. If he is aggressive, angry, or envious, he creates disharmonies in the universe and within himself.

Discussion with ritual experts indicates that certain entities in popular religion may be related to man's immoral actions in two ways. Five demons (*ng̃-kwái*) are portrayed as noncivilized men (wearing loin cloths) on commonly used charm-papers. This kind of demon may be seen as a metaphorical counterpart of man acting in an uncivilized, i.e. disturbing, manner, the five as a group being a metonym for all kinds of disturbing activity. On the other hand, the demon itself may be thought of as activated or conjured up by disturbing human activity and itself an independent agent of disease and misfortune. On the charms are also portrayed a tiger, eagle, wild pig, and snake. They are termed "improper" (*ts'e*). Again they are metaphorical counterparts, this time of disturbed forces of nature and as a group a metonym for all such disturbed forces. At the same time they are also malevolent entities activated by these forces, and have an independent role. But gods defend men from them. The White Tiger, Cock, and Dog (the tiger in this context has been tamed by a Taoist Immortal) quell the demons, and the killing and improper creatures. Other gods, symbolizing culture and its values, are dressed as officials. They do for man as part of nature what literal officials do for him as a member of society.

Buddhism introduced to China another conception of man and nature different from the cosmic theory we have discussed so far. According to formal Buddhism, man is part of a natural order governed by moral law. If he complies with this law, he works out his fate in this life and dies a completed individual. But if he acts unnaturally, he activates principles inherent in the law of nature (*karma*) which cause him to be reborn. One important difference between the Buddhist and Chinese cosmic view is that in Buddhism natural law may sometimes be in opposition to the customs and laws of society. It is unnatural to kill pigs for ritual purposes, for example, although it may be demanded by Chinese custom (e.g., ancestral rites). A Chinese view, and one certainly accepted by the politically dominant Confucian philosophy, is that culture and nature can never be in opposition, since one is the morally correct method for approaching and understanding the other. The conflict of nature and culture is resolved to some extent in popular Buddhism by introducing sins against society and culture as additional causes for rebirth (cf. Eberhard 1967). Approximately, the Buddhist position may be depicted as in Figure 2.

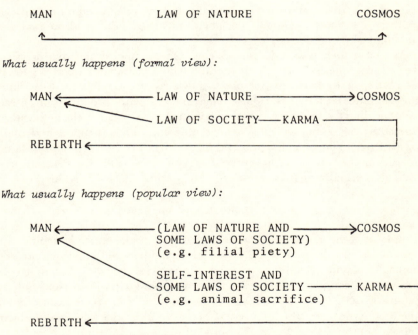

FIGURE 2. The Buddhist view of nature and the cosmos.

The Buddhist theory of rebirth affects ideas about health and sickness in several ways. Some souls are antipathetic to their mothers or fathers because of some bad relationship in a former life. In the eyes of my informants, an antipathetic soul in a child, and an incompatible horoscope between mother and child, are directly correlated. A moral conception is added to the amoral one of cosmic clash by the notion that an infant with an antipathetic soul may urinate or have a bowel movement on leaving the womb "to show contempt." I was told that in former times when this happened boys would be given away and girls "thrown on the rubbish heap." Nowadays children are born in hospitals and "it is difficult to know of such things." Some souls are so resentful they go on being born in the bodies of successive children in a family, only to die soon after birth. This is a *lóh-kwái tsái*, "child drawing after it spirits of the dead." Traditionally, it was said, mothers would beat the corpses of children in anger at them for dying for this reason.

Buddhism also contributes to the theory of homeostasis. Souls, whatever their previous connections, do not take kindly to birth, and the mongolian spot (*tache mongoloid*) on the infant's lower back was said to be the mark where a reluctant soul was kicked into new life by the authorities of the Buddhist underworld. Any disturbance in the family or immediate environment, any aggressive activity on the part of the mother or a demon, and it might depart, or the whole constitution may become disbalanced. This syndrome is known as "injury by fright" (Topley 1970).

We have then two major subsystems. One is amoral and matter of fact. It includes quasi-science, both literal (medical) and nonliteral (symbolic) activities, and mystical science—again, as we will see, with literal and nonliteral activities. Quasi-science deals with problems of internal balance directly, and mystical science with internal balance through external adjustments. The other subsystem is religion, which is moral and matter of principle. The specialist in literal quasi-science is the "orthodox" Chinese physician. The specialist in symbolic quasi-science is the diviner and priest, who also specialize in mystical science and in ritual acts of religion.

THE INTEGRATION OF PRACTICES

People in Hong Kong may wander in and out of these idea systems or subsystems, using different specialists and techniques for handling problems of health. Some techniques may be alternatives to each other, but many are used as complementary ways for coping with a problem from different points of view. I will give hypothetical examples of the relationships among these activities (see also Figure 3). My examples are children's problems, but part of the pattern I describe would also apply to an adult's illness.

A child becomes sick after attending a wedding feast or a funeral. The mother decides it has a medical symptom, *hot air* (*ît hei*), an imbalance of the hot and cold ethers in the body. *Hot air* is not serious in itself, but it may be regarded as an initial stage in a more serious disease. Its symptoms are a sore throat, an ulcerated tongue, and a slight temperature. It is often attributed to the patient's having eaten too much hot food. Mothers usually treat *hot air* themselves with cooling herbal teas and other brews. If they are anxious,

MYSTICAL SCIENCE

Literal-Social Act	Ritual	Literal-Mystical Science Act	Diagnosis	Symbolic Act
		Comparing horoscope with almanac	*laū-nin*	avoidance of frying food
adoption of child by another (alternative)	adoption of child by its own mother (*rite de passage*)	comparing horoscopes of mother and child	mutual incompatibility of horoscopes	-
-	child wearing jade bangle or pendant on chain	-	'injury by fright' cosmic imbalance	-

QUASI SCIENCE		RELIGION		SYMPTOM
Literal	Diagnosis	Ritual	Diagnosis	
avoidance of fried food cooling diet	'hot-air'	-	-	ulcerated tongue sore throat slight fever
-	-	*Sip T'aai-Sui* ('propping up')	non-affinity of souls	" plus irritability (mother also ailing) refusal to feed
medicine: *po-ying taan* crushed pearl powder	instability	*haam-king* — rites to lift (parent's) offence - if syndrome prolonged	soul instability or separation	crying; slight fever; irritability; convulsive jerking refusal to feed

FIGURE 3. Diagnoses of Symptous of ill health seen in terms of various etiological explanations, and showing the different classes of activity associated with these explanations.

they may also consult a traditional doctor. They may even consult a modern doctor if the child has a fever. Modern doctors remark on the frequency with which mothers bring children with common "colds" to see them.

The mother might consult a horoscope reader if she associates the *hot air* illness of her child with having attended the transitional rite. Comparing the child's horoscope with the almanac, he may find that it is indeed "out of phase" with events that year (*laū-nīn*). This means that the child is in an unbalanced relationship with the universe for one whole year, and is likely to ail. Events that are out of balance are more likely to aggravate internal imbalance during this time. Having failed to avoid this danger, the child has developed *hot air*. The external imbalance cannot be treated, since there is no technique for rebalancing weddings and funerals. If the mother consults a traditional doctor for the internal correction of her child's illness, he will usually recommend a cooling diet and no fried foods. As part of her own traditional knowledge, she will avoid frying foods in the presence of the child. This is a metonymical act—frying standing for fried foods, which are metaphysically heating substances. These are actions of literal and symbolic quasi-science.

Suppose the child continues to be sick, and becomes fractious. The mother will then consider other possibilities. Perhaps she had a difficult pregnancy. She may suspect a mutual incompatibility. Her horoscope may be compared to the child's, and her diagnosis confirmed. She may then perform an act of mystical science to neutralize the unhealthy effects of this clash. She might literally have the child adopted by another, thus directing its incompatible forces away from her; or she might become the child's adoptive mother herself, through the performance of a *rite de passage*. For this ritual the child is wrapped in a blanket and taken to the fishing people whose homes are their boats. They take the child on a journey by rowing around the harbor. It is brought back in a new status position, this ritual adoption similarly neutralizing the cosmic incompatibility revealed by the horoscopes.

In addition, the mother may use quasi-science by continuing to consult practitioners of Chinese medicine for remedies for particular symptoms, or she might consult a modern doctor for "quicker results," as it was explained to me. In this case she will usually ask for an injection.

If the mother is inclined to seek a moral explanation for her child's illness, she may consult a priest who will explain it as the consequence of past lives and antipathy between souls. She might consult a Buddhist or a Taoist priest, or even a spirit medium. All of these religious specialists deal with souls and the problems of rebirth. As a consequence of these consultations, the mother may perform a religious ritual. A God called *T'aaì-Sui* is believed to control time. Since he is the "Minister of Time" who decides when one is to be reborn, he determines one's horoscope. Because he makes his decision on the basis of performances in other lives, the cosmic processes at the time of birth and the karmic processes—that is to say, Chinese cosmology and

Buddhist cosmology—are unified. The rite which might be performed is called *sìp T'aaì-Suì* (propping up *T'aaì-Suì*). His image is raised by placing a large wad of mock money under it.

I will give a final example. If a child cries and jerks convulsively, particularly during sleep, has a slight temperature, is irritable, and refuses to eat or to be left alone, a mother will suspect that it is suffering from *haàk-ts'an* (*injury by fright*). This illness is caused by an imbalance among the animating forces, including the Buddhist soul. In severe cases these forces may be separated from the body. The mother might consult a modern doctor for a sedative to "restore balance" and medicines to treat the accompanying fever. She might alternatively, or additionally, take it to a Chinese doctor for some rebalancing medicine. Or she may purchase a medicine herself from a Chinese chemist shop without any consultation. The most common remedies in Hong Kong are crushed pearl powder and "protect infant pills" (*pó-ying taan*). The mother may also give the child a jade bangle or pendant on a chain to wear, since jade is regarded as a perfectly balanced stone. These objects are believed to "incorporate" the constitution or lock in the animating forces, but their potency is questioned by orthodox practitioners of Chinese medicine.

The mother might perform a ritual called a *haàm-king*, "calling out against fear," particularly if she suspects the animating forces have left the body. Notions of immorality and symbols for dealing with it are involved. It is immoral of the soul to wish to leave the body of the child, and it may be reprimanded. Leaving may cause the child's death. The soul will be told to come back and "obey people's instructions," and the Jade Emperor may be evoked to aid in this task. He is the head of the Chinese pantheon and the ultimate religious symbol of cosmic harmony.

The soul and other animating forces may have been disturbed by a demon, or one of the "improper" creatures referred to. Or one of these demons or creatures may have taken advantage of the situation to make away with the soul, or to take its place in the child's body. *Haàm-king* rites to expel these malevolent spirits may be performed by Taoist priests, by female ritual experts, or by the mother or another female member of the family. They generally take place at an altar to the White Tiger, Cock God, and Stone Dog God, who protect people from immoral disturbances.

If these rituals are not successful, additional consultations may be necessary to discover other causes of the fright. Perhaps the soul does not want to return because of some misdemeanor on the part of one or both of the parents. If further complications are diagnosed by a priest, additional rites are necessary: propitiations of *T'aaì Suì* again, or rites to lift the offense of the parents. I have discussed *haàk-ts'an* in detail in another paper (1970), but we can see from this brief account that many causes of the condition may be uncovered, and treatments used. Some of the treatments are quasi-science, some are mystical science, and some are religious in the sense that they seek to fix moral responsibility for the illness.

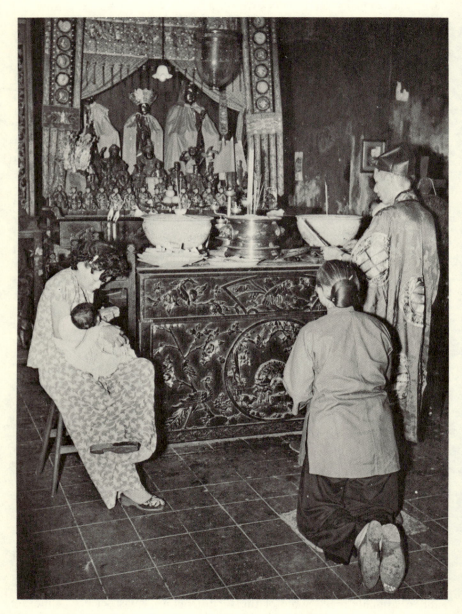

PLATE 1. Taoist priest performing a ritual to cure a sick infant, with the mother and paternal grandmother in attendance.

We have then an etiology of disease related to a theory of internal and external balance. Its core is the Chinese theory of *yin*, *yang*, and the Five Elements. Buddhism, incorporated into this etiology, explains why children might die prematurely or be sick, and helps explain difficulties in maintaining homeostasis. It relates the individual to one law of nature, while Chinese cosmology relates him to the Will of Heaven. Buddhism introduces moral attitudes toward sickness in the concept of *lōh-kwái*, "children drawing spirits of the dead," and in the concept of souls reluctant to assume a relationship with a parent who has "behaved badly." In contrast, the Chinese theory of balance and imbalance provides a view of sickness as an amoral, matter-of-fact event. This allows for therapy that does not consider morality. Such activities are notably restrained. They do not deal with the anger a mother may feel when a child dies, or is sick, or the frustration and guilt she feels when she fails to get on with her child. No blame is defined by these therapeutic activities. They dramatize no benevolence or forgiveness, and evoke little moral and emotional catharsis.

However, nature humanized by values and symbolized by gods and demons provides a moral explanation of sickness. In the amoral universe, people maintain stability by avoiding incompatible relationships, and therapy corrects instability by acts of quasi-science and mystical science. In the moral universe, sickness is caused by immoral changes in man and nature, and ritual therapy propitiates the gods, or treats demons and souls in a hortatory manner. These rites deal with anger, frustration, and guilt; they define responsibilities, appeal to benevolent forces, and seek forgiveness; and they provide a degree of catharsis. In Figure 3 I plot the activities I have described so far in a diagram.

PATIENTS AND SPECIALISTS

Patients

To what extent do people explain health problems in moral ways, seeking to blame themselves or someone else for illness, and to use emotional non-sacramental rites for therapy? And to what extent do they look for amoral explanations? The people I talked to said that they were prepared to consider all possibilities, although some said they usually went first to a doctor while others went first to a diviner or priest.

Clearly such decisions depend on economic and other social circumstances, and on individual temperament. The situation is complicated by the fact that modern and traditional medical knowledge may come from advertisements in newspapers and magazines, or on radio and television programs. Television has a half-hour program each morning with a practitioner of traditional Chinese medicine.

I found many mothers in my sample were using modern medicines in response to advertising, and sometimes for categories of illness peculiar to

Chinese culture. Several modern patent medicines are advertised in Hong Kong as cures for conditions such as *hot air*, or as having traditional properties such as *nourishing the blood (pó-huèt)*. Education fosters the development of modern attitudes toward health, and many of my informants were aware of modern methods of treating children's complaints. They had learned about them in the hospitals where they gave birth, in the clinics they attended with their infants, from their older children who were more modern in outlook than themselves, and, occasionally, through being urged by their husbands to seek advice from a modern specialist. But what Yap (1969) called a *culture-bound syndrome*, or, in the present volume Obeyesekere calls *cultural disease*, was important in the health concepts of these women. The reality of the two I have discussed, "mutual incompatibility" and "injury by fright," is often confirmed by kinsmen and neighbors. Though they were exposed to modern knowledge, they expressed a very strong feeling that old people know about children's complaints, and they indicated willingness to take advice from them.

While the mothers recognized the association of symptoms in culture-bound illnesses, their major concern in scientifically recognized diseases was often with single symptoms. When I asked them to list common childhood diseases, four listed chickenpox, two listed mumps, but all listed high temperature and sore throat (which are also *hot air* symptoms), diarrhea, and runny nose. For high temperature, diarrhea, and runny nose, they went to either modern or Chinese doctors. Members of a family often consult different modern and traditional doctors, on the ground that one doctor suits one member and one another. In addition, an ill person may consult several cures. Of the 20 mothers interviewed, 12 claimed to consult more than one doctor in the modern or traditional field, and one regularly consulted as many as 8 modern doctors.

The division between medical and ritual specialists is sometimes difficult to draw, and so is the distinction between doctor and patient. Many families claim to be specialists in the cure of certain diseases, particularly those of childhood. The more educated families own prescription books passed down over the generations, which are only available to family members and friends. A recent movement in China has been to persuade families to give up their secrets to the *barefoot doctors* who now practice at the village or commune level. These family traditions are partly a heritage from the distribution of doctors in the homeland. And here is another territorial factor influencing choice of specialist: Most doctors practiced in towns. At the village level people often had to be content with the medical-*cum*-ritual services of priests and other religious specialists, or develop their own family expertise. Anthropologists working in Hong Kong's rural areas have also observed that people make much use of ritual specialists (Potter 1974). This may be partly due to "faith"; but again, one should note the rarity of doctors of either modern or traditional medicine in the villages.

Ordinary people in urban Hong Kong know the names and properties of many medicines and have considerable knowledge of therapeutic practices and rituals of cure. I recorded the contents of the medicine chests (usually a tin or cardboard box) of the women I interviewed, and they had four kinds of items. The first was traditional drugs. Only 4 mothers had none of these, and one said she lived near a chemist and could buy them at any time. The most common was *pó-ying taan*, "protect infant pills" used for "injury by fright." One mother had crushed pearl powder, which is used for the same malady. Other common traditional medicines were for diarrhea and vomiting, and medications for boils or other skin complaints. The second category of items in the medicine chests one might call modern traditional medications. It includes oils and ointments for skin trouble, stomachache, headache, and toothache. Many of these preparations are produced by a Burmese Chinese whose medicines are popular throughout Southeast Asia. All but two mothers had at least one of these. The third category was modern medicine, including penicillin ointment, iodine, and other preparations for wounds, aspirins, and cold cures; 14 mothers had at least one of these.

Finally, 6 mothers had an interesting intermediary category of drug: traditional substances packaged to look like modern medicine, with the formula printed on the outside like a modern drug, or a modern drug named and packaged like a traditional medicine. Numerous modernized traditional medicines produced in China are sold in Hong Kong, including herbal remedies now manufactured in pill form. This makes them more convenient than traditional medicines, which are usually brewed for several hours; but traditional doctors in Hong Kong claim that their efficacy is reduced by the preservatives which are added. Other modernized traditional medicines and traditionalized modern medicines are made in Singapore, Korea, Japan, and Taiwan. Many of them are panaceas.

Formal and Informal Ritual-cum-Medical Specialists
Between the ordinary housewife and formal specialist is the female ritual expert who often knows a lot about herbs. These experts are usually widowed or unmarried, and take up their specialty as they get older. They perform rites for payment, and their performances include not only rites of sickness, but those connected with misfortunes and with death. Thus, they cut across the system, providing a degree of continuity. This is also true of Taoist priests, and occasionally of Buddhist priests, though the latter specialize more in rites of repentance and placation. Priests may play several curing roles, performing acts of mystical science, administering herbs of quasi-science, and performing religious rites.

One kind of specialist is often both priest and doctor. This is the high-ranking member of one of the flourishing syncretic sects of Hong Kong. These sects, often politically militant in nineteenth-century China, claim to combine the ethics of Confucianism, the hygiene and meditation of Taoism, and the prayers and self-cultivation of the Buddhist monk. Today in Hong Kong they are often concerned with charity and care of the aged (Topley 1963). Those who reach the top levels of administration are often traditional scholars, and some have studied Chinese medicine seriously under masters.

Formal Medical Specialists

The traditional doctor may be a general herbal practitioner or a specialist in acupuncture or bone-setting. He is often attached to a Chinese chemist shop, and may be the proprietor. But some doctors are well-known throughout Hong Kong. They have their own consulting rooms hung with mirrors upon which messages have been written by grateful patients. Some doctors have two practices: one where they see patients without charge, and another in which patients pay high fees. Even so, it is said that their paying patients outnumber their charity patients, and a successful traditional doctor may earn HK$18,000 per month if he has a medicine shop attached to his practice.

Many doctors were trained by their fathers or by masters to whom they were apprenticed, but a movement is emerging in Hong Kong to train traditional doctors in schools. Little is yet known about these schools, but more than 20 of them existed in 1966 (Choa 1967). A few only taught acupuncture, and several claimed to be postgraduate institutes.

The calendar of one school stated that it offered a two-year course, and that anybody over 18 who had attended senior middle school could enroll. The fee was HK$240 in 1966, plus $60 for notes and another $60 for accommodations. Classes were held from 8 to 10 P.M., which indicates that the students worked in other occupations during the day. Every summer the school ran free clinics where practical clinical instruction was given. Apparently this was the only way that students received clinical instruction.

The post-graduate "institutes" offer one-year courses in various specialties. The fees are about the same as those for undergraduate courses. Anyone who has completed undergraduate studies, or practiced traditional medicine for three years, is eligible to enroll.

In 1971 I visited an acupuncture night school in an office suite in Kowloon, and met a group of students. Some of them were physiotherapy students during the day at a nearby government hospital, and they intended to combine physiotherapy with knowledge of acupuncture. Others intended to use their knowledge within their families. Several were office workers, who noted the convenience of part-time study and said that they would take up practice when they retired from their present occupations. They regarded medicine as a profession that would increase the security of old age. These students believed that Chinese medicine would continue in popularity in Hong Kong. A herbalist student I met elsewhere explained that modern medicine was good for critical conditions, but that traditional medicine was essential to strengthen the constitution of people who were subject to frequent illness. He maintained that modern medicine was often debilitating, and one needed

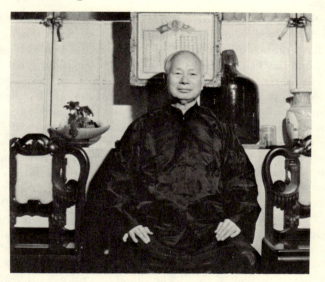

PLATE 2. Portrait of a Chinese bone-setter, with his certificate to practice issued by the government in Taiwan in the back-ground.

to follow its use with revitalizing medicine from a traditional practitioner. He explained the tendency for northerners to go to northern doctors and southerners to those from the south by differences in body types and in the regional use of herbs.

A pharmacist may sometimes fill almost the role of a doctor, recommending prescriptions as well as filling them, and even having his own private remedies. The training of a pharmacist or dispenser is by apprenticeship and takes many years. For three years he works as cook and cleaner in a medicine shop, also drying herbs. He learns to prepare herbal prescriptions for another two or three years, meanwhile looking after the bottles, boxes, and storage areas. He then becomes a counter-helper. During these occupational grades he earns no more, usually, than $400 a month. By the time he reaches the next status, that of counter-server and pharmacist, he may be middle-aged. By then he is supposed to know all the properties of medicines, and be able to dispense prescriptions with speed. Dispensing a prescription is highly skilled work: the pharmacist's hands move rapidly, opening and shutting the many drawers in the cabinet where the ingredients are stored and a mistake could be serious. Yet he earns only $500–$600 a month for this skilled performance.

Because the Chinese medical profession has not been subject to governmental control, many newcomers have set up as doctors, particularly since the war. They include not only traditional pharmacists seeking a better reward for their years of training, but others with no training at all. Properly trained practitioners often criticize the lack of supervision. More recently, a concern for status has caused them to break away from other associations which include doctors with dubious qualifications, and organize their own. Several have branch offices, along with elected and honorary sections—for example, one has 14 permanent honorary advisors and a great many other positions for various departments and committees. In this, of course, they follow a typical pattern for overseas Chinese associations. Unlike the medical profession itself, the use of medicants and the treatment of certain diseases has been subject to increasing restrictions. Sometimes the more orthodox associations cooperate with those of the unqualified doctors, as well as with dealers and sellers of medical herbs, to protest the new restrictions. This has happened several times during the last decade. Two examples will illustrate their methods.

One protest took place in 1958 over restrictions on the treatment of eye diseases. Representatives from ten associations of traditional practitioners and of medicine-shop owners sent a delegation to the Secretary of Chinese Affairs. The Secretary pointed out that the restriction was introduced to control untrained doctors, and not to "wipe out Chinese medicine." The effect would be felt, nevertheless, by all traditional practitioners. The doctors tried to mobilize public support through press conferences and talks to trade unions, clansman's associations, and other groups. But it could not be disputed that blindness was caused by unqualified persons who called themselves traditional doctors, and nothing came of these protests. However, an outcome of this effort was a loose federation of medical associations, and the date of the protest was annually celebrated as the "integration festival" for Chinese doctors in Hong Kong.

Another issue arose in 1960 concerning a Chinese medicant containing arsenic pentasulphide. This medicant, called *hung-wong*, is put on children's heads at the Dragon Boat festival, when epidemics caused by seasonal disbalance and demons are likely to occur. And it is used on many other occasions. It is not generally absorbed, but when breathed down the throat it may be transformed into white arsenic, which can be lethal. Following deaths from its usage, the government proposed to ban *hung-wong*. The association got together and composed a letter on the long and proud history of *hung-wong*, and again met with the Secretary for Chinese Affairs. As a result of their protest, and because the medication was only dangerous if used in a particular way, *hung-wong* was not made illegal.

Qualified Chinese doctors are anxious to have their associations recognized as legitimate bodies for setting legally enforced standards. The constitution of one association gives its aims as "concern with integrating Chinese doctors, research into Chinese medicine, improving the efficacy of Chinese medicine, helping the poor, helping to maintain public health and sanitation, and working for the betterment of the members' welfare." Although the associations are divided by the medical qualifications and ethnic differences of their members, many are registered with the Overseas Chinese Commission of the Nationalist Government in Taiwan and claim official recognition from that body. As a result, most traditional doctors in Hong Kong are rightist in sympathy.

It is generally recognized that without official enforcement of standards, and official definition of status of *bona fide* doctors, malpractice and misuse of herbs and other medical substances will continue. For this reason, some Chinese practitioners of modern medicine support the traditional doctors' desire for an official association similar to their own British Medical Association and the Hong Kong Medical Association. These modern doctors believe that traditional medicine has an important role in the Colony's medical system, even though some treatments are dangerous.

Among the traditional medical treatments modern physicians consider to be dangerous is the ritual of measles. The Chinese have traditionally believed that everyone must have measles, and that it is necessary for future health. It is therefore treated as a transition from one equilibrium of the body to another, and the occasion for a *rite de passage*. I have described measles rituals elsewhere (1970). The point is that the mortality rate has been high, in part because of the way it is treated in traditional Chinese health culture. Some of the herbal treatments administered by traditional doctors are also considered harmful by physicians of modern medicine. One of these is called *ch'uen-lin*. Mothers who follow traditional medical ideas avoid cooling foods during pregnancy. But this is believed to cause the baby to be born hot. *Ch'uen-lin* is given to cool the infant, but its use seems to cause jaundice.

Modern doctors who urge traditional physicians to press for governmental recognition may be influenced by the favor shown to Chinese medicine on the mainland. However, I find that traditional doctors are often cynical about mainland policy. Many modern doctors, whatever their convictions, recognize the placebo effect of traditional consultations, and in some cases also the use of ritual in treating traditionally-minded patients. Some feel that a course in Chinese medicine should be taught at the University medical school, so that modern doctors will understand their patient's conceptions and the supplementary therapy they are inclined to use.

A former leading psychiatrist in Hong Kong was convinced that it is essential to understand traditional views of illness to deal with mental disturbances involving notions of spirit possession, or anxieties about physiological changes such as *kuro*, penis shrinking. He pointed out that culture-bound syndromes cause very real problems of clinical practice and should be subjects for extended cross-cultural epidemiological research (Yap 1969:219). It is fallacious to think, as some people apparently do, that culture-bound syndromes are rare (Yap 1969:223). In this essay I have shown that "injury by fright" and the metaphysical notion of mutual incompatibility of mother and child were taken quite seriously by my informants.

CONCLUSION

I have suggested that a process of conceptual differentiation in medical thinking started in early times in China and continues in present-day Hong Kong. Different contemporary approaches and methods of cure may centuries ago have formed a unitary system. I distinguished quasi-science, which deals with internal cure, from mystical science, where internal imbalance is related to external cure. And I have distinguished these categories from religion. While these distinctions suggest processes of specialization, the actual situation is ambiguous. Patients use different methods of cure in complementary and supplementary fashion, and specialists themselves do not adhere to a single specialty.

Hong Kong is undergoing rapid change, and large numbers of young people have received a modern education and pay little attention to Chinese customs. A superficial glimpse may incline the visitor to believe that Hong Kong is a thoroughly cosmopolitan city. But at festival times the entire pattern of life is rearranged to expose its Chinese nature. We have come a long way from the belief that science, rationalism, and empiricism would drive out "superstitions." When the pressures of urban life and new ways place intolerable burdens on individuals, they seek comfort in practices and ideas that are centuries old.

Literature Cited

Anderson, E. N., Jr., and Marja L. Anderson
  1968 "Folk Medicine in Rural Hong Kong." *Etnoiatria* 2: 22–28.
Choa, Gerald
  1967 "Chinese Traditional Medicine and Contemporary Hong Kong," in Marjorie Topley, ed., *Some Traditional Ideas and Conceptions in Hong Kong Social Life Today*. Hong Kong: Royal Asiatic Society, Hong Kong Branch.
Eberhard, Wolfram
  1967 *Guilt and Sin in Traditional China*. Berkeley and Los Angeles: University of California Press.
Freedman, Maurice
  1967 *Rites and Duties, or Chinese Marriage*. London: Bell.
  1968 "Geomancy." *Proceedings of the Royal Anthropological Institute of Great Britain and Ireland*, pp. 5–15.
  1970 "Ritual Aspects of Chinese Kinship and Marriage," in Maurice Freedman, ed., *Family and Kinship in Chinese Society*, pp. 163–187. Stanford: Stanford University Press.
Hon Ch'in-wen
  1970 "Mao Tse-Tung Thought Lights Up the Way for Advance of China's Medical Science," trans. in *Selections from Mainland Magazines*, nos. 675–755: 49–63. Hong Kong: American Consulate General.
Lévi-Strauss, Claude
  1962 *The Savage Mind (La Pensée Sauvage)*. London: Wiedenfeld and Nicolson.

Meyer, B. F., and T. F. Wempe
  1947 *The Student's Cantonese English Dictionary*. New York: Field Afar Press.
Needham, Joseph
  1969 *The Grand Titration: Science and Society in East and West*. London: George Allen and Unwin.
  1970 "Medicine and Culture," in *Clerks and Craftsmen in China and the West: Lectures and Addresses on the History of Science and Technology*, pp. 263–293. Cambridge, England: Cambridge University Press.
Potter, Jack
  1974 "Cantonese Shamanism," in Arthur P. Wolf, ed., *Religion and Ritual in Chinese Society*, pp. 207–231. Stanford: Stanford University Press.
Simpson, G. G.
  1961 *Principles of Animal Taxonomy*. New York: Columbia University Press.
Survey
  1971 "Medical Work in East China *hsien* Advances Rapidly," trans. in *Survey of China Mainland Press*, no. 5003: 114–115. Hong Kong: American Consulate General.
Topley, Marjorie
  1963 "The Great Way of Former Heaven: A Group of Chinese Secret Religious Sects." *Bull. of the School of Oriental and African Studies* 26: 362–392.
  1970 "Chinese Traditional Ideas and the Treatment of Disease: Two Example from Hong Kong." *Man* (N. S.) 5: 421–437.
  1974 "Cosmic Antagonisms: a mother-child syndrome," in Arthur P. Wolf, ed., *Religion and Ritual in Chinese Society*, pp. 233–244. Stanford: Stanford University press.
Welch, Holmes
  1957 *The Parting of the Way: Lao Tzu and the Taoist Movement*. Boston: Beacon Press.
Yap, P. M.
  1969 "Classification of the Culture-Bound Reactive Syndromes." *Far East Medical Journal* 7: 219–225.

PART V

The Ecology of Indigenous
and Cosmopolitan Medical Practice

T he essays in this and the preceding section all deal in one way or another with the question: How are different medical traditions related to each other in contemporary Asian societies? The authors in the preceding section were primarily concerned with explicating the views of participants in those societies, translating their categories and habits of mind so that others will understand them. In contrast, the authors in this section interpret their data to emphasize their own categories and goals. Thus, the essays in Part IV described different medical systems from emic, or inside, perspectives, while those in the present section describe them from etic, or outside, perspectives.

In the first essay, Edward Montgomery sets out to use "a rigorous concept of system" in defining variables for comparative research on medical practice. The variables that he proposes are the rates of changes in the populations of practitioners and patients, the rate of consultations, and the set of medications accessible for prescription. He may seem to propose a simple push-pull equilibrium model when, for example, he reasons that "a high rate of change in the practitioner population" could be "a response to the collective consultation rate's having exceeded the limits which maintain system stability"; yet this interpretation would misconstrue his argument, for his variables summarize complex phenomena. He conceives of them as composite scales of numerous observations. Thus, he includes in the rate of change in the patient population items such as changes in concepts of disease and in "awareness of the availability of treatment," along with the incidence of illnesses and differential access to care. In the rate of change in the practitioner population, he includes changes in the numbers and proportions of physicians according to sex, age, birthplace, education, religion, caste, language, and so on. The fee-for-service solo practitioners he interviewed in the city of Vellore were trained in Āyurveda, Siddha, Yunānī, homeopathy, and cosmopolitan medicine, but in practice two-thirds of them reported that they mixed these traditions. Thus, Montgomery's data and ideas challenge new researchers to employ a set of complex parameters for describing the structure of practice in pluralistic medical systems.

Recommending that cosmopolitan medical specialists accommodate to medical pluralism, the sociologist Anselm Strauss wrote:

Especially I would emphasize that plural systems of medical belief and practice exist in all countries, and at every class level; hence the conclusion that health officials and personnel everywhere would do well to come more directly—and imaginatively—to grips with the problem of meshing their own systems of medical care with the plural medical observations and life-styles of all segments of their populations. (quoted by Weidman and Egeland 1973:846)

The great difficulty in following this kind of advice is that pluralism favors the autonomy of laymen to diagnose their own health problems and decide which specialists they should consult. Paul Unschuld emphasizes this point in the following pages, where he describes the dual system of Chinese and cosmopolitan medicine in Taiwan; and essays in the preceding pages showed how ideas alien to cosmopolitan medicine often guide laymen in making these decisions. Specialists in cosmopolitan medicine draw upon the authority of modern science to claim knowledge beyond the comprehension of laymen, and superior to that of all other practitioners. Their professional demand is that these practitioners and laymen should delegate to them the right to diagnose all health problems, giving doctors and paramedical workers under their control exclusive authority to define medical situations, and on the basis of these definitions to direct proper courses of action. Health officials committed to professional cosmopolitan medicine are not likely to surrender this demand to the exigencies of medical pluralism.

Another difficulty of medical pluralism for health officials is that the high status of cosmopolitan medicine causes specialists who have not been trained in this system to borrow from it. One might think that this is a good thing, and feel a surge of approval for Man Aher, the folk doctor in Sumatra, when Jaspen describes his open-minded empiricism and desire to learn from patients who had consulted cosmopolitan physicians how they had been treated. Evidently Man Aher had borrowed little, though Jaspen says that he and other members of the community knew that some illnesses were caused by viruses. In contrast, the physicians in Vellore, the Punjab, and Taiwan, whose practices are described in essays in the present section, have considerable access to medications and knowledge developed in cosmopolitan medicine, though they may have little or no formal training in this system. Carl Taylor shows that indigenous medical practitioners in the Punjab borrow a great deal, and Paul Unschuld reports that many practitioners of Chinese medicine in Taiwan advocate combining diagnostic techniques from cosmopolitan medicine with traditional therapy. According to Unschuld, this program is "largely impossible" because "no terminological bridges . . . connect the system of modern medical diagnosis to the Chinese conceptions of therapy." On the same grounds, critics have objected to similar proposals by Āyurvedic and Yunani physicians in Sri Lanka, Pakistan, and India.

Finally, an important aspect of pluralism for health officials, one that anthropologists and sociologists should study, is the practice of "pharmaceutical medicine." Indigenous and cosmopolitan medicines are manufactured by private companies on a large scale in many Asian countries. Marjorie Topley described the variety of these preparations in the medicine chests of women she interviewed in Hong Kong in her essay in the preceding section, and in the following pages Carl Taylor and Paul Unschuld discuss their dissemination in Taiwan and the Punjab. Taylor writes that some practitioners of indigenous medicine whom his research team observed are part of "an underground system of health care that provides the bulk of medical treatment for the people in India."

The system Taylor describes is not peculiarly Indian, nor are its practitioners limited to physicians registered as indigenous medical practitioners. It evolved in Europe during the seventeenth and eighteenth centuries with the commercial manufacture of medicines, many of them "galenicals," and it spread around the world in the nineteenth century, when patented and widely advertised medicines made many "toadstool millionaires" (Young 1961). The system thrives today wherever fee-for-service practitioners and the capitalistic system of drug manufacture encourage entreprenuerial medical practice. The underground sector of the system may violate laws regulating the prescription and sale of modern drugs, but where those laws are not enforced it is only nominally "underground." It is, in fact, part of the normative system of many Asian and Western societies. Paul Unschuld criticizes "the commercialization of health" and the massive use of chemotherapy in this system, referring to licensed practice in Taiwan and Germany. Among other Western countries, he might add the United States to this list (Muller 1972). Carl Taylor's sketch of commercial pharmaceutical medicine in India indicates the need for new research on this system and on its relationship to other forms of practice.

CHARLES LESLIE

Literature Cited

Muller, Charlotte
    1972 "The Overmedicated Society: Forces in the Marketplace of Medical Care." *Science* 176 (May 5): 488–492.
Weidman, Hazel Hitson, and Janice A. Egeland
    1973 "A Behavioral Science Perspective in the Comparative Approach to the Delivery of Health Care." *Social Science and Medicine* 7, (11): 845–860.
Young, James Harvey
    1961 *The Toadstool Millionaires: A Social History of Patent Medicines in America Before Federal Regulation.* Princeton: Princeton University Press.

Systems and the Medical
Practitioners of a Tamil Town

EDWARD MONTGOMERY

Generic concepts of medical systems are a focal point of the present volume. Comparative studies will largely depend upon specifying the systemic nature of medical traditions and practices. I will use one way of conceiving the medical system to discuss a study of medical practitioners in southern India, and must begin by explaining my concept of *system*. The term can be applied to diverse phenomena. Certain usages facilitate operational specificity in analyzing the static, dynamic, regulated, homeostatic, or hieratic properties of systems. If the logical relationships of a rigorously defined system are adequately explicated, the values of some of the system's variables may be deduced from information about the values of other variables (see Rapoport 1970). A central task of my essay is to utilize a rigorous concept of system with reference to the practice of medicine in India.

SYSTEMS AND MEDICINE IN INDIA

Among the ways in which the system concept can be used to discuss medicine and medical practice in India, two emphases deserve mention. First, by emphasizing the organizational and ecological aspects of medical practice, one can speak of a medical system or health-care system which deals with illness and disease in a population or community. Within India, the diversity of medical practice indicates the utility of speaking of not one, but several, medical systems (Alexander and Shivaswamy 1971; Leslie 1967; Singh et al. 1962). The notion of a single system may only be appropriate for analyzing practices in limited sectors of local populations. The various medical systems of India seem to manifest different organizational and ecological features, in that their practitioners may be consulted for different diseases or by different sectors of the population (Madan 1969; Singh et al 1962; Lozoff, Kamath, and Feldman, in press). Second, to emphasize the cultural, ideological, national, and ethnic aspects of medical practice, the medical traditions of India can be considered systems. Thus, common speech refers to the Hindu and Muslim traditions of Ayurveda, Siddha, and Unani medicine as "indigenous medical systems." This usage identifies these traditions in contrast to the "allopathic" or "modern" system of medicine.

Two problems that these or any other concepts of the medical system raise are: How can the boundaries of the system be determined? How can changes in the system be analyzed? Recent research in India magnifies these questions. For example, transformations in the organization and ideology of the Indian medical systems have been occurring over the past two centuries (Leslie 1968, 1969). Medical practitioners who claim to preserve the classical textual traditions have innovated changes that can be described as processes of professionalization, politicization, and alienation.

In order to investigate at least some of the theoretically significant aspects of changes in Indian medicine in greater detail, we need a precise definition of system. Paul W. Collins has demonstrated that a logically sound explanation can be given for the ways that cultural variables or traits work within a functional system. His analysis has focused new research on the operation of variables as an independent endeavor from attempting to explain the origin, presence, or necessary conditions of these variables (see Collins 1965, 1969; Collins and Vayda 1969).

The definition appropriate to this task is that *a system is a set of variables having ranges of values or states with specified limits,* and these variables are interrelated in such a manner that, if one is displaced from the specified range, one or more of the other variables will change to permit the return of the displaced variable to within the limits. The variables comprising such a system may be from the cultural, social, biological, or environmental domains. The strengths of this definition are that it makes it incumbent upon the investigator to specify the range of system-maintaining values or states for any variable, and it effectively tests the systemic qualities of variables by requiring that changes in one variable be related to changes in another.

I will organize data from a recent study in southern India, using this framework to illustrate the questions which should be asked and the observations which need to be made if the practitioners and practice of medicine are to be discussed in a precise manner. While the data do not prove system dynamics, they do yield interesting tentative generalizations concerning system variables. Since the data are new, I will provide descriptive material before analyzing the systemic aspects.

THE STUDY

I studied medical practitioners in Vellore, Tamil Nadu, in 1968 and 1969, as part of a broader study of sociocultural and ecological aspects of disease and treatment.[1] My interest in studying the medical practitioners developed

1 Field work in North Arcot District extended from December 1967 to May 1970. Financial support of the study, under the sponsorship of Dr. Alexander Alland, by the National Institute of Mental Health (Research Grant No. MH-13811–01) and by the Department of Anthropology, Columbia University, is gratefully acknowledged.

after recognizing their considerable importance as treatment sources for villagers in the surrounding rural settlements, as well as for townsfolk. After surveying the different sources of medical treatment in and about Vellore, I organized part of my research to investigate the conspicuously large number of medical practitioners in private practice. Numerous other medical specialists in Vellore are also significant as sources of treatment, but will not be considered here. They include the doctors and staff of the Christian Medical College Hospital and the Government Hospital in Vellore, local trance curers and exorcists, and various sidewalk and village herbalists.

A total of 77 private medical practitioners cooperated in the research, and 11 others have been left out of the study: I was unable to contact 3 of these practitioners, 6 were co-resident relatives in families of practitioners already studied, and 2 preferred to remain outside the study. In the course of the research I found that 29 other practitioners who were listed on a government register compiled about three years earlier had apparently left Vellore. Some of these may have only listed their parents' address for the purpose of registering to practice, but others were reported to have definitely moved to another location.

The setting within which these physicians practice has been described in recent biostatistical and morbidity studies in the Vellore municipality (Christian Medical College 1968; Feldman, et al. 1969). The town is about 135 kilometers west of Madras city. It has long been a regional administrative center, and now serves as a hub for North Arcot District, particularly for agricultural marketing. A census by the Christian Medical College (1968) showed that Vellore had grown from about 50,000 people in 1921 to about 127,000 in 1965. In-migrations are important, since about 15 percent of the 1965–66 population had been resident within the municipality less than ten years. About 75 percent of the population is Hindu, 20 percent is Muslim, and 5 percent is Christian. Located in the northern part of Tamil Nadu, only 69 percent of the Vellore families speak Tamil at home, while 14 percent speak Telugu and 15 percent speak Urdu.

Although such statistics on Vellore are relatively good, and the patterns of disease are unusually well-documented, it is difficult to estimate the number of persons who may require medical treatment—for, in addition to the continual influx of villagers, local concepts of illness cause families to avoid medical treatment for diseases like smallpox, chickenpox, and mumps, and to quarantine and care for the affected individuals within their households; other illnesses, such as some childhood diarrheal episodes, may be treated in the home or at temples by chanting (Lozoff, Kamath, and Feldman, in press).

The 77 private practitioners I studied were contacted by mail or an initial visit to their homes or places of practice. I gave them a statement of the purposes and asked for an interview appointment. In the interview I asked about their background and training, the nature of their current practice, relationships to other practitioners, satisfactions in medical practice, and their future plans. Since there was one issue which I learned was sensitive, I assured them that as a foreign researcher I had absolutely no interest in learning about secret medicines or herbs. The interviews were conducted in English or Tamil, and were done by me or by two experienced co-researchers.[2] An average interview took about an hour. The size, furnishings, arrangement, and locations of the places of practice were separately recorded. Further details were gained by informal visits to the homes and clinics of some of the practitioners, and tape-recorded biographical interviews were conducted with 10 of them.

DESCRIPTIVE DATA

My argument is that certain points of similarity in medical practice systematically unite these practitioners in Vellore, even though there are many specific characteristics which can be used to identify contrasts within the group. By "medical practice" I mean regularly receiving and responding to patients seeking medical aid. By this broad definition, only one of the 77 private practitioners was not practicing daily, and hence he has not been included in the following discussion. Apparent diversity within the group can be seen in terms of background, education, and training: They belonged to at least 22 castes (*jātis*), and spoke 6 different "mother tongues"; there were 72 men and 4 women; 9 were Muslim, 7 were Christian, and 56 were Hindu; 51 were born in Vellore, 19 were born elsewhere in Tamil Nadu and 6 had migrated from other states.

The formal educational backgrounds ranged from fifth-standard (the fifth elementary year) schooling to postgraduate training in an American medical school. Only slightly more than half of these physicians had completed high school. Their ages ranged from 26 to 68, with the average age about 45. Years of practice ranged from 1 to 48 years, with the average about 13 years. Of these 76 practitioners, 56 engaged in full-time practice, whereas 8 of them had another secondary occupation; 12 were predominantly involved in other work but practiced some medicine every day. The occupations that supplemented part-time medical practice included selling drugs in a chemist's shop, managing a pharmacy, teaching high school, selling life insurance, driving a taxi, managing agricultural lands, and serving as a social worker in a children's home.

The most interesting variation among these practitioners was in their modes of training. A few of them reminisced about family legacies of generations of hereditary medical practice, and about successful careers based upon secret medicinal preparations—29 had fathers who practiced one of the indigenous traditions: 8 Ayurveda, 13 Siddha, and 8 Unani. Of these, 28

2 An expression of my appreciation for their outstanding efforts is due to T. Vasanth Kumar and Joseph Jeyaraj Walser. Special thanks must also be given to P. S. Sunder Rao for his many contributions to the planning and data analyses for the study.

recalled a period of filial apprenticeship, but only 13 went into medical practice with just that background; 8 had attended a college of indigenous or integrated medicine, and 1 had attended a college of "Western" medicine, another had studied pharmacy, and 6 had taken training in homeopathy.

The majority of these physicians (47) had parents in occupations other than medical practice, including business (12), government (10), teaching (5), artisan's work (5), clerical work (4), agriculture (3), and others (1 lawyer, 1 Army man, 1 mechanic, 2 evangelists, and 3 nonhereditary practitioners). Of the practitioners with such backgrounds, 10 had received their medical training at one of the colleges of "Western" medicine which gave the L.M.P. (Licentiate Medical Practitioner) and M.B.,B.S. (Bachelor of Medicine, Bachelor of Surgery) degrees; another 5 had attended one of the colleges of indigenous or integrated medicine. Nearly 40 percent (30) of the total group had received their training from a homeopathic institute by a period of postal correspondence courses, usually about one year, followed by a briefer period of practical training, a week to a month, at the institute.

To understand the diversity of training among these physicians, I must explain the circumstances requiring and permitting the legal registration of medical practitioners. This is a subject on which my information is limited, but I hope that the brevity of my discussion will stimulate a more adequate treatment of the topic. Provision for the registration of medical practitioners in Madras dates from the enactment of the Madras Medical Registration Act in 1914. The Act established a provincial medical council to register physicians and regulate their practice. Only degree and diploma holders from certain institutions were eligible for registration. Similar enactments were made in other parts of India about the same time—the Bombay Medical Act of 1912, the Bengal Medical Act of 1914, the central government's Indian Medical Degree Act of 1916, and the United Provinces Medical Act of 1917. The British Medical Act of 1858 served as a model for these laws. Such legal manipulations were just part of the broader colonial strategy, and some of the far-reaching consequences for medical traditions in India were soon perceived. An English-language newspaper in Madras published the following story from Bombay in 1918:

The eighth session of the All-India Ayurveda and Unani Tibbi conference began today, the Hon'able Sir Fazulbhoy Curimbhoy presiding. ... Sir Fazulbhoy, in his presidential address, referred to the usefulness of the conference and said he felt sure that the Government would be ready to give a sympathetic hearing to any suggestions for the reform of the Medical Registration Act if it was properly represented to them that the measure was calculated to strike at the root of the Indian medical science. He warned them that it was not enough to move the Government for an amendment of the Act and make no effort on their part in improving the standard of education of the practitioners of indigenous systems of medicine.

In 1933 the Madras government issued rules to register practitioners of indigenous medicine. In the following years pressure groups lobbied to change these rules to extend or further limit the legal status of physicians other than those trained in modern medical schools, and to distinguish various grades of practitioners. The rules changed back and forth, and the administrative interpretation and enforcement of them varied from year to year. This

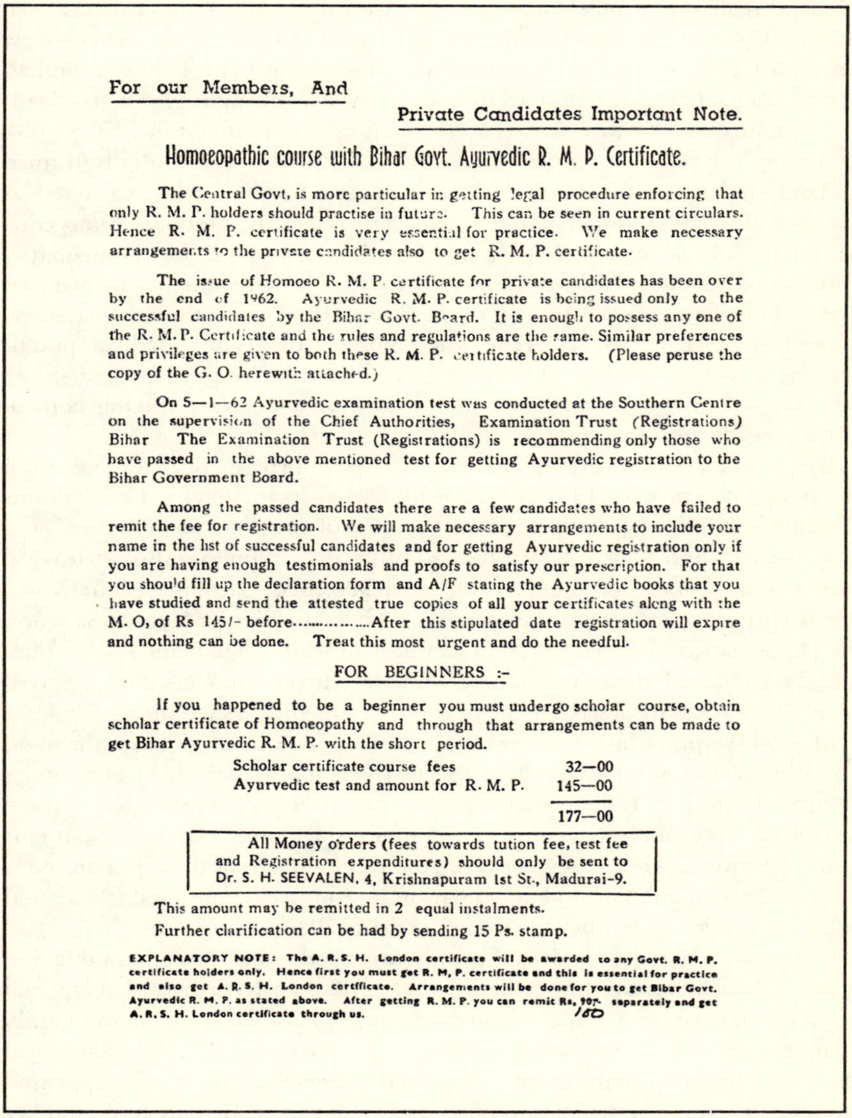

For our Members, And

Private Candidates Important Note.

Homoeopathic course with Bihar Govt. Ayurvedic R. M. P. Certificate.

The Central Govt. is more particular in getting legal procedure enforcing that only R. M. P. holders should practise in future. This can be seen in current circulars. Hence R. M. P. certificate is very essential for practice. We make necessary arrangements to the private candidates also to get R. M. P. certificate.

The issue of Homoeo R. M. P. certificate for private candidates has been over by the end of 1962. Ayurvedic R. M. P. certificate is being issued only to the successful candidates by the Bihar Govt. Board. It is enough to possess any one of the R. M. P. Certificate and the rules and regulations are the same. Similar preferences and privileges are given to both these R. M. P. certificate holders. (Please peruse the copy of the G. O. herewith attached.)

On 5—1—62 Ayurvedic examination test was conducted at the Southern Centre on the supervision of the Chief Authorities, Examination Trust (Registrations) Bihar The Examination Trust (Registrations) is recommending only those who have passed in the above mentioned test for getting Ayurvedic registration to the Bihar Government Board.

Among the passed candidates there are a few candidates who have failed to remit the fee for registration. We will make necessary arrangements to include your name in the list of successful candidates and for getting Ayurvedic registration only if you are having enough testimonials and proofs to satisfy our prescription. For that you should fill up the declaration form and A/F stating the Ayurvedic books that you have studied and send the attested true copies of all your certificates along with the M. O. of Rs 145/- before................After this stipulated date registration will expire and nothing can be done. Treat this most urgent and do the needful.

FOR BEGINNERS :-

If you happened to be a beginner you must undergo scholar course, obtain scholar certificate of Homoeopathy and through that arrangements can be made to get Bihar Ayurvedic R. M. P. with the short period.

Scholar certificate course fees	32—00
Ayurvedic test and amount for R. M. P.	145—00
	177—00

All Money orders (fees towards tution fee, test fee and Registration expenditures) should only be sent to Dr. S. H. SEEVALEN, 4, Krishnapuram Ist St., Madurai-9.

This amount may be remitted in 2 equal instalments.

Further clarification can be had by sending 15 Ps. stamp.

EXPLANATORY NOTE: The A. R. S. H. London certificate will be awarded to any Govt. R. M. P. certificate holders only. Hence first you must get R. M. P. certificate and this is essential for practice and also get A. R. S. H. London certificate. Arrangements will be done for you to get Bihar Govt. Ayurvedic R. M. P. as stated above. After getting R. M. P. you can remit Rs, 90/- separately and get A. R. S. H. London certificate through us. 150

FIGURE 1. Advertisement for a course in homeopathic medicine.

complex history has special significance here, because a large number of the practitioners in this study had received registration and training in homeopathic medicine. Apparently it has not been unusual for homeopathic institutes to assist their students to obtain legal registration. Figure 1 reprints a passage from the advertisement of a homeopathic institute advising potential students of a way to become registered under the laws of another state. Medical registration under any of the reciprocally valid state laws has been accepted and, in the case of homeopathy trainees in Tamil Nadu, is necessary, since no legislation for the registration of homeopaths in Tamil Nadu had yet been enacted at the time of this study. A law setting uniform standards for the entire country was passed by the Central Government in 1970.

Among the practitioners in this study were 30 who were initially trained and registered as homeopathic physicians, and 8 others who registered as homeopathic practitioners after first registering as Siddha, Ayurvedic, or Unani physicians; 7 hereditary practitioners opted for homeopathy registration, including one of the two men who were originally trained and licensed as pharmacists. Only 10 of the 29 hereditary practitioners we interviewed were registered as Ayurvedic, Siddha, or Unani medical practitioners; 3 each of whom had practiced in Vellore for over twenty years, had long refused to register with the state, but 2 of them were seeking homeopathic registration in 1968.

Registration alone did not distinguish these private practitioners from the trance curers, exorcists, and sidewalk herbalists in Vellore. Other points of contrast were the location and clinic style of practice, the types of cases they treated, and their relationships to other practitioners. Also, at least in earlier years, many of the private physicians had participated in North Arcot District practitioners' associations such as the Siddha Vaidya Sangam, the Homeopaths' Association, the Licentiate in Indian Medicine Association, and the Indian Medical Association. Many of the practitioners made references in 1968–69 to the local decline of voluntary medical associations.

Most of the practitioners we interviewed had clinics with signs on the main or easily accessible side streets of the town. Roughly one-third had clinics separate from their residence. Those who practiced at home tended to use a separate front room or part of the varanda for the clinic; 3 consulted patients at the pharmacy where they worked. About one-fourth of these practitioners had clinics both at home and at a separate location; 11 commuted to a second place of practice in another town or in nearby villages.

Clinics were usually small and simply arranged, with a wooden table and chair, a bench for waiting patients, and prominently displayed medicinal bottles on shelves or a table. Pictures of deities, national leaders, and family members decorated the whitewashed walls. Occasionally an anatomical chart or a framed certificate was displayed. In general, the clinics appeared modest, or even plain. The younger practitioners tended to have smaller clinics, while a few of the well-established men and women had considerably larger setups. The largest was a row of houses effectively organized into a small hospital. Two other clinics also maintained beds for patients.

Estimates of the average number of patients per day were obtained from the practitioners. Some of them said that the number of patients was greatest in the cool, rainy months (October–January), but I have averaged these reported seasonal variations to calculate year-round daily figures: 20 of the practitioners reported a daily average of less than 10 patients; 31 reported between 10 and 25 patients per day; 14 said they saw between 26 and 50 patients a day; and 9 reported that their daily average was greater than 50 persons. Only 2 of the 76 preferred not to discuss this aspect of their practice.

Though incomes of most of these practitioners could not be documented, many of those with smaller practices lived in modest houses and perhaps owned a bicycle. Fewer than 10 of the most prominent men and women in the group owned large homes and had a telephone and car. The great majority said that the average fee they charged a patient was one rupee, roughly the equivalent of one-third of a day's earnings for a male agricultural laborer, or one-sixth to one-eighth of one day's pay for an elementary school teacher. Most physicians also reported that they reduced their charges or waived them entirely for very poor patients. Usually they charged an additional two rupees for an injection.

Most of the physicians in the group managed their practices by themselves. A few were helped by their wives, a son, or a brother. One practitioner said that the presence of a woman assistant or nurse greatly improved communications with all patients, and 20 physicians among those with larger practices employed a nurse or other attendant.

Only about one-third of the practitioners in this study utilized medicines which were specific to the medical tradition in which they were trained. The greater number utilized "indigenous" and "Western" medicines as seemed appropriate to them for each patient. Medications for Ayurvedic, Siddha, and Unani treatments were personally prepared, purchased locally, or bought from outlets in Madras or Bombay. One Vellore shop exclusively sold raw ingredients for preparing these medicines, and though about half of the practitioners prepared some medicines themselves, only 6 relied solely on their own preparations. Homeopathic medicines were usually purchased from the homeopathic institutes where training was received, or from cities like Kumbakonam, Madras, and Calcutta. Vellore pharmacies and chemists' shops sold "allopathic" or "English" medicines to the practitioners, who gave them directly to their patients much more commonly than writing prescriptions for them. Since direct distribution of medicines was so common, maintaining a supply of these medications was of special importance to most of the practitioners, and 9 of them had ties to a pharmacy or chemist's shop through close kin, employment, or ownership.

A large number of the physicians in this study reported that they would not take certain kinds of cases. Apart from patients with advanced illnesses which were believed to be beyond treatment, four of the cases most frequently said to be refused were leprosy, fractures, tuberculosis, and patients requiring surgery. On the other hand, some of these practitioners claimed to have reputations for special skills. These claims included menstrual disorders, children's disease, venereal diseases, eye infections, cancer, and nervous and mental disorders. I could not judge the validity of these claims, but we did ask about how referrals of patients were made.

The patterns of referrals seemed to be consistent with the information on training and patient loads. Most of these practitioners said they referred certain cases to other physicians, and slightly more than half of them claimed to receive referrals. Those who said they did not refer their patients seemed to be less prestigious practitioners, with less training and smaller daily patient loads. Some of the more highly-trained physicians emphasized the number of patients they received from younger homeopaths and village curers. Several homeopaths sent many of their patients to certain of the well-established individuals in the group, and they received a commission or share of the consultation fee. Some of the prominent physicians expressed a strong sense of competition with other private practitioners, and said that they referred patients to one of the two hospitals in Vellore. However, the hospitals were thought of by most physicians in this study as places to which difficult and hopeless cases should be sent, and apparently many townsfolk and villagers held a similar view. Reciprocal relationships among the private practitioners and the hospitals were almost nonexistent.

SYSTEMS

I will abstract four sets of information from the data I have summarized. First, the described group of persons practicing medicine in Vellore are part of the local *practitioner population*. A complete account of the practitioner population would include data on physicians at the hospitals, and on the various other curers and healers. I have provided information on the ways in which these men and women became private medical practitioners. Entry into the profession was gained through parental training, apprenticeship, study at schools, or correspondence courses. Efforts to regulate medical practitioners influenced the routes of entry into practice. The number of practitioners was greater than might be expected if practice had been limited to those for whom it was a family heritage, or who had earned a degree from a medical college. A measure of the number of men and women entering and leaving the practitioner population over a given time period could be called *the rate of change of the practitioner population*.

Second, I have mentioned the diverse medications which are employed in practice. I did not enumerate the items in use or describe how they were used, but asserted that a tendency to dispense medicines was important. A general *set of medicines* can be said to be available to these practitioners.

While changes in this set have undoubtedly been important, I am presuming here that the way available medications are used is more important than precisely what is used, and I have described how most of the private practitioners utilize both "indigenous" and "Western" medications.

Third, I have assumed that a *population of patients* requiring and seeking medical treatment exists. I have not specified any characteristics of the patient population, except to indicate that many villagers are included. Good statistics on morbidity patterns and some preliminary data on utilization of health services in Vellore are available.

Fourth, I have described several aspects of private medical practice. My definition of "practice"—*regularly receiving and responding to patients who seek medical aid*—refers to a series of consultations, so that medical practice over a period of time or among a number of practitioners at one point in time is a sum of consultations. The data on the number of patients of the private practitioners I have described permits calculation of a *collective consultation, or medical practice, rate.*

To analyze the systemic aspect of the data, I believe that the most interesting event to explain is "medical practice." The collective rate of consultations can be considered a maintained variable in a system. Specifying this rate would be a starting point for analysis. If this variable operates within a functional system, other related variables must be specified. Three supporting variables may be postulated as parts of the system. These are: the rate of change in the practitioner population, the rate of change in the patient population, and the set of medications. Diagrammatically, this system may be represented in Figure 1.

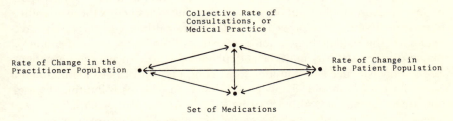

Collective Rate of
Consultations, or
Medical Practice

Rate of Change in the
Practitioner Population

Rate of Change in
the Patient Population

Set of Medications

FIGURE 2. The system of medical practice.

To demonstrate that these variables constitute a functional system, ranges of values for each of the variables need to be specified, and change in the values beyond the specified ranges or limits of the maintained variable must be demonstrated to cause changes in values of one or more of the supporting variables. My quantitative data do not permit this kind of analysis, but the model is useful to make several points.

The measurement of first importance is to specify the maximal and minimal rates at which the present practitioner population must practice to maintain the system without change. If the rates are above or below this system-main-taining range, responsive changes will hypothetically occur in one or more of the other variables. While some of the practitioners I have described had as few as 4 to 6 patients per day, the collective rate of consultations was sizable. The sum of reported figures was over 2,400 patients daily, a number roughly equal to the combined daily totals at the outpatient clinics of the town's two hospitals. Direct observation of practices would yield a better measure than interviews in which physicians estimate their own practice, but 25 percent of the respondents in the study stated that they were not satisfied with the size of their practices. Few indicated that the demand for their services was below their expectations, and over half expressed hopes of improving the location or size of their clinics. The strikingly modest size of many of the individual practices may permit a larger practitioner population.

Of the physicians we interviewed, 25 percent had entered medical practice after 1960, suggesting that there has been a high rate of change in the practitioner population in recent years. Certainly this would have been possible, given the multiple routes of entry into medical practice and the opportunities for migration. In terms of the model, such change would be seen as a response to the collective consultation rate's having exceeded the limits which maintain system stability, and indicating unmet demands for medical services. The popularity of homeopathy needs to be studied in this regard.

The model also specifies a direct relationship between the collective rate of consultations and the rate of change in the patient population. About 70 percent of the practitioners in the present study described seasonal differences in their patient loads. The highest daily averages for the cooler, rainy months were often double or triple those for the hot, dry months. Over a longer span of time, increases in the total population, growing awareness of the availability of treatment, and the improved accessibility of health services probably have expanded the patient population proportionally, despite the eradication of major diseases such as malaria and plague. Measurements of the patient population will need to consider local concepts of disease and treatment. Special attention should be given to the ways in which self-limiting diseases and anxiety about ill health are managed (see Alland 1970:Chap. 6).

For a population like the present one, the most difficult measurement will be with regard to the set of medications. Traditionally, the preparation and dispensing of medicines have been important to physicians in India, and the continuing emphasis on this practice was shown by my study. The expansion of the set of medications available to physicians needs documentation. In Vellore, the number of pharmacies had increased from one or two a generation earlier to over 10 in 1968–69. During the same period, new factories for indigenous and "English" medicines have been constructed across India. The systemic significance of the greater availability of a variety of medications deserves further investigation.

The model I have presented of a medical system invites a large number of basic empirical observations. Detailed research on the consultation or practice capacities will refine the concept of "medical practice." The model is intended to encourage studies of the ways in which changes in medical practice are causally related to equally important changes in other aspects of the medical system.[3]

Literature Cited

Alexander, C. Alex, and M. K. Shivaswamy
    1971 "Traditional Healers in a Region of Mysore," *Social Science and Medicine* 5(6): 595–601.
Alland, Alexander, Jr.
    1970 *Adaptation in Cultural Evolution: An Approach to Medical Anthropology*. New York: Columbia University Press.
Christian Medical College, Dept. of Biostatistics
    1968 *Household Survey of Vellore Town, Parts One and Two* (mimeo.). Vellore: Christian Medical College.
Collins, Paul W.
    1965 "Functional Analyses in the Symposium 'Man, Culture, and Animals,'" in Anthony Leeds and Andrew P. Vayda, eds., *Man, Culture and Animals*. Washington, D. C.: Am. Assn. for the Advancement of Science, Pub. no. 78.
    1969 *The logic of Functional Analysis in Anthropology*, Ann Arbor: University Microfilms.
Collins, Paul W., and Andrew P. Vayda
    1969 "Functional Analysis and Its Aims." *Australian and New Zealand J. Sociology* 5(2): 153–156.
Feldman, R. A., K. R. Kamath, P. S. S. Sunder Rao, and J. K. G. Webb
    1969 "Infection and Disease in a Group of South Indian Families: I. Introduction, Methods, Definitions, and General Observations in a Continuing Study." *Am. J. Epidemiology* 89(4): 364–374.
Hindu, The
    1968 "Fifty Years Ago: May 17, 1918," in *The Hindu*, Madras, May 18, p. 2.
Leslie, Charles,
    1967 "Professional and Popular Health Cultures in South Asia: Needed Research in Medical Sociology and Anthropology," in *Understanding Science and Technology in India and Pakistan*. New York: State University of New York, Foreign Area Materials Center, Occasional Publications no. 8.
    1968 "The Professionalization of Ayurvedic and Unani Medicine." *Transactions N. Y. Acad. of Sciences, Ser. II* 30(4): 559–572.
    1969 "Modern India's Ancient Medicine." *Trans-action* 6: 46–55.
Lozoff, Betsy, K. R. Kamath, and R. A. Feldman
    In press "Infection and Disease in a Group of South Indian Families: VII. Beliefs About Cause and Cure of Childhood Diarrhea." *Human Organization*.
Madan, T. N.
    1969 "Who Chooses Modern Medicine and Why," *Economic and Political Weekly* 4(37): 1475–1484.

3 In preparing this paper I have benefited from numerous suggestions, though this presentation hardly reflects all of them. My greatest debt is to Charles Leslie, for having encouraged and helped to develop this study from a point early in the research in 1968 up to its present form.

Rapoport, Anatol
    1970 "Modern Systems Theory—An Outlook for Coping with Change." *General Systems* (*Yearbook of the Society for General Systems Research*) 15: 15–25.
Singh, Sohan, John E. Gordon, and John B. Wyon
    1962 "Medical Care in Fatal Illnesses of A Rural Punjab Population: Some Social, Biological, and Cultural Factors and Their Ecological Implication." *Indian J. Medical Research* 50(6): 865–880.

The Place of Indigenous Medical Practitioners in the Modernization of Health Services

CARL E. TAYLOR

More than half of my life has been spent in the villages of developing countries, and some of my best friends have been Vaids, Hakims, and other indigenous practitioners. My boyhood was spent in the villages of North India where my father practiced rural medicine as a medical missionary. Our three-month winter vacation from school in the Himalayas was spent living in tents, touring from village to village in the Siwalik foothills. Our relationship with village people could not have been more intimate. Twenty-five years ago I started the first of two terms as a medical missionary in the U.P. and Punjab states of India. Since then, my academic research at Harvard and Johns Hopkins has concentrated largely on rural health services and the health team.

It was not until five years ago, however, that I realized how little I knew about indigenous practice. We had been doing research on the preparation of doctors for rural work and on ways of improving health center services. For years I had tried to manipulate indigenous practitioners into cooperating with our programs. We had shown that a health center that offers good services can replace a Vaid in the health-care pattern of a village. But there was always an ethical ambivalence in trying to maneuver relationships so as to keep the friendship and cooperation of indigenous practitioners, while deliberately working them out of their livelihood. This personalized relationship, however, provided no appreciation of their overall role in the health system. I have always held that some sort of synthesis between modern medicine and Ayurvedic medicine is desirable. (Taylor 1952).

INDIGENOUS PRACTITIONERS' SURVEY

More detailed understanding of the indigenous practitioner's present contributions came out of our research projects on functional analysis of local health services five years ago. We had completed four macroplanning projects on national health manpower in Turkey, Taiwan, Peru, and Nigeria. We decided to concentrate next on determining local health manpower mix and

285

the development of a microplanning methodology of functional analysis by measuring total community morbidity, who provided what care, how much did this care cost, and what might be done with actual and potential health center resources. We studied 2 community development blocks in North India, 2 more in South India, and 9 health center units in Eastern Anatolia. We found that in India organized health services provide only 10 percent of the medical care. Another 10 percent is provided by qualified physicians in towns and cities. The balance is split between home medical care and indigenous practitioners. This led to intensive study of the health coverage provided by the indigenous practitioners.

Indian social scientists in both Punjab and Mysore undertook to track down and interview all indigenous practitioners in a community development block with 80,000 people. In Pakhowal Block in the Punjab, 59 full-time indigenous practitioners were found by making detailed inquiries in every village. This represents a practitioner–population ratio of 1/1400. In addition, there were over 300 part-time spiritual healers and specialized practitioners focusing on particular conditions. Preliminary visits gained the cooperation of all the full-time practitioners; in fact, they proved to be almost grateful that someone was interested in them. A detailed questionnaire provided data (Neumann et al. 1971). For instance, most had been trained in various kinds of apprenticeship relationships (Table 1).

TABLE 1

Apprenticeship Training of 59 Indigenous Practitioners
in Pakhowal Block, Punjab, India, 1965

Type of Apprenticeship	Number	Percentage
Ayurvedic	21	36
Unani	9	15
Homeopathic	2	3
Modern	9	15
Combination of modern with one or more indigenous schools	13	22
No apprenticeship	4	7
No information	1	2
Total	59	100%

Then our social scientist arranged to spend three days sitting in the office of each full-time practitioner with a check list which was filled out describing the practitioner–patient interaction (Tables 2 and 3).

TABLE 2

Nature of Physical Examination Conducted by 59 Indigenous Practirioners in Pakhowal Block, Punjab, India, 1965

Type of Examination	No. Examined	Percentage
No physical examination	182	47
Physical done, but without "Western" instruments	81	21
Physical done using "Western" instruments appropriately	13	3
Physical done using "Western" instruments inappropriately	47	13
Observed without physical contact with patient (usually skin pathology)	53	14
Uncodable, no information	3	1
Total	379	99%

TABLE 3

Type of Medication Prescribed by 59 Indigenous Practitioners in Pakhowal Block, Punjab, India, 1965

Type of Medication	No. Treated	Percentage
None	0	0
Modern only	312	82
Mixed modern and indigenous	21	5
Indigenous only	46	12
Total	379	99%

The great use of modern medicine surprised us. It showed that when we used the term "indigenous practitioner," we were really talking about indigenous practitioners of medicine, and not practitioners of indigenous medicine.

Some other generalizations are that Punjabi practitioners were visited mainly (71 percent) by patients traveling less than half a mile; they charged small fees (51 percent charged less than 1 rupee, and 77 percent, less than 2 rupees); more than half of the patients paid cash; and the more traditional a practitioner was, the more likely he was to spend more than ten minutes with each patient.

In Mysore, many more part-time practitioners were found, 656 in a taluk of 120,000 population. But only 30 were full-time, and of those only 7 were registered. The median fee was 1.50 rupees for full-time practitioners, and 0.50 rupees for part-time. As in the Punjab, 80 percent of drugs given were allopathic, with about 50 percent of the patients getting injections of penicillin (Alexander and Shivaswamy 1971). Since the bulk of the care was provided by full-time practitioners, there was a much greater tendency for them to use modern medicines.

A casual episode opened up a whole new range of inquiry. As a patient was going out, Mr. Bhatia, our social scientist in the Punjab, said to a Vaid, "What was that medicine you gave him?" The practitioner handed the bottle to him, saying, "I can't read English. Why don't you read the label and tell me what it is?" Bhatia saw that it was one of our most powerful and potentially dangerous antibiotics, but written in Punjabi across the top of the label was "Bukhar de liye," or "for fever." He was then shown other bottles of standard drugs with similar punjabi inscriptions specifying diarrhea, conjunctivitis, or cramps. When Bhatia asked the Vaid where he had gotten his medicine and learned how to use it, the practitioner said, "Oh, my friend the pharmacist in Ludhiana keeps me up to date."

In following up this lead, we uncovered not only an underground system of health care providing the bulk of medical treatment for the people of India, but also a widely pervasive and previously unrecognized separate system of medical education. The professors are the drug-detail men from pharmaceutical companies, often the largest and most reputable companies in the world. The junior faculty are the pharmacists in the cities. Each pharmacist has a continuing class of practitioners scattered throughout the neighboring villages. The practitioner will drop into the pharmacist's shop and say, "I am seeing a lot of conjunctivitis these days. What do you have that's good?"

The indigenous practitioners of Ludhiana District have organized an association and have monthly meetings to discuss clinical cases and new treatments. The government has set up a registration system, but essentially no control.

When we told the health authorities of India about our findings, it was apparent that few had realized the extent to which the new pattern had spread. The general stereotype was that indigenous practitioners were still dealing in "jari-booties," herbs and roots which can safely be considered innocuous, even if not beneficial. One Vaid in our area has developed a tremendous reputation and is reputed to make an income of 200,000 rupees a year. As I watched him practice, it was apparent that his reputation was built on penicillin. A large syringe was used to inject a sizable dose into successive patients, the only gesture toward sterilization being that he would wave the needle through a dirty pan of weak antiseptic. Health officials are shocked; but the reality is that until something better is provided, such practices will continue to respond to existing demand. The greatest source of hazard is the tendency of such pseudo-indigenous practitioners to use the most powerful drugs possible in order to get quick results. For instance, one of the most commonly used drugs is chloramphenicol, with no realization of its toxicity.

HISTORICAL SEQUENCE OF HEALTH-SERVICES DEVELOPMENT

The role of the indigenous practitioner in a country such as India may be placed into perspective in a sequence of five stages in the natural history of health-services development.

1. *Traditional System of Care*: No country has a vacuum of health care. There are always traditional methods which have evolved within the local culture. These are often associated with religious beliefs.

2. *Elite Medical Care*: Regardless of political theory or claims about equality, it is always true that high-quality care will be provided first for the elite, whether indigenous or colonial. This is not completely irrational, since the leadership of a country can consider itself an important investment. A fascinating phenomenon in India is the carry-over of a high-class Ayurvedic medicine as a component of elite medicine. Particularly among the conservative upper classes, cultural pride leads to great reliance on indigenous practitioners.

3. *Mass Development of Curative Service*: Political insistence that there be some sort of care for the masses leads most developing countries to devote a large part of health expenditures to public medical care. In the early stages of development, such services tend to be so overwhelmed by expanding demand that they become more of a gesture than a reality. They will gradually replace the indigenous system, except for the usual residue of practitioners caring for conditions such as arthritis that do not respond to any treatment.

4. *Mass Preventive Services*: Public-health measures have frequently started mainly because the elite needed to protect themselves from mass epidemics. Increasing health sophistication and international pressures lead to general application of preventive measures as the only long-range and economically rational method of controlling diseases.

5. *Comprehensive Care*: The traditional dichotomy between curative and preventive services is not only inefficient but also leads to major gaps in health care. Especially where resources are limited, a more rational aproach is to provide comprehensive care by a health team under the leadership of a doctor, but with most services being carried out by auxiliaries and paramedical workers. Each individual's role should be clearly defined, and each activity actually carried out by personnel with the minimum level of preparation appropriate for a particular task. During the transitional stage of developing such rationalized services, it is particularly important to plan deliberately for as much cooperation as possible with indigenous practitioners.

A classical case of a drastic approach of trying to eliminate indigenous medical practice abruptly is provided by Turkey. Under Ataturk, legislation was passed outlawing Hakims' practicing the ancient Persian and Arabic system of medicine. Legal pressure was sufficiently great to eliminate overt practice and preceptorship training, so that the system gradually disappeared. Since government health services did not develop to fill the need, a spontaneous solution appeared in a new group of practitioners—the needlemen. In the National Health Manpower Study that we did in 1963, there were 30,000 needlemen, as compared with 10,000 doctors. Even more numerous were the *ebe annes*, or indigenous midwives. Then there were also assorted bone-setters, circumcisers, tooth-pullers, lead-pourers, umbilicus-setters, and coccyx-pullers, so that every village averaged one practitioner and one traditional midwife (Taylor et al. 1968).

In India since independence, by contrast, official policy has been to promote a revival of traditional Ayurvedic medicine. With the passing of the British raj, there was great emotional appeal in trying to revive the ancient glories of Ram Raj, with Ayurvedic medicine as a symbol. Increased status and recognition were given to Ayurvedic practitioners, and more than 100,000 have been registered. Ayurvedic medical schools were opened, and efforts were made to synthesize scientific modern medicine with the Ayurvedic system. About ten years ago, many of these schools were closed by student riots, because graduates wanted the same recognition and salaries as MBBS graduates. Now many of the Ayurvedic medical colleges have been converted to regular medical colleges, giving the MBBS degree. Others are trying to go back to Shudh Ayurveda, or the pure traditional system.

RELATIONSHIP OF AYURVEDIC MEDICINE TO POPULAR BELIEFS

"Start where the people are" is a generally accepted axiom of health education. Scientifically trained health personnel working with traditional populations typically have difficulty communicating with rural people. Even in such everyday matters as explaining a therapeutic regimen, both practitioners and patients continue to experience great frustration. Each blames the other—doctors say that patients are stupid and superstitious, and patients say that doctors just do not care. All too often the professionals never bother to find out if their patients have understood an explanation or instruction. In addition to problems in understanding words and phrases, a more fundamental issue is that the basic patterns of meanings, interpretations, and expectations are different.

Many times I have heard village patients say to an Indian physician after treatment has been prescribed, "*Aur kya parhez hai?*" which means "And what is forbidden?"—referring to dietary prohibitions which are important in Ayurvedic practice. When the doctor says "Nothing," the patient walks away shaking his head, baffled, with his confidence shaken.

It is not easy to find out what people believe. Most doctors come from elite groups and pride themselves on having given up the old superstitions, or at least the most obvious ones. Their science-oriented education creates ambivalence and a superficial rejection of the old traditions, with a complex and erratic holding to select beliefs from their childhood.

In trying to improve understanding of local beliefs, a possible short-cut to be explored was that popular notions might be derived from Ayurvedic traditions. If so, the best way of finding out what people believe would be to ask the practitioners and study the classics. When we tried this, however, we were baffled by the lack of uniformity in present interpretations of the Ayurvedic classics, and the multiple contaminations from Unani and Siddha medical systems. The wide variations led us to inquire if there were any uniform patterns in belief in the various parts of the country.

From 1962 to 1966, we had Indian social scientists living in villages in widely distributed geographical areas as part of a study of the adaptation of doctors to rural services. We decided to inquire into popular beliefs about the causation, prevention, and treatment of specific diseases, and beliefs about diet. We worked first with open-ended depth questionnaires, then with a more structured general survey, and finally with a carefully structured questionnaire asking carefully selected random samples of village people about 7 common diseases and 50 common foods.

The most dramatic finding was the tremendous variation in beliefs in different parts of India. The disease most often attributed to the wrath of a goddess was cholera, with this causation considered important by 49 percent of people from villages near Vellore; 34 percent from near Lucknow; 31 percent from Purulia in Western Bengal; and 21 percent from near Nagpur. Eating bad foods was thought to be the major cause of cholera near Lucknow, Ludhiana, and Trivandrum (Table 4).

Leprosy was also considered to be caused by divine wrath or by past sins, by people in Nagpur, Purulia, and Vellore (Table 5).

In most places, diarrhea was thought to be caused by eating spoiled foods, but in some states there was more concern about eating incompatible foods according to the hot and cold categorization. One-fifth of the people near Nagpur thought diarrhea was caused by dislocation of the umbilicus, and more than half of the response from Vellore attributed it to "eating hair unknowingly." About half of the people near Ludhiana, Nagpur, and Vellore also thought that heat was important in the causation of diarrhea (Table 6).

Tuberculosis was thought to be caused by infection in most places; however, 77 percent of the people in villages near Trivandrum said that it was caused by "trauma to the chest" (Table 7).

Roundworms showed particular variation, with people near Ludhiana and Bengal saying that this malady was caused by eating mud; near Bombay it was attributed to too much sweet food; whereas near Vellore it was related to eating raw rice (Table 8).

Respondents were asked what type of practitioner they would prefer for particular conditions. Vaids and other indigenous practitioners were most preferred for rheumatism by 87 percent of people near Trivandrum; 59

TABLE 4

Beliefs About Causes of Cholera
from Interviews of 100 Households in Each of 7 Indian Village Areas, 1965
(in percentages)

	Bombay	Lucknow	Ludhiana	Nagpur	Trivandrum	Vellore	Purulia
Wrath of goddess	—	34	—	21	—	49	31
Stale food	18	44	42	10	20	—	30
Flies	—	—	11	16	—	—	19
Personal contact	31	—	24	—	26	18	17
Eating dirty food	—	23	40	—	52	—	12
Sudden climate change	35	—	—	—	—	—	—
Overeating rich foods	—	—	45	—	—	—	—
Heat exposure	—	—	31	—	—	—	—
Water after eating melons	—	—	31	—	—	—	—
Don't know	—	—	—	35	22	18	—
Other causes	12	11	22	33	33	43	—

TABLE 5

Beliefs About Causes of Leprosy

from Interviews of 100 Households in Each of 4 Indian Village Areas, 1965
(in Percentages)

	Nagpur	*Trivandrum*	*Vellore*	*Purulia*
Contagion (contact)	15	10	18	27
Infection	20	38	17	—
God's wrath	34	—	16	24
Bad condition of blood	—	14	—	10
Past sins	19	—	—	30
Heredity	—	10	23	19
Don't know	44	31	20	—
Other causes	10	21	24	—

percent near Purulia; and 57 percent near Bombay (Table 9). For most other conditions, Ayurvedic practitioners tended to be much less popular than doctors.

Beliefs about hot and cold foods are so widespread in India that it seemed reasonable to think that there might be some uniformity in these patterns. These distinctions are supposed to be based on how specific foods are thought to affect bodily functions, and not on temperature or spiciness. Eating patterns seem to be related to ideas about hazards of eating hot foods in summer or cold foods in winter, or in association with fevers, diarrheas, or rheumatism. We thought it would help physicians if we could provide an overall classification of those foods which were considered hot, cold, or neutral.

Dramatic geographical differences became apparent. Many foods that were considered hot in the North were thought to be cold in the South. It seemed apparent that any possible empiric validity underlying the concept of hot and cold foods could not be substantiated. We have not been able to define a basic principle underlying local beliefs such as Foster. (1962) said he had found in similar investigations in Latin America. If there were any consistent underlying effect, there should be more uniformity. These findings should at least help doctors understand their patients' beliefs and help them to define local patterns in their own areas.

DELIBERATE ADAPTATION OF TRADITIONAL PRACTICES

Scientific medicine has developed its own accretion of rituals and dogma. Much that doctors now do has evolved into a tradition by historical accident and has continued because there have been no good reasons for changing.

TABLE 6

Beliefs About Causes of Diarrhea

from Interviews of 100 Households in Each of 7 Indian Village Areas, 1965

(in percentages)

	Bombay	Lucknow	Ludhiana	Nagpur	Trivandrum	Vellore	Purulia
Dislocation of umbilicus	12	—	13	21	—	18	—
Eating too much	12	21	65	39	30	46	54
Eating spoiled food	60	48	37	12	25	18	47
Eating wrong type of food	38	38	36	14	32	15	—
Eating incompatible food	—	20	16	10	50	—	—
Don't know	—	—	—	18	—	—	—
Other causes	—	—	56	36	36	47	—

TABLE 7

Beliefs About Causes of Tuberculosis

from Interviews of 100 Households in Each of 7 Indian Village Areas, 1965

(in percentages)

	Bombay	Lucknow	Ludhiana	Nagpur	Trivandrum	Vellore	Purulia
Infection	27	27	26	13	32	18	—
Contagion (contact)	15	10	53	—	12	—	32
Germs in lungs	14	10	17	14	—	—	—
Neglected fever	14	19	32	—	77	—	—
Trauma to chest	—	—	—	—	—	11	18
Unbalanced diet	20	—	34	14	—	—	18
Overindulgence (sexual)	12	—	—	23	—	—	17
Heredity	—	—	16	—	14	10	—
Inpurity of blood	14	18	—	—	—	—	11
Worries	12	10	10	10	—	—	—
Don't know	—	13	—	41	14	37	—
Other causes	—	—	28	24	16	22	—

TABLE 8

Beliefs About Causes of Roundworms

from Interviews of 100 Households in Each of 7 Indian Village Areas, 1965

(in percentages)

	Bombay	Lucknow	Ludhiana	Nagpur	Trivandrum	Vellore	Purulia
Children eating mud	18	24	62	10	—	10	58
Too many sweets	77	17	30	17	—	—	—
Eating dirty Vegetables	—	18	—	—	—	—	—
Germs	10	—	—	30	—	—	—
Eating raw rice	—	—	—	—	—	59	54
Don't know	—	25	—	41	34	—	12
Other causes	—	17	27	31	45	32	—

TABLE 9

Type of Practitioner Preferred for Treatment of Rheumatism

from Interviews of 100 Households in Each of 7 Indian Village Areas, 1965

(in percentages)

	Bombay	Lucknow	Ludhiana	Nagpur	Trivandrum	Vellore	Purulia
Doctor	44	54	67	72	15	30	24
Vaid (Ayurvedic)	57	20	21	26	87	—	59
Home treatment	—	43	21	80	—	71	25
Other	—	—	—	—	—	10	—

Unfortunately, most established routines are more for the convenience of the practitioner than to help the patient.

In adapting scientific medicine to local needs, a particularly challenging opportunity for innovative thinking is the prospect of divesting medical practice of its Western rituals and adjusting basic scientific principles to local cultural practices. This pattern of synthesis is clearly desirable.

Our population and nutrition action-and-research projects in the Punjab require the development of new comprehensive-care patterns for rural India. In integrating scientific measures into the matrix of traditional practice, we have been analyzing the detailed steps in providing specific services such as obstetrics. We do not try to replace the indigenous *dai*, since it will be many years before qualified health workers will be available to assist in all deliveries. Our auxiliary nurse-midwives try to become friends of the dais and support them in their work. The dai is trained to improve her handling of normal deliveries and encouraged to refer problem cases, via the ANM, to the health centre.

We have analyzed the dais' normal practices, classifying each activity under three headings: those that are dangerous; those that are beneficial; and those that are neutral. We try to change only those that are clearly dangerous. An example is the use of cow-dung ash on the umbilical stump, since its use leads to neonatal tetanus, which is the fourth cause of death in the Punjab. Massaging with oil, however, may be beneficial. We are not sure yet about the squatting position for delivery; but the modern practice of having the woman on her back, with her legs dangling in the air, is clearly designed mainly for the convenience of the doctor.

During the years that family planning has been building up to become the highest priority and largest health program in India, there has been continuing speculation but little precise information about the possibility of using indigenous practitioners in the National Family Planning Program. One of our doctoral candidates, Mr. Sunny Andrews, comes from Kerala, an area where Ayurvedic medicine is particularly strong. He has just completed field work exploring the attitudes of indigenous practitioners, village people, and government health personnel on the possibility of incorporating indigenous practitioners into the National Family Planning Program. He found out what these practitioners were already doing and saying about family planning.

The data are encouraging, first of all, in that there is very little overt opposition and considerable spontaneous support. The busiest practitioners said they could not take on added responsibility. Most indigenous practitioners, however, seemed delighted that an effort was being made to ask their opinions. It would apparently take only a small financial incentive to get their cooperation and active participation. The personnel of government health centers have experienced so much frustration in trying to increase family-planning acceptance in villages that they seemed eager for any contribution by indigenous practitioners. In any trials that are developed, it will be particularly

important to distinguish varied roles, depending on the type and preparation
of the practitioner.

The experience and specific findings of our various research teams suggest the
following propositions relating to the future of indigenous medicine. Although
we have gathered considerable theoretical data from field studies, it must
be realized that we have little evidence from actual trials of program alternatives.

1. Indigenous medical practice will probably fade slowly into a general
synthesis with scientific medicine. Practitioners will not disappear as long as
the present vacuum of health care in villages persists, but as organized health
services expand, they will gradually be reduced in number. In the first village
near Ludhiana where we started a teaching health center, the leading Vaid
became a member of our health committee. As his own clinical practice
vanished, he converted his office into a grocery store. In Narangwal village,
where we have our major research base and a teaching health center for a rural
intership program, the Vaid stopped me on the street one day. Catching my
lapels, he shook me hard, saying, "You have ruined my practice, now you must
find me a job!" He finally moved to another village, because we could not
work out a sufficiently prestigious position for him. However, in the last few
years a young man with basic pharmacy training has started a shop in the
village, building a lucrative clinical practice using more powerful Western
drugs than we dare to use in our rural practice.

2. India will continue to officially sponsor the indigenous systems and promote research to discover the empiric preparations that can scientifically be
demonstrated to be clinically effective. Several institutions, such as Lucknow
and Jamnagar, are continuing methodical testing of Ayurvedic herbs for
their pharmacological effects.

3. We can learn from indigenous practitioners much that will help us to
design better health systems for rural areas. Particularly important could be
incorporating into medical and nursing education an increased understanding
of and adjustment to the beliefs of people about health and disease. Health
personnel will then be able to make more understandable explanations to their
patients and to provide more effective health education. It is also important
to synthesize scientifically-derived health measures with locally acceptable
health practices.

4. During the transitional period, when serious shortages of trained health
personnel in countries such as India will be most acute, the possibility of
bringing indigenous practitioners into the health system will continue to be
evaluated. Around the world, the most successful such integration has been
in the use of indigenous midwives. In many countries domiciliary midwifery
has been raised to acceptable levels by training the women who have traditionally filled this role. We have not had any success, however, in using
practitioners of indigenous medicine for organized medical care, and control
of their private practice will continue to be difficult. However, there is an

opportunity for innovative thinking in the increasingly important area of family planning. Not only indigenous midwives, but also other types of indigenous practitioners, might participate effectively. Cooperation rather than competition between indigenous and scientific systems of health services may then increase our ability to meet the urgent challenges of reducing population presure in developing countries.

Literature Cited

Alexander, C. A., and M. K. Shivaswamy
    1971 "Traditional Healers in a Region of Mysore (India)." *Social Science and Medicine* 5(6): 595–601.
Foster, George
    1962 *Traditional Cultures and the Impact of Technological Change.* New York: Harper and Row.
Neumann, A. K., M. A. Bhatia, S. Andrews, and A. K. S. Murphy
    1971 "Role of the Indigenous Medicine Practitioner in Two Areas of India— Report of a Study." *Social Science and Medicine* 5(2): 137–149.
Taylor, Carl E.
    1952 "Hindu Medicine and India's Health." *Atlantic Monthly* 190: 51–53.
Taylor, Carl E., Rahmi Dirican, and Kurt N. Deuschle
    1968 *Health Manpower Planning in Turkey: An International Research Case Study.* Baltimore: Johns Hopkins University Press.

The Social Organization and Ecology of Medical Practice in Taiwan

PAUL U. UNSCHULD

How to develop a public health service in keeping with the modern age is a problem for all countries. It is complicated for states within the Chinese and Indian cultural sphere by the fact that they have ancient healing systems which are still part of their cultures. These medical systems are linked to profoundly valued religious and philosophical traditions; yet for over a century now, Asian governments have been forced to acknowledge Western leadership in medical science and technology. To adapt modern Western medicine is an integral part of building a modern state, for it alone is effective in controlling or preventing epidemics, and its superiority is especially evident for treating acute illness. Nevertheless, the Western medical system has not been accepted without great internal struggles.[1]

In conflicts over medical policy, three factions can be identified: There were those who demanded the radical takeover of a Western-oriented medical system, with the abolition of most things connected with tradition as showing superstition and ignorance. In opposition there appeared, often after a long period of silence, those who advocated rejecting Western medicine in its entirety. Between these two extremes were a broad gamut of those who

1 The term "medical system" will be used to refer to both a traditional Chinese healing system and a modern Western medical system. The term "system" is appropriate, because in both cases there exists a consciously-worked-out "edifice" of medical care covering all aspects from prevention to actual treatment, and ranging from a theoretical basis to practical use.

Different opinions were expressed during the Symposium at Burg Wartenstein about the appropriate term to signify what is called "modern, Western medicine." One suggestion was that it be called "international medicine," because it is practiced all over the world. Chinese medicine is not restricted to Chinese soil, but is practiced in many other Asian countries, and Chinese drugs and acupuncture have reached Africa, Europe, and America. But this healing system could not be properly called international. The term "modern, Western medicine" indicates the place of origin and the fact that there were and still are pre-modern Western medicines such as phytotherapy, homeopathy a la Hahnemann, or water-curing a la Kneipp, which are integrated parts of Western medical practice in Germany and other European countries.

Thus, according to our observations, Western medicine in Taiwan is quite different from that conducted in Germany—and, according to the publications which reach us from Communist China, Western medical practice there is different again from that in Germany or Taiwan. Perhaps we should call the Communist Chinese model of combining traditional elements and Western imports into a completely new medical system "modern Chinese medicine."

wanted to combine a greater or smaller proportion of both systems, either by fusing them into a new system or by allowing them to exist side by side. The real problems of adopting Western medicine were not taken into account in these discussions, and to some extent can only be analyzed now that first experiences have been gathered.

The most important problem to be encountered in transferring Western medicine to Asian cultures having ancient medical traditions of their own is the profound difference in role expectations of medical personnel and patients towards each other. It has been observed frequently, that Western-type physicians can replace traditional practitioners only to a limited extent, no matter how sophisticated their knowledge and facilities are. Subsequent parallel existence of two or more medical systems within one country may be a reason for great uncertainty and discomfort among the people.

A further problem is whether the medical systems in industrialized nations should be models for countries of the third world. Partly due to modern therapy, a large number of the people in highly develop-ed countries now live longer, but the population as a whole has become more ill in the sense of being more dependent on medicines. This dependency has been brought about by a variety of factors. One of the most influential factors in this regard has been the commercialization of health which pervades almost all levels of Western medical systems. Health has ceased to be an ordinary condition and has become something that must first of all be bought. The ability to prevent morbidity and to lower mortality has often enough been based on a heavier and continuous intake of costly modern medicines where other methods or programs, including social change, might have been at least equally successful.

We will analyze these problems in Taiwan, as we learned about them during field research in 1969 and 1970.

JAPANESE HEALTH POLICY IN TAIWAN

When the Japanese incorporated Taiwan into their sphere of administra-tion in 1895, the tendency in Japan was to place great value on using the achievements of modern science and technology, including Western medicine. In 1897, two years after their arrival in Taiwan, the Japanese authorities held an examination for doctors of traditional Chinese medicine. The only condition for participation was practice as a traditional physician. It was not in fact an examination, but the registration of practitioners of traditional medicine. Every candidate passed the examination and received official permission to continue carrying out his professional duties. During the period which followed, no further examinations for traditional doctors were held, and no more permits issued. After two or three decades, death had caused a sharp decline in the number of officially practicing doctors of traditional medicine, and by 1945 only 30 or 40 were left on the whole island.

Permission to continue their work was given to traditional chemists in 1895, without any formalities. Subsequently, a new traditional pharmacy could be opened, subject to certain restrictions, by qualified druggists who had received a Western education or by traditional doctors. Examinations were held at irregular intervals for the druggists; sometimes every year, then again after a period of up to five years. These examinations were independently given in every administrative district, and a candidate's success depended almost entirely on whether or not the officials who gave them considered that new druggists were needed.

In 1925 the Japanese announced that the system of Western medicine in Taiwan was sufficiently advanced to take the dominant role in caring for the population. At the same time, the Japanese began a drive to make Taiwan an integrated part of their cultural sphere. In the course of this drive, they exerted great pressure on the traditional physicians and chemists. Although the number of doctors who officially practiced Chinese medicine had been restricted, one tradition it was impossible for the Japanese to suppress helped preserve traditional medicine. Everyone who wanted to fulfill a child's duties to his parents, according to the teaching of Confucius, had to possess some knowledge in the medical field. Thus, a potential doctor was latent in every "well-educated" Chinese. The result was that a number of doctors practiced in secret. The Japanese attempted to identify these illegal practitioners after 1925 through spies and by other means. Traditional chemists were only allowed to dispense licensed prescriptions, and a Public Health Police Organization was created.

This severe policy was not relaxed until the war with China broke out. Then personnel was not available to supervise medical practices, and to meet military demands the export from Japan to Taiwan of Western-type medicaments was reduced. Also, the supplies of traditional druggists had previously come from China, and now during the war the costs of importing these drugs came to be considered too great by the Japanese, who urged people to make use of indigenous Taiwan remedies.

The aim of Japanese policy in Taiwan had been to establish a public health service run by qualified physicians whose modern training included knowledge of traditional drugs. The war and the capitulation of Japan prevented this aim from being realized. Nevertheless, when the Chinese Nationalists took over the island, a Western-type health service which exerted great influence on the population had been developed, and the reliance on traditional therapy and drugs had been reduced, although it had not been completely suppressed.

After their arrival in Taiwan, the Chinese did not continue this policy (Croizier 1968:210–228). They released Taiwanese traditional doctors and chemists from all existing laws, and admitted to the medical profession numerous people who had never acted as physicians on the mainland, but who lacked employment and wanted to try their hand at medicine by claiming family skills or knowledge from independent reading. This policy has led to a dual system of modern and Chinese medicine. Both are equal according to law; but while traditional physicians are legally tolerated, they are not actively supported by the state health system.

THE SUCCESS OF WESTERN MEDICINE

The use of Western medicine has dramatically improved some health problems in Taiwan. In 1954, more than 60 percent of the schoolchildren in Taipei suffered from trachoma. This was reduced to less than 5 percent by 1969. Venereal diseases became a great danger in Taipei with the influx of tourists and American servicemen from Vietnam. Since 1969 the Venereal Disease Control Institute has worked successfully to provide facilities to diagnose and treat persons at special risk. Poliomyelitis has been controlled by a preventive oral vaccination campaign for children. Other illnesses which the public health authorities are concerned with on a large scale are tuberculosis, diphtheria, dysentery, paratyphoid, epidemic meningitis, tetanus, and malaria (Taipei City Health Bureau 1970). Even so, a critic of Western medicine has written:

Many foreigners look upon the Chinese as a people who ignore the rules of hygiene in their living habits and food. The Chinese nation has a history of . . . great length . . . and a population of a colossal size; while other ancient peoples . . . have dwindled into insignificance . . . the Chinese continue to be powerful and numerous. For the Chinese possess a secret for the promotion of their physical well-being in the system of spiritual hygiene (that is, mental hygiene). The system does not consist of superficial practices of disinfection and outward cleanliness, but advocates the practice of "cultivating calmness of the heart, and nurturing of mind." In the United States, medical science has been so well developed that most contagious diseases are now preventable. But in that country today there are reported exceptionally high incidents of nervous weakness, mental ailments, high blood pressure, cardiac diseases, cancer, nephritis, and diabetes. The Chinese people, excepting those in larger cities, seldom contract these diseases. (Chen Chan Yuen 1968:14–15)

Traditional Chinese medicine is in no position to take over the public health service of Taiwan. But even in the realm of the individual's health it could not respond successfully to the impact of recent changes in economy and other aspects of society. Traditional physicians who suffer from diabetes, for example, or who need rapidly effective treatment in acute illness, resort to Western medicine as the more reliable system with regard to these kinds of problems.

ADVANTAGES OF CHINESE MEDICINE

What major advantages exist today in traditional Chinese medicine? Originally this system had a strongly preventive character. The old theories were less relevant to cure a disease which was already manifest than to forestall the outbreak of illness. To prevent disorders, the theories of the Five Evolutive Phases (*wu-hsing*) and *yin-yang* were applied to the organism. The idea that the complementary and mutually destructive powers in the body should be in equilibrium aimed at prevention. Thus a proverb says:

The ancient sages did not treat those who were already ill, they instructed those who were not ill (*ku sheng-jen pu chih i ping chih wei ping*).

According to the theoretical texts, curing was not the ideal of medical practice. The good physician prevented his patients from becoming ill in the first place. A second-century author wrote:

When the five body spheres are without any defect, when the six organs are not yet exhausted, when blood and the arteries are still in order, and the spirit is not yet perplexed, then medicine will be effective. If the disease is manifest, one may cure it in 50 percent of the cases. But if the disease has overcome the patient, it will be very difficult to save his life. (Okanishi 1964:32)

However, the famous Taoist author T'ao Hung-ching pointed to the difficulties of preventive medicine in 500 A.D.:

Who, except a brilliant physician, can recognize a disease which is not yet a disease by listening to the tones of the patient's voice, examining the colors of the face, or feeling the pulse? (Okanishi 1964:32)

A real advantage of the Chinese system of healing lay in the fact that it embraced, theoretically at least, the patient's whole way of life. It began with everyday food, which formed a part of the medical system, acting as it were as preventive dietetics. Then it considered regular sleep, sexual intercourse, physical exercise, and other activities as a comprehensive system of health practices. In Western societies this need to treat the mind and body of healthy as well as sick people has been neglected under the impact of new findings in chemotherapy and surgery, combined with exact diagnostic techniques. Although in recent years attempts are being made to resurrect a concern for the patient's way of life, and psychotherapy is stressed quite a lot, there is still too much reliance in Western society on taking drugs, compared to providing the psychological treatment and nonpolluted environment people need to stay healthy or to recover from illness.

Alongside the theoretical tradition of medical learning, a true and effective tradition of healing developed among the people. It was based on experience with herbs and other drugs, and with acupuncture, massage, and other therapeutic techniques, but also upon philosophical deductions and magic ideas. The successes of traditional practitioners in Taiwan today are mainly based on acupuncture—which is useful, for example, in treating rheumatic and nervous diseases—and the use of a large variety of more or less effective drugs from the traditional Chinese pharmacopoeia.

THE DANGERS OF TWO HEALTH SYSTEMS

It would appear that where Chinese and Western medicine exist side by side, the individual would use the traditional system until he suffered an acute illness, and only in extreme distress would he resort to Western chemotherapy. In reality this is not the case. Chinese medicine abandoned its preventive character long ago, and has joined in senseless competition with Western medicine; and patients in Taiwan are as impatient as those in other modern industrial states, and have no wish to submit to protracted medical treatment. They hope that by taking a few pills they can have a rapid recovery from every disease.

The non-supervised parallel existence of two medical systems endangers the welfare of patients by stressing self-diagnosis by laymen. A layman does not know whether his malady can be cured by traditional methods which use drugs supported by remedial techniques that require a long period to take effect. He could avoid chemotherapy with all its side-effects and the influence of foreign substances on the organism if he resorted to traditional therapy, but he must himself decide whether his illness is so severe that it can only be treated by a doctor with Western training who will use chemotherapy or surgery. The decision about which system to turn to does not lie with an expert who after an exact examination stipulates phytotherapy or chemotherapy. Not infrequently, a layman will avoid Western medicine through misunderstanding and prejudice. Yet the traditional practitioner he consults may not be capable of properly diagnosing his illness.

Diagnosis is the weakest link in the traditional system, and very few practitioners today master even a reasonable proportion of what is required of them. Thus, precious time may be lost in a serious illness before the patient realizes that the treatment he is receiving is not helping him, and goes to another traditional physician or to a Western-style doctor.

On the other hand, patients will go to a Western-trained doctor with a mild digestive ailment or insomnia. They are then treated quite unnecessarily with chemotherapeutica. The result may often be headaches and stomach complaints, among other things, for people with a low irritant level for these foreign substances. What is more, patients of the modern doctor are soon raised to a level of insensibility which the mild traditional drugs that are efficacious for everyday ailments would not induce. These patients then find themselves irrevocably in the clutches of Western medicine.

Medical care in Germany and some other European societies presents the opposite picture. Here, too, a wealth of drugs were handed down through the centuries, many of them with very effective components. However, the development of chemotherapy emanated from the same people who had the monopoly of traditional medicines, so that the traditional German system, as an example, was enriched from the center outward by chemotherapy. In this system, new understanding and possibilities of treatment were assimilated without a break in the training of doctors and chemists. Traditional drugs and modern chemotherapeutica are all used within one medical system, and the decision about which type of treatment is applied rests with the specialist, the doctor.

THE POSITION OF WESTERN MEDICINE IN TAIWAN

In 1969 Taiwan imported the equivalent of 13 million American dollars' worth of Western medicines. There were approximately 700 registered legal manufacturers of pharmaceutical preparations on the island. Western medicine was represented in the city of Taipei, which had a population of 1,700,000 people in 1970, by 1,862 doctors, 1,090 pharmacies that stocked Western medicines, and 737 trained pharmacists (Taipei City Health Bureau 1970). In addition to the legally registered pharmacies, numerous unlicensed retail shops sell Western medicines, as do many traditional druggists.

No statistics were available for rural districts, but our observations and inquiries indicated that shops for Western medicines were much more numerous than those for traditional drugs. In one village, which was said to have about 2,000 inhabitants and was about forty miles from the city of Tainan, we counted 14 Western-supplied chemists and 4 traditional druggists. We often found villages with less than 2,000 inhabitants that lacked any traditional pharmacy but had one or two shops for modern medicines. We never encountered a place with traditional druggists but no Western-oriented pharmacy.

When we ask who represents Western medicine to the population, we must mention the relatively small group of foreign missionary doctors who work in Christian and other hospitals. They or their institutions are often known over a wide area. The Christian Clinic in Taipei, for example, is a reputable institution that attracts patients from many parts of the island. But the most numerous and influential representatives of modern science to the common people are Chinese physicians trained in Western medicine. Since the 1920's, when Western-educated doctors were concerned in the struggles of *jen-sheng-kuan* or *k'e-hsueh* (philosophy of life versus science), Western medicine has been a synonym for "science." The prestige of science is so great in the popular culture of Taiwan that practitioners of Chinese medicine attempt to attain equal status with Western medicine by trying to prove that the traditional system is also scientific (Unschuld 1973).

This faith in "science" involves a belief in miracles, so that patients expect doctors of Western medicine to produce clearly visible successes as rapidly as possible. To meet this expectation, many doctors take great pains to make their successes public. This may take the form of photographs showing the naked bosom of a young woman before and after plastic surgery, or showing all the phases of an operation for hemorrhoids in color and more than life-size. It may also take the form of a collection of bottles in which the development of the fetus is shown, along with miscarriages and deformed cases from the physician's own practice. Expectant mothers look at these bottles in Chinese maternity clinics, and are persuaded that the doctor treating them is skillful.

Rapid results are necessary for the doctor to maintain his "scientific image" and to keep patients from seeking relief from another doctor. The custom of changing doctors after a short time, if dissatisfied with his therapy, is widespread, and can be historically documented for earlier centuries. Two possible courses of action may be followed to achieve rapid cures. One consists of using rapidly-acting antibiotics, spasmolytics, and analgesics. The utilization of this possibility is reflected in the high volume of imports of these drugs. A second possibility consists in giving the patient a false diagnosis, to persuade him that he has a disastrous illness. Thus, patients may wrongly be told their pains or swellings of the stomach or breast indicate cancer. If the illness is treated successfully, the doctor may claim to be a great therapist. If the patients of such doctors do become dissatisfied and resort to traditional physicians, then these curers may later point to their letters of thanks for a successful cure, together with an attached diagnosis of cancer by a Western doctor.

As an aside, it should be pointed out that modern doctors in Taiwan acquire their knowledge to a large extent from American books. It is our firm belief that the study of medicine in a foreign language but in one's own language environment must have a negative effect on the standard of training. Other questions about their cultural position, besides those of language, arise for indigenous practitioners of Western medicine in many third-world countries. A problem for further research will be to investigate the degree to which the practitioner's medical concepts are influenced by the categories of his own tradition.

A third group of people representing Western medicine to laymen in Taiwan are workers in shops for Western medicines; and a final group is composed of traditional chemists who also sell Western medicines. In Taipei alone, no trained pharmacists are available in approximately 250 of the registered Western pharmacies. Completely untrained personnel, without any apparent restrictions except for opiates and narcotics, sell Western drugs in both the licensed shops of traditional chemists and the countless unlicensed shops. We visited these shops to ask for sun cream and were given cortisone ointments; we affected illness and after two or three questions were confidently diagnosed and recommended some kind of medicine. In the shop of a traditional chemist who illegally sold Western medicines, we observed a hospital-sized pack of a drug used with great caution by Western doctors to treat rheumatism, which in Germany can only be obtained on prescription. The proprietor of this pharmacy asked us, since we were Europeans, whether he was right to use it as a remedy for coughs and colds, instructing the sick person to take one tablet every four hours for several weeks.

Newspaper articles reported that the market was flooded by drugs illegally produced in Taiwan under the name of Western medicines, but containing no effective constituents. The government halted this practice, but unsuitable handling and storage damages the efficacy of many chemotherapeutica. Only a few registered chemists and scarcely a single illegal one are fully air-conditioned and can offer perishable drugs the conditions of storage they require. Remedies that sell well are displayed in glass cases in the blazing sun. The printed English instructions "Store in a cool place" cannot save them.

The first drug law came into force in 1970, to eliminate the abuses we describe; but we did not have an opportunity to observe its effects.

THE POSITION OF THE
TRADITIONAL CHINESE SYSTEM OF HEALING

Approximately 3,000 registered practitioners and 7,300 traditional pharmacies served Taiwan's population of 14 million people in 1970. The city of Taipei had 348 registered Chinese medicine practitioners and 515 traditional pharmacies.[2] Four distinct groups of doctors use traditional drugs or therapy: Some doctors consider medicine to be their main profession. A second group consists of government officials, businessmen, and others who possess a few effective formulae handed down in their families, or who have some knowledge from reading about Chinese medicine in their spare time— these people may demand high prices, or they may treat people without charge, especially their kinsmen and friends. The third group consists of so-called druggist-doctors, traditional chemists who claim to have accumulated knowledge through practical experience in their shops, and who may write prescriptions themselves. The fourth group is composed of itinerant traders who extol the virtues of individual remedies at festivals or other gatherings. The first three groups claim to represent the traditional Chinese medical system and its theories, while the fourth group has only marginal influence on medical care.

The education of professional practitioners was begun by the China Medical College in Taichung in 1958, with the aim of training doctors to be equally proficient in both Chinese and modern medicine. This aim was later modified, and at the time of our visit in 1970 a department of traditional medicine with approximately 200 students existed alongside a department of Western medicine with 700 students. Many of the teachers were experts in their fields, but most of the traditional practitioners we interviewed had a negative opinion of the school. One of the chief criticisms was that traditional doctors trained there lacked practical experience.

Another way of being trained in Chinese medicine was to become the pupil of a good doctor, learning the theory from him and gaining experience in his

2 The exact numbers were received from the Taipei City Health Bureau. The approximate numbers are from the National Druggists Association and National Physicians Association.

practice. But few members of historical chains of traditional practice reside in Taiwan today, and this is prerequisite to being a good doctor. So many pupils flock to the few good teachers that they must be taught in classes, and the tradition of individual instruction suffers. Self-instruction forms a large part of the training of traditional doctors in Taiwan. These autodidacts search for remedies for certain diseases in the old texts, and attempt to acquire knowledge of diagnosis from the sections on treating diseases according to their symptoms.

It may be doubted whether more than a very few traditional doctors in Taiwan can be called true representatives of a theory-based level of traditional Chinese medicine. Such a representative should have mastered the theories of *wu-hsing* and *yin-yang* and their relevance for classical physiology. He should have the classical diagnostic skills, which include forecasting illness. He should use drugs by referring to the ancient theoretical pharmacology, and he should have practical experience.

It is extremely difficult, if not impossible, to achieve a deep understanding of the old theories, to say nothing of diagnosis, by self-instruction. The classical texts are fully comprehensible to very few scholars. Even graduates of the China Medical College whom we met in Taichung were unable to explain the classical sections on pharmacology. The theory alone, even supposing someone can understand it, is not a sufficient medical training without the clinical experience which relates it to the practical side of medicine. This experience must be accumulated and handed down through generations. Only a sustained line of people who have had the meaning of the old texts made clear to them, who have had diagnosis explained to them in a lengthy process that combines theory with personal experience, and who have inherited the long experience of their predecessors, may truly be said to represent the traditional art of theory-based Chinese medicine. Those who try to force their way into this system from outside are powerless to do more than select cures for certain illnesses out of old books of remedies. In the process, it is quite likely that they will become victims of terminological confusion. They might, for example, find remedies in the texts for a *kan* disease, which today means a disease of the liver, but which were intended to be used in cases of madness. In the classical understanding of medicine, the term *kan* conveyed something quite different from its meaning today.

Diagnostic skills cannot be of a high standard when they are self-taught through reading texts which describe how to cure illness according to the symptoms. Many traditional doctors assert that although Chinese drugs are better than Western medicines because they have no side-effects, the Western methods of diagnosis are more exact. They therefore want to diagnose illnesses by means of Western apparatus, and then cure them by traditional methods. We consider this to be largely impossible. There are simply no terminological bridges to connect the system of modern medical diagnosis to the traditional Chinese conceptions of therapy. If we observe what happens in traditional practice today when drugs are prescribed according to the symptoms, it is often a kind of phytotherapy such as is also used in Germany. The claims of the traditional system of healing are accordingly largely untrue, and cannot be supported by objective study of contemporary practices.

To be sure, non theory-based forms of traditional Chinese medicine have existed alongside theory-based traditional Chinese medicine all the time of the latter's long history. Medical practice outside the theoretical framework has probably even formed the major part of health care in imperial China; the bequest of the Yellow Emperor as the alleged founder of theoretical Chinese medicine has most likely guarded the health of only some small proportion of the upper class in old China, and this proportion may have further shrinked under the impact of this century's changes.

However, the justification for traditional Chinese medicine to survive as a separate system today and in the future is entirely based on its theoretical claims. Effective drugs and useful techniques could easily—and this has often been the case—be integrated into a modern health care delivery system, even without understanding how they work. It is the theory which cannot be integrated and forms the bastion of defence by traditional Chinese practitioners and some Western scholars to keep traditional Chinese medicine separately alive. We feel that Chinese medicine should survive in a modern health care delivery system in effective drugs and treatments and, more important, in basic concepts like the indivisibility of body and mind, to mention only one example. These are not incompatible with Western medicine, in fact they should act as stimuli to Western medicine to abandon certain biases and to find its way back to comprehensive care.

THE INTERACTION OF THE TWO SYSTEMS

The two systems have influenced one another. We have mentioned that many traditional doctors use Western methods and aids to diagnosis. The measuring of temperature and blood pressure, X-rays, and blood, stool, and urine tests are carried out partly by the traditional doctors themselves, and partly in the laboratories of friends. We also found that highly efficacious Western medicines were on rare occasions used by traditional practitioners. While many traditional doctors and pharmacists complained that the market for traditional medicine was going downhill because more and more people were turning to Western drugs, a smaller number insisted happily that trade was growing again as people became disillusioned by Western medicine and returned to the Chinese system. Druggists said that they had incorporated Western medicines into their collections when their sale of traditional medicine declined. And they obviously believed that far less knowledge was necessary when selling Western medicines than when selling traditional drugs. Often the instructions for use are printed on the box, so that they only have to sell it.

One handicap for traditionalists has been the inconvenience of administering their preparations. The usual method is by *t'ang* decoction, which normally takes fifteen to twenty minutes and is usually done at home. In contrast, modern pills or drops can be taken quickly and unobtrusively. Several firms in Taiwan now manufacture soluble powders, or special products with traditional drugs as a base, but of Western appearance. These medicines are advertised as "Chinese drugs with all the benefits of modern science."

We have already described the most far-reaching change in the Chinese medical system caused by its competition with Western medicine, and this is the transfer of attention away from its real task of prevention to that of treating illness. This, together with the kind of phytotherapy we have described, means the greatest possible alienation from and adulteration of the theoretical claims of classical Chinese medicine.

The practice of Western medicine has not remained untouched by traditional influence, though very few doctors with Western training show any interest in traditional drugs, quite apart from the traditional methods of diagnosis and treatment. The great majority of them regard everything connected with the old system as "quack medicine." They refuse to recognize the healing qualities of herbal medicines. Yet in a traditional manner, the patient who buys tablets from a Western chemist will take only a day's supply. In the traditional system, only a day's supply is prescribed, except in chronic illness.

Another habit which has been passed on from the traditional system is the reliance on experience. The untrained personnel in many chemist shops have no scientific knowledge, yet without hesitating they use whatever experience they have. The chemist who prescribed the strong rheumatism drug as a cold cure did so because a customer had assured him that his cough disappeared when he took the remedy. Another traditional chemist near Taipei, who said that he was forced to incorporate more and more Western medicines into his stock because his shop was in a very small village, had developed a system for testing the effects of these drugs. According to the meager information he gained from sales representatives or from leaflets, he prepared compounds of Western medicines or sold them individually. He then asked his customers to describe the effects. These accounts both guided his future action and raised the level of his experience.

THE ATTITUDE OF THE PUBLIC
TOWARD THE TWO MEDICAL SYSTEMS

To analyze the attitude of the public, we used questionnaires and also conducted individual interviews with 250 college and university students in Taipei and among 60 rural people in the southern part of the island, near Taiwan.[3]

3 The surveys were conducted in the spring of 1970. In Taipei we used 17 questions to interview 250 college and university students—all between 20 and 26 years old, from middle-class families, and from various localities. The people interviewed in the south all lived in a village with about 2,000 inhabitants. These employees of a rural cooperative association and various other villagers were interviewed by indigenous assistants, to avoid the notion that respondents would try to appear to Westerners in a better light by reporting more "scientific behavior" than they actually practiced.

TABLE 1

Resort to Western and Traditional Chinese Medical Systems Indicated
By College Students, Workers and Peasants in Response to a Survey
Questionnaire in Taiwan, 1970
(in percentages)

	250 students in Taipei	60 workers and peasants in the south
First call on the Western medical system	31.1	63.8
First call on the Traditional Chinese system	0.8	—
Resort to both, but predominantly Western	46.4	28.4
Resort to both equally	17.8	7.3
Resort to both, but predominantly Chinese	3.6	—

Table 1 shows the response to one question: "When someone in your family is ill and outside help is needed, do you first call on the Western medical system, the traditional system, or both at the same time?"

In contrast to the widely-held opinion that traditional medicine is particularly deep-rooted in the rural areas, our finding was that it is less popular there than in the city. Besides the influence of the Japanese policy of suppressing Chinese medical practice, other far more influential factors explain the popularity of Western medicine. A basic reason for resorting to Western medicine is that it is more effective than traditional medicine for treating trachoma, diphtheria, typhoid, and numerous other acute and childhood diseases. Also, an overwhelming proportion of television advertising in Taiwan is for Western medicines. The largest amount is commissioned by Japanese companies. In Japan itself, these pharmaceutical firms have created, largely by advertising, the highest per capita consumption of medicines in the world. And advertisements for medicines from Europe and the U.S.A. are so successful that in Taipei 60 percent of the people we interviewed were able to name straightaway one or more manufacturers of American or European drugs.

The relative cost of Chinese and Western medicine is another basic factor influencing patient's decisions to use them. Apart from the enormous cost of hospital treatment—no hospital for traditional therapy exists in Taiwan as yet—it is not clear that therapy in one or other of the two systems will be more expensive. This uncertainty was expressed by respondents in Taipei; 35 percent held that Western medicine was generally more expensive, 20 percent considered the traditional methods to be generally more expensive, and 37 percent were undecided. Comments revealed highly differentiated opinions. For example, the costs of diagnosis and of kinds of therapy were distinguished. Diagnoses by Western doctors were stated to be generally more expensive than those of traditional physicians. Tonics and the treatment for asthma were said to be more expensive in the traditional system. In fact, the normal costs for a traditional medication in a Taipei shop is between 20 and 30 NTD (40 NTD = one U.S. dollar); in the country it averages 25 percent cheaper. If the patient asks for a tonic—and tonics are used throughout the winter as a surviving preventive characteristic from the earlier Chinese medical system—he will pay considerably more: a tonic may cost 50 to 100, and not infrequently 200 to 300, NTD. It must be remembered that a one-day supply is involved, so that the cost rises proportionately as treatment is repeated.

The society of Traditional Doctors advises its members to charge 20 NTD for each examination and prescription, and half this amount from soldiers and policemen. Poor people are supposed to be treated without charge. A home visit usually costs 100 NTD. These rates represent the low fees, however. Acupuncture treatment by a well-known doctor would cost more. Yet the traditional idea that medicine should be practiced whenever possible without charge is remembered by physicians and laymen. One famous doctor of acupuncture makes a gesture toward this ideal by charging no more than 50 NTD for acupuncture therapy, but varying the fee for the medicine he prescribes as part of the treatment from 20 to as much as 800 NTD, according to his estimate of the patient's means.

As a rule, resort to the traditional medical system involves a doctor's examination; resort to Western medicine may simply be to a pharmacy, following the recommendations of advertisements. The pharmacist is very willing to give advice, and the patient may select medicines according to his own diagnosis and the pharmacist's recommendations. In this way, patients avoid expensive consultations with doctors of Western medicine, and themselves try out various Western medicines to form their own opinions about their efficacy.

The population is encouraged to move toward Western medicine by state health insurance policies, which exclude the therapies of traditional Chinese medicine. Approximately 790,000 workers in Taiwan pay social insurance contributions. Civil servants and employees in public services receive assistance in the case of illness. Relatives are included when costly hospitalization is required for a member of the worker's immediate family. But the only therapy provided to state employees or by insurance programs is through personnel and institutions of the Western medical system.

A common behavior pattern according to the ideas we have just described proceeds in the following manner. When resort to outside help in treating illness seems desirable, the first resort will be to a Western pharmacy to try out a few highly advertised medicines. If these do not help, the person goes to a Western-trained doctor for treatment. Perhaps after only one, but usually after two or three trials of the doctor's therapy which seem to the patient to have had no effect, the force of tradition takes over and the patient begins changing doctors as often as possible. We found this ancient custom practiced by nearly 44 percent of the students we interviewed, and by 75 percent of those interviewed in country districts. This custom is explained by comments such as "You have to change doctors frequently to discover which one can help, so that you can remain with him." This is the reverse of the German ideal of relying on one doctor from childhood to old age, so that the physician knows his patient thoroughly. In China the doctor and patient traditionally expect to be complete strangers.

Apart from dissatisfaction with the physician's treatment, patients change from one doctor to another because they feel ill but are diagnosed to be well. The Chinese people are very concerned with their physical condition, which includes everything from extremely intensive cosmetic care to personal hygiene. Patients often come to a doctor with apparently trivial or non-existent illnesses. This may be a consequence of being trained in the preventive medical thought of the Chinese system. In these cases, placebo treatment has been adopted by many Western-style doctors. At least, this is how they explain their excessively high consumption of solvents for antibiotic injections. Finally, women go to traditional practitioners more frequently than men. Two-thirds of their patients were women—which fact one elderly doctor accounted for by saying that a women's build is more complicated, and therefore more susceptible to illness.

Thus, patients travel from one doctor to another, and from one system to another. In the case of certain diseases, however, set patterns have developed. Western medicine is allegedly unable to cure a cold. The term "one-hundred-day cold" is the name which modern doctors are said to have invented for an incurable illness which traditional doctors are supposed to cure without difficulty. Western medicine is always resorted to for acute, serious illness, while traditional medicine is said to work well for rheumatism and gynecological complaints. Painful diseases and surgery are put in the hands of Western practice; but bone damage, high blood pressure, and diseases of the liver and kidneys, as examples, are allegedly in safer keeping in traditional hands. Doctors who rely mainly on acupuncture are considered to be experts in the treatment of rheumatic complaints and nervous diseases.

CONCLUSIONS

After this very condensed study of the medical system in Taiwan, we can recognize the following problems: We do not find in Taiwan a full system of traditional medicine, nor a full system of Western medicine. This may be attributed to the standards of training and to lax legislation. The existence of two systems side by side is not advantageous to the population at large, although nearly everyone we interviewed wanted to keep both systems in the future. This is due to their experience that advantages are to be found in both systems, while they cannot imagine any alternative to or synthesis of the two existing systems.

A glance at the latest developments in Mainland China shows that there, too, similar problems have had to be contended with. The number of trained Western doctors was too small to provide care for the whole population. The number of traditional doctors was large enough, but the Communists did not want to entrust the care of the population to them. The mutual integration of both systems was doomed to failure, for reasons which we have indicated: despite the claims of traditional physicians, there are no terminological bridges to link the categories of modern diagnoses to traditional Chinese forms of philosophy related therapy.

In the last few years, a new kind of practitioner has been developed in Mainland China: the so-called "barefoot doctor." He has been equipped with many ideological accessories by Communist China, and was described in the West in many contemptuous articles until recently. If we look at what the barefoot doctor represents, however, we find that an earlier attempt to integrate the Chinese and Western medical systems on the level of fully trained physicians has been abandoned and replaced, instead, by cooperation. On a primary care level, however, young people who are free from the traditional patterns of thought are now being trained. They are instructed in Western methods of diagnosis and in the use of efficacious traditional drugs. They are trained to examine patients and to treat harmless cases by means of phytotherapy and simple chemotherapy. They must have a sufficient sense of responsibility to refer cases which they cannot cure to fully qualified doctors without dangerous delays. Even so, fully-trained doctors are relieved of part of their burden. Barefoot doctors also help to educate the population in matters of hygiene. In this way, the excellent Chinese techniques of acupuncture, dietetics, and massage, and some effective drugs, are not sacrificed.

In addition, through the barefoot doctors, the use of expensive and possibly harmful chemotherapeutica in treating a wide range of illnesses has become unnecessary. The import of such drugs places a heavy burden on foreign exchange in countries of the third world. Perhaps this new type of doctor can serve as a model for countries which have their own reserves of efficacious drugs to fall back on, but which suffer from a deficiency of highly qualified physicians. This new type of doctor possesses some knowledge of Western diagnosis and uses the old effective drugs and healing techniques of his own country, yet he is free from the ballast of traditional terminology. Even more important seems to be the fact that the barefoot doctors are peasant workers in the first place; this implies that they remain with their people and cannot be subject to brain drain from rural to urban areas and from less to highly industrialized countries.

As the feldshers are gradually replaced in the Soviet Union by fully trained physicians now, it is likely that the barefoot doctors will become superfluous at some time in future. The tendency goes toward the construction of one integrated medical system, possibly structured in levels of primary, secondary, and tertiary care but based on one single body of knowledge. The ecology of medical practice seems to be quite similar in many countries of the southern hemisphere. It is the differences in health politics which account for the variation as to how difficulties are conceived and dealt with.

Literature Cited

Chen Chan Yuen
    1968 *History of Chinese Medical Science Illustrated with Pictures.* Hongkong: Hsiang-kang Shang-hai yin-shu-kuan.
Croizier, Ralph C.
    1968 *Traditional Medicine in Modern China: Science, Nationalism, and the Tensions of Cultural Change.* Cambridge: Harvard University Press.
Okanishi, Tameto
    1964 *Ch'ung-chi Hsin-hsiu pen-ts'ao.* (*A scientific Reproduction of the* Hsin-hsiu pen-ts'ao *from 659* A.D.). Taipei: Kuo-li chung-kuo i-yao yen-chiu suo.
Taipei City Health Bureau
    1970 *Public Health in Taipei.*
Unschuld, Paul U.
    1973 *Die Praxis des traditionellen chinesischen Heilsystems—dargestellt unter Einschluß der Pharmazie an der heutigen Situation auf Taiwan.* Wiesbaden: F. Steiner Verlag.

PART VI

Medical Revivalism

F ROM THE Renaissance to the present day, the world has been awash with
revival movements. They occur in virtually all spheres of activity—in
art, religion, the family, language, politics—wherever people desire to reform
their lives. A vast literature describes incidents of such movements, ranging
from the enthusiastic religious cults anthropologists study in tribal societies
to nationalistic revivals that affect the highly differentiated institutions of
complex societies.

Medical revivalism in China and India is clearly an aspect of cultural
nationalism in these societies. However, Dr. Yasuo Otsuka's essay on Japan
in the present section does not suggest that medical revivalism is related to
Japanese nationalism—and since it is Chinese medicine that is being revived,
this is understandable. Earlier in the present volume, J. Christoph Bürgel
reasoned that medicine played little role in the revival movements of Islamic
countries—except in South Asia, where it has symbolic value in contrast
to Hindu and Buddhist revivals of Āyurveda—because it is called "Greek
medicine," and thus clearly labeled as a foreign import.

Dr. Otsuka's essay provides a valuable beginning for this section, not only
because the existence of medical revivalism in Japan is not as well known
to the outside world as that of China and India, but also because it may
correct an inclination to overemphasize the nationalistic aspects of medical
revivalism in those countries. Medical revivals are movements to correct
perceived faults in the existing forms of education and care. Thus, they are
modes for professionalizing traditional practice, and should be understood
as sociological as well as cultural phenomena.

The professionalization of occupations is a long-term process transforming
the organization of work in modern societies. It involves the creation of new
institutional arrangements to cultivate technical knowledge, train workers
with special skills, regulate standards of practice, exclude the unqualified,
and improve the status of qualified practitioners. In Western society these
activities were initiated by associations that originated in medieval guilds
and universities, but great advances were not achieved until the Industrial

319

Revolution (Carr-Saunders and Wilson 1933:295). As the effects of industrialization spread through the world, changes in economic, political, and educational structures alter the division of labor, creating new jobs and elaborating the technical competence of traditional occupations. Scientific work, in particular, acquires new significance for the rest of society, and medical practitioners gain respect as they are progressively more successful in applying scientific knowledge to alleviate individual suffering.

We learn in the following pages that in Japan during the eighteenth century, a revival movement known as the Kohoha school advocated "classicism in medicine" through return to the empirical, clinical spirit of Chang Chung-ching's ancient text on fever. This revival occurred while the country maintained an almost complete social isolation, but responded to new scientific knowledge from the West. By encouraging the acquisition of new knowledge and a skeptical approach to traditional concepts, this revival movement in Chinese medicine prepared the intellectual climate in which cosmopolitan medicine was made the only state-supported form of legal practice during the nineteenth century.

A second revival movement in Chinese medicine gained momentum in Japan after the Second World War. Earlier in this volume, William Caudill illustrated how closely "traditional medicine in Japan is tied to the everyday ideas and feelings of people." This relationship may facilitate the contemporary revival; for, according to Caudill, "traditional medicine and general cultural belief blend into one another, and both are strongly influenced by very old ideas stemming from Shintoistic and Buddhistic thought about the position of man in the environment." Dr. Otsuka, a leading practitioner and scholar of the revival, records that most users of Chinese medicine in Japan belong to the middle class, and that two-thirds of them are women. This fact deserves comparative study. Middle-class women are said to be the main clients for "irregular" health practices in other industrial countries where cosmopolitan medicine is preeminent. Their interests in herbal medicines, health foods, Christian Science, and so on, may indicate that women are more conscious of the dehumanizing effects of bureaucratic cosmopolitan medical practice than other categories of people in these societies, and in a better position to utilize alternative forms of health care. Although the revival of Chinese medicine in Japan does not have the nationalistic resonance of medical revivalism in China and India, its advocates criticize the monopoly of state support for cosmopolitan medicine and the technological orientation that neglects the pastoral functions of medical care. The revival stands symbolically and practically for the humanization of medical practice.

The essays on China and India by Ralph Croizier, Brahmananda Gupta, and myself describe revival movements that have gained considerable attention in recent years. Medical revivalism began in China as a middle-class movement in the 1920's and '30's, and it has been turned to revolutionary ends by the Communists. In both its early and present phases, it inculcates cultural pride in opposition to the humiliation of Western imperialism. But as a revolutionary revival, it is being used for drastic changes in the social order. It symbolizes the new egalitarian ethos based on folk and popular culture traditions. It is used to humble the pride of "experts" who claim professional autonomy to make decisions that affect the welfare of laymen. And it symbolizes the pastoral functions of medicine, which make it a calling to serve humanity rather than a self-serving career. Medical revivalism in China is a fundamental ingredient in a radical program of modernization that seeks to use the resources of indigenous medicine in creating a comprehensive system of health care.

The medical revival in India resembles the bourgeois phase of the movement in China, except that it began in the first quarter of the nineteenth century and thus has a longer and more complex history. By the time of independence, it had built a much larger infrastructure of professional institutions than existed in China; yet, since it has never been the instrument of a strong governmental health policy, it has evolved in a pluralistic context of competing interest groups (Brass 1973). In doing so, it has created a dual system of professionalized medicine in which the Āyurvedic and Yunānī practitioners and their institutions are in an ambiguous paraprofessional relationship to cosmopolitan medicine.

Movements to revive and professionalize Asian medicine exist in Pakistan, Sri Lanka, Burma, Korea, and perhaps other Asian countries, but they have not been studied. They may not have had the consequences in these countries that they have had in eighteenth-century Japan, or in contemporary China and India, where they have played a fundamental role in transforming medical systems. We do not know. Future research on medical revivalism in Asian societies will extend and deepen our knowledge of the processes by which modern forms of knowledge and professional organization are related to ancient scientific modes of thought.

CHARLES LESLIE

Literature Cited

Brass, Paul
    1973 "The Politics of Ayurvedic Education: A Case Study of Revivalism and Modernization in India," in Lloyd and Susanne Rudolph, eds., *Politics and Education in India*. Cambridge: Harvard University Press.
Carr-Saunders, A. M., and P. A. Wilson
    1933 *The Professions*. Oxford: Clarendon Press.

Chinese Traditional Medicine in Japan

YASUO OTSUKA

The medical sciences made great progress in Japan during the 1950's and 1960's. Many new drugs were developed and brought into use, including new antibiotics, hormone preparations, and psychotropic drugs. It may therefore sound strange that Kanpo medicine, Chinese traditional medicine in Japan, has gained increasing strength parallel with the development of modern medicine. I believe that this phenomenon has three causes:

1. *The increasing incidence of serious side-effects from synthetic drugs*
Kanpo medicine uses only crude drugs or crude extracts from them, and most of these drugs have been used for more than a thousand years. People are convinced that they are relatively secure from the adverse effects of chemo-therapy.

2. *The analytic nature of modern medicine*
Increasing knowledge and the division of labor have separated medical practice into ever-smaller divisions. Thus, internal medicine has been divided into cardiology, neurology, hematology, etc. This tendency comes from the fundamental character of modern medicine's relationship to basic scientific research. But in clinical practice, a patient is ill always as a whole body. In Kanpo medicine, a patient is always examined and treated as a whole body, even if he suffers from a nose or eye disease. Abdominal palpation is indispensable, for example, in a case of ear disease.

3. *Disregard of patients' complaints in modern medicine*
The greatest interest for physicians of modern medicine tends to be the cause and nature of the disease. The biopsy represents this tendency. The complaints of patients are less interesting; they will often claim, "Every doctor says that I am healthy. But I really suffer." In Kanpo medical practice, the cause and nature of the disease are relatively unimportant, while the complaints of the patient are highly important. In modern medicine, the basic sciences have made great progress, but the therapeutics remain rather poor. In Kanpo medicine the reverse is true.

322

HISTORY OF CHINESE TRADITIONAL MEDICINE IN CHINA

Manfred Porkert's essay in the present volume outlines the history of Chinese medicine, but I would like to review this history briefly to provide a background for my discussion of the medico-historical relationship between China and Japan.

The oldest and most important medical text is *Huang-ti nei ching* (*The Yellow Emperor's Classic of Internal Medicine*). The author is not known, but the text was presumably written in the course of the last two centuries B.C. This work considered anatomy, physiology, hygiene, and the basic knowledge of acupuncture and moxibustion, but treatment with drugs was less frequently described.

Materia medica was called *Pên t'sao* (*Honzo* in Japanese pronunciation), which means "nature of plants." The oldest text on this subject, *Shen-nung pên t'sao ching* (*Materia Medica of Shen-nung*), was also by an unknown author and seems to have been written before 220 A.D. This book described 365 drugs and classified them in three ranks: the upper-rank drugs number 120, and were said to nourish life; the 120 middle-rank drugs were supposed to nourish nature; and the 125 lower-rank drugs cured disease. I believe the mode of thought in this classification is inherently Chinese (Otsuka 1968). For the Chinese, who were interested primarily in man, drugs should be valued according to their effects on human beings. Whether or not one of them belonged to the vegetable kingdom was relatively unimportant. The Occident was different—Dioscorides, for instance, classified drugs according to their botanical nature.

Besides these two works, *Shang han lun* (*Treatise on Shang han*, a typhoid-like acute febrile disease) was one of the most important and influential medical texts in ancient China. The author of this work was Chang Chung-ching, and the date of issue is thought to be about 200 A.D. Chang Chung-ching also wrote *Chin kuei yao lüeh* (*Important Prescriptions Worth Treasuring in the Golden Chamber*). This work classified different kinds of diseases according to their chief symptoms.

Shang han lun described the whole process of the disease in six stages: T'ai-yang, Shao-yang, Yang-ming, T'ai-yin, Shao-yin, and Chüeh-yin. The first three categories belong to Yang, while the others belong to Yin. *Yang* means sunny, bright, hot, dry, positive, active, acute, etc. *Yin* means shadowy, dark, cold, wet, negative, passive, chronic, etc. Regarding the human body, the surface belongs to Yang and the inside to Yin. Among the inside organs, the hollow organs belong to Yang and the parenchymatous organs to Yin. Yang and Yin are relative notions; there are neither absolute Yang nor absolute Yin. If a person has caught a cold and has a high fever and a strong headache, he should be treated as a patient in Yang-state. But if another patient has caught a cold and has no remarkable symptoms or complaints except a slight loss of appetite, he may be in Yin-state.

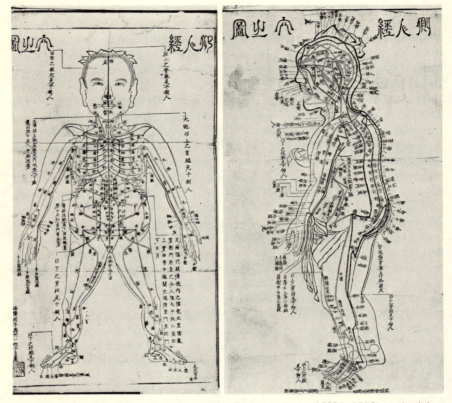

PLATE 1. A set of meridian charts drawn by Okamoto Ippo (1655?–1716), a physician of the Goseiha school.

A *T'ai-yang* state is one in which hot-natured reactions take place at the outside region of the body—that is, headache, fever, or chilliness. A *Shao-yang* state is one in which hot-natured reactions take place in the half-outside-and-half-inside region—that is, vertigo, nausea, or loss of appetite. A *Yang-ming* state is one in which hot-natured reactions take place in the inside region—that is, continuous fever, constipation, or delirium. In these three Yang states the power of body resistance is superior to the power of disease—in T'ai-yang to the highest degree, then in Shao-yang and in Yang-ming to the lowest.

The three Yin states—*T'ai-yin*, *Shao-yin*, and *Chüeh-yin*—are those in which cold-natured reactions take place in the inside region of the body—that is, diarrhea, abdominal pain, coldness of extremities, or sleepiness. In these three Yin states, the power of body resistance is inferior to that of disease—in T'ai-yin to the lowest degree, then in Shao-yin and in Chüeh-yin to the highest.

Thus the body is grossly divided into three parts—the outside (*Piao*), the half-outside-and-half-inside (*Han piao han li*), and the inside (*Li*). Roughly speaking, the outside contains skin and neighboring tissues, the inside contains the digestive system, and the half-outside-and-half-inside contains organs between the outside and the inside.

Shang han lun contains 113 prescriptions, and *Chin kuei yao lüeh* contains 262. A great many of these prescriptions are still effectively used, so that these two works are not only important classics for medical historians but also indispensable textbooks for contemporary medical practitioners.

The greatest change in the history of medicine in China occurred after the fall of the Northern Sung dynasty in 1127 A.D. Ch'êng Wu-i was the first who advocated that *Shang han lun* should be reorganized with the logic of *Huang-ti nei ching*. His theory was set forth in *Chu chieh shang han lun* (*A Commentary on Shang han lun*), published in 1172, and in *Shang han ming li lun* (*Logic of Shang han lun*), published in 1157. It has been thought that *Shang han lun* and *Huang-ti nei ching* were formed on a different basis and represented two different schools of medicine: *Shang han lun* was above all a practical textbook of pharmacotherapeutics; it contained few philosophical and speculative expressions. *Huang-ti nei ching* was, in contrast, full of philosophical or speculative expressions. It contained the basic knowledge of acupuncture and moxibustion, but only a few fragments on pharmacotherapeutics.

Ch'êng Wu-i tried to combine these two classics and the different sorts of Chinese therapeutics they represented, pharmacotherapy and acupuncture–moxibustion. His followers came to think that each drug had a selective effect on one or more meridians. As for the five elements theory, *Shang han lun* is scarcely influenced by this speculative logic, while *Huang-ti nei ching* is largely influenced by it. Ch'êng Wu-i and his followers made use of this theory to explain pharmacology. The aim of their medical reformation was to rearrange the highly extended content of medical knowledge by inductive reasoning. But the whole process of this reformation was laden with speculative thought.

China's twelfth-century medical reformation occurred in the field of pharmacotherapeutics and did not succeed, while Europe's in the sixteenth century occurred in the field of anatomy, and succeeded. Here we see again a difference between these two civilizations (Otsuka 1970a).

A school of physicians followed Ch'êng Wu-i and flourished in the Chin (1115–1234) and Yüan (1271–1368) dynasties. The school of Chin–Yüan medicine had a great influence on Japanese medicine after the sixteenth century. Medicine of the Ming (1368–1662) and Ch'ing (1662–1911) dynasties was generally a continuation of Chin–Yüan medicine.

CHINESE MEDICINE IN JAPAN

The history of Chinese traditional medicine in Japan can be divided into the following five periods:

1. Early period (6th–15th century): from faithful imitation to the first attempt to attain independence.
2. Goseiha school (16th–19th century): the influence of Chin–Yüan medicine,
3. Kohoha school (17th–19th century): the Japanization of Chinese traditional medicine.
4. Competition with Western medicine (16–19th century).
5. Revival of Chinese traditional medicine (20th century).

The Early Period (6th to 15th Century)

As early as 689, the first health-services law (*Omi-ryo*) was proclaimed in Japan, following the example of *T'ang lü*, a famous law of China in the T'ang dynasty. But this law was completely lost. The second such law (*Taiho-ryo*) was made in 702, and the third (*Yoro-ryo*) in 718; these two were said to be almost the same. Today we can see a part of them through the fragments cited in later literature. According to the book *Ryo no gige* (*A Commentary on Yoro-ryo*), the following staff members and students belonged to the Ministry of Health (*Tenyaku-ryo*) in the early 8th century: one minister of health (*Kami*), one vice-minister (*Suke*), one secretary (*Jo*), one senior assistant (*O-sakan*), one junior assistant (*Ko-sakan*), 10 physicians (*I-shi*), one doctor of medicine (*I-hakase*), 40 students of medicine (*I-sei*), 5 acupuncture practitioners (*Hari-shi*), one doctor of acupuncture (*Hari-hakase*), 20 students of acupuncture (*Hari-sei*), two massagists (*Anma-shi*), one doctor of massage (*Anma-hakase*), 10 students of massage (*Anma-sei*), two magicians (*Jugon-shi*), one doctor of magic (*Jugon-hakase*), 6 students of magic (*Jugon-sei*), two herbalists (*Yakuen-shi*), 6 students of herbal lore (*Yakuen-sei*), and some nonacademic staff members. The 40 students of medicine were divided into four sections: 24 students of internal medicine (*Tairyo*), 6 students of pediatrics (*Shosho*), 6 students of surgery (*Soshu*), and 4 students of diseases of the ears, eyes, mouth, and teeth (*Ji-moku-ko-shi*).

The introduction of Chinese medicine created the problem of how to get the drugs necessary to prepare prescriptions from the texts. Many of these drugs can hardly be cultivated in Japan, including very important ones such as cinnamon, licorice, rhubarb, and ephedra. These drugs had to be imported; and this has remained a problem for the Japanese right up to the present time. Great efforts were always made to keep a good supply on hand.

Circumstances of the drug supply during the 8th to 10th centuries are revealed by the drugs preserved in Shosoin (treasure house in Todaiji temple), and by a list of drugs in a book called *Engishiki*. A former emperor, Shomu, died on June 3, 756, and 49 days after his death many things were dedicated to Todaiji temple in his memory, including 60 kinds of drugs. These drugs have been preserved for more than 1200 years. They were examined carefully for the first time by a group of scholars in 1948, and the results of an extended study were published in 1955 (Asahina et al. 1955). These drugs were all imported from China, although some of them were products of more remote lands which had been brought to Japan via China.

Engishiki describes formal customs in the Imperial Court during the period of Engi (901–922). Book 37, *Tenyaku-ryo* (*On the Ministry of Health*), contains a list of 209 drugs which had been presented by local authorities to the Imperial Court. Most of these drugs seem to have been produced in Japan, but some plants are listed which do not grow or can hardly be cultivated in Japan today. We do not know whether these drugs were imported or cultivated in Japan—and of course it is possible that some botanical identifications were incorrect.

The oldest medical text now in existence was written by Tanba Yasuyori (912–995). This 30-volume work, called *Ishinpo*, was dedicated to the Emperor in 984. It was a sort of medical encyclopedia containing various sorts of knowledge: prescriptions of drugs, herbal lore, hygiene, acupuncture, moxibustion, alchemy, magic, directions for sexual life, regimen, and others. All of the descriptions, however, are quotations from Chinese texts.

Following *Ishinpo*, other important works were written, including *Iryakusho* (*Select First-Aid Treatments*) by Tanba Masatada, published in 1081; *Kissa yojoki* (*Healthy Life Through Tea Drinking*) by Eisai, published in 1211; *Ton-i sho* (a medical encyclopedia) by Kajiwara Shozen, published in 1302–04; and *Man-an po* (a medical encyclopedia) by Kajiwara Shozen, published in 1315–27.

The Goseiha School (16th to 19th Century)

The literal meaning of the Goseiha school is "the school of the latter-days' medicine." The name was adopted from the necessity to distinguish this school from the Kohoha school, which means "the school of classicism in medicine." "The latter-days' medicine" referred to Chin–Yüan medicine in China, because the Chin and Yüan dynasties were much later than the Han dynasty, in which *Shang han lun* was produced. The Goseiha school was composed of sympathizers of Chin–Yüan medicine, while the Kohoha school, which emerged about 150 years later, was in opposition to Chin–Yüan medicine and advocated a "return to *Shang han lun*."

The pioneer of the Goseiha school was Tashiro Sanki (1465–1537), who stayed in China for twelve years (1487–98) to study medicine, and met there a Japanese physician, Gekko, who is known as the author of two medical books, *Zenkushu* (1452) and *Saiinho* (1455). Tashiro brought these two books, together with other materials, to Japan when he returned in 1498.

Manase Dosan (1507–1594), the most important member of the Goseiha school, studied medicine under Tashiro. After Tashiro's death he returned to his home in Kyoto, where he set up medical practice and built a private medical school. He left many publications, *Keitekishu* (a textbook of internal medicine) being the most important. Goseiha scholars adopted the logic of Chin-Yüan medicine, which was based on the Neo-Confucianism of the Sung dynasty. But they were not always restricted by this speculative logic. They valued their own practical experiences, and tried to create their own methods of treatment. Manase Dosan said: "The dialogue between Huang-ti and Ch'i Po shows us the general rule of medicine, but we should take measures suited to the occasion; therefore a proverb says that *medicine* ("I" in Chinese as well as Japanese) is *will* (also "I" in Chinese as well as Japanese)" (Otsuka 1967a). "The dialogue between Huang-ti and Ch'i Po" referred to the classic *Huang-ti nei ching*.

The Kohoha School (17th to 19th Century)

This school advocated a "return to *Shang han lun*" or to its author, Chang Chung-ching. This group of reformists denied all authorities but Chang Chung-ching—and what is more, they sometimes even criticized his work. No corresponding movement occurred in China, so we may say that Chinese traditional medicine was Japanized by this school.

Nagoya Geni (1628–1696) was the first to oppose the speculative tendency of the Goseiha school by advocating a "return to Chang Chung-ching." His opinion paralleled the new movement in Confucianism led by Ito Jinsai, who called for a "return to the original work of Confucius." This classicism in Confucianism was in opposition to the so-called Neo-Confucianism of Chu Hsi and other scholars of the Sung dynasty in China. Neo-Confucianism was strongly connected with Chin–Yüan medicine, and therefore with the Goseiha school.

Goto Gonzan (1659–1733) developed the logic of Nagoya Geni, and pushed forward the theory of *Ikki-ryutai-setsu*—that is, only the stagnation of Ch'i was responsible for the occurrence of disease. *Ch'i* literally and phenomenally means "air." But it also referred to the most important substance to maintain the organized function of the universe (macrocosmos) as well as of the human body (microcosmos). In this respect it is similar to *pneuma* in Greek. According to one of his pupils, Goto Gonzan said:

All diseases occur from the stagnation of Ch'i, and not from anything else. Wind and cold cause the stagnation of Ch'i, food and drinks cause the same, and seven kinds of emotions do the same, too. If the stagnation of Ch'i takes place in one meridian or somewhere in the skin, it finally always infiltrates into the viscera. (anonymous ca. 1780)

The theory of pathogenesis in this statement attributed to Goto Gonzan was first made by Ch'ên Yen, a Chinese physician of the Sung dynasty, and had a great influence on Chin–Yüan medicine and the Goseiha school. Ch'ên Yen explained that there were three kinds of pathogenesis: intrinsic, extrinsic, and non-intrinsic-non-extrinsic. *Intrinsic* causes were the seven kinds of emotions: joy, anger, sorrow, worry, grief, fear, and terror. *Extrinsic*

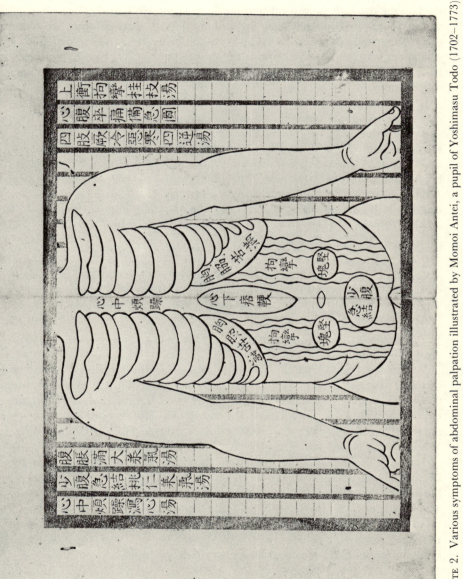

PLATE 2. Various symptoms of abdominal palpation illustrated by Momoi Antei, a pupil of Yoshimasu Todo (1702–1773).

causes were the six climatic conditions: cold, warmth, dryness, wetness, wind, and heat. *Non-intrinsic-non-extrinsic* causes were those which man brings on himself through unnatural actions such as inadequate diet or excess of venery. Thus we could say that the Kohoha physician Goto aimed to unify the pathogenetic pluralism of Chin-Yüan medicine. The principle of Goto's treatment was therefore to remove the stagnation of Ch'i. For this purpose, he especially recommended the bathing cure, internal use of bear gall, and moxibustion.

Kagawa Shuan (1683–1755), a pupil of Goto Gonzan, developed the theory of his teacher and denied all authorities except *Shang han lun*; Goto had also valued classics such as *Huang-ti nei ching* and *Nan ching* (*Difficult Problems*). Kagawa even criticized *Shang han lun*, insofar as it was influenced by *Huang-ti nei ching* and contained speculative concepts like Yin and Yang. Nevertheless, he claimed that it was the most important and trustworthy classic (Kagawa 1788: preface). Ippondo was another name for Kagawa, who wrote two important books, *Ippondo gyoigen* (*Ippondo's Notes on Medicine*) and *Ippondo yakusen* (*Ippondo's Notes on Drugs*), in which he expounded his theory:

Generally speaking, a disease always concerns one's body as a whole, and not any special part of it. There is no disease of one special meridian or of one special organ. If the outside of the body suffers, so does the inside, and vice versa. All parenchymatous organs and hollow organs connect with each other. If any part suffers, the whole body suffers, because it is filled in every nook and corner with Ch'i, which is by no means separable. (Kagawa 1734)

Very importantly, Kagawa depended on his own clinical experiences and on nothing else.

Yoshimasu Todo (1702–1773) was an important and influential character of the Tokugawa period (1603–1867). After many difficult years, he one day by chance met Yamawaki Toyo, a famous physician, and soon became famous himself as a physician at the age of 45. His revolutionary theory denied all authorities except *Shang han lun* and its author, Chang Chung-ching. While Kagawa had criticized this work for the few speculative notions it contained, Yoshimasu held that these passages had not been written by Chang Chung-ching, but had been added by other people in later ages. He argued that Chang Chung-ching could not have written such silly things. Yashimasu was a profilic author, publishing *Idan* (*Organon of Medicine*) in 1747, *Ruijuho* (*Indications of Recipes*) in 1762, *Hokyoku* (*Chief Indications of Important Recipes*) in 1764, *Yakucho* (*Characteristics of Drugs*) in 1785, and many other books. He rejected all speculations, saying:

It is for me nonsense to discuss the pathogenesis of a disease, because pathogenesis is more or less a product of speculation. For instance, it is held that a patient with purulent stool is suffering from intestinal abscess, and another patient with purulent spit is suffering from lung abscess. But how is it possible to know that these patients suffer from intestinal abscess or lung abscess unless the chest or abdomen are opened?

So these so-called pathogeneses are products of speculation. Purulent stool and purulent spit are not to be doubted. We therefore depend on what we have really seen and examined, and nothing else. (Yoshimasu 1785)

Yoshimasu proposed the theory of *Manbyo-ichidoku-setsu* ("All diseases result from one and the same poison"). In *Idan* (*Organon of Medicine*) he wrote:

All diseases result from one and the same poison. All medicines are poisons. We attack poison with poison. The body gets well, after the poison goes away. The volume of Ch'i remains unchanged during this process. What does it mean to compensate Ch'i, when Ch'i remains unchanged? (Yoshimasu 1747)

The poison was in the belly, according to Yoshimasu, so that the abdominal examination must be done most carefully.

Competition with Western Medicine (16th and 19th Century)

The Portuguese, the first Europeans in Japan, landed by accident in 1543. After that the Portuguese and Spanish came to Japan frequently, and the physicians among them introduced Western medicine to the country. This school, which the Japanese called *Nanban-igaku* ("Southern-barbarian medicine"), flourished for a short period. But the policy of national isolation which began in 1639 caused it to be replaced gradually by a new school identified with the Dutch. The Dutch were the only Europeans permitted to continue commerce with Japan, and they were restricted to the harbor of Nagasaki. Thus, from the beginning of the 17th century until national isolation ended in 1854, Western medicine came to Japan primarily through the Dutch. This school of European medicine was first called *Komo-igaku* ("medicine of red-haired people"), but as it gained importance it was called *Ranpo* or *Ranpo-igaku* ("school of Dutch medicine").

The event which marked an epoch in the history of Western medicine in Japan was the publication of *Kaitai-shinsho* (*New Book of Anatomy*) by Sugita Genpaku and others in 1774. This was a translation of the *Anatomische Tabellen* of Kulmus. Sugita Genpaku and Maeno Ryotaku had observed the dissection of an executed criminal in 1771, and they were much moved by the accuracy of the anatomical pictures in the Western medical text. Chinese anatomy seemed in comparison to be primitive and inaccurate. This was the direct motive that drove them to begin the translation: They aimed to reject speculations and to increase regard for direct experience. In this respect, the Ranpo school and the Kohoha school connect with each other.

A distinguished physician of the Kohoha school, Yamawaki Toyo, had dissected an executed criminal as early as 1754, and had published *Zoshi* (*On the Internal Organs*) in 1759. It is said to have been the first human body dissection in Japan. Nagatomi Dokushoan, one of Yamawaki's pupils, was much interested in Western medicine and went to Nagasaki to learn it. His work, *Manyu zakki* (*Notes of a Journey*), published in 1763, described some

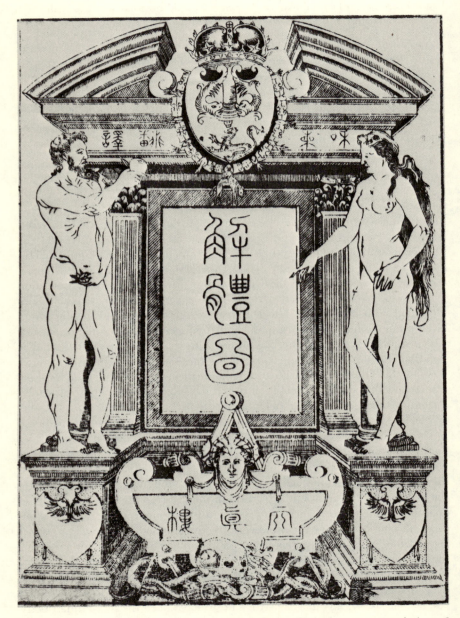

PLATE 3. Title page from *Kaitai-shinsho* (New Book of Anatomy), a translation of J. A. Kulmus' *Anatomische Tabellen* by Sugita Genpaku, Maeno Ryotaku and others, published in 1774.

aspects of Western medicine—e.g., the surgical treatment of cancer of the breast. Koishi Genshun first studied Kohoha medicine under Nagatomi, and after the early death of his teacher he studied the Ranpo school and became one of its most famous physicians after Sugita Genpaku.

Otsuki Gentaku (1757–1827), one of Sugita's pupils, established the Ranpo school through his many-sided academic and political activities. He thought that one should set off the merits of Ranpo against the faults of Kanpo; but he appreciated Kanpo, especially in the field of internal medicine (Otsuka 1967b).

Utagawa Genzui (1755–1797) published *Seisetsu naika senyo* (*Western Internal Medicine*), the first work on Western internal medicine in Japan, in 1793. The first edition of this book contained a preface by Taki Genkan, a famous contemporary physician of the Kanpo school. In the second edition, this preface was removed, probably because younger practitioners of Kanpo and Ranpo stood against such a cooperative—or, from another point of view, conciliatory—attitude. Apparently the competition between the Kanpo and Ranpo schools was not serious in the eighteenth century. The real collision took place in the nineteenth century.

At this point I would like to mention some influential foreign physicians who stayed in Japan in this period and were therefore much involved in the evolution of Ranpo medicine (Bowers 1965, 1970):

Willem ten Rhyne (1647–1700) came to Japan in 1674 and stayed about two years. We have a very interesting document of a dialogue between him and a Japanese physician, Iwanaga Soko, though the interpretation is perhaps not always correct (Otsuka 1967c). In his *Dissertatio de arthritide* (1683), two Japanese drugs, *Puerariae radix* and *Cnidii rhizoma*, were mentioned, and acupuncture–moxibustion was elucidated with four charts of meridians and a picture of a needle (Otsuka 1967c, 1971:251–259). He also included some Japanese drugs and prescriptions in another book, *Verhandelige van de Asiatise Melaatsheid* (1687).

Engelbert Kaempfer (1651–1716), a German physician, stayed in Japan from 1690 to 1692. He introduced the Japanese flora and medicine in his works, *Amoenitatum exoticarum* (1712) and *The History of Japan* (1727).

Carl Peter Thunberg (1743–1828), a Swedish physician, was in Japan 1775–76. Katsuragawa Hoshu and Nakagawa Junan, both able physicians and co-translaters with Sugita of *Kaitai-shinsho*, were pupils of Thunberg. He himself collected material about the Japanese flora and fauna, as well as Japanese medicine, and published much of this work after returning to Sweden.

Philipp Franz von Siebold (1796–1866), a German physician, stayed in Japan from 1823 to 1829 and from 1859 to 1862. As the most influential foreigner in the period of national isolation, he has been commented upon often. He published *Nipponische Archiv zur Beschreibung von Japan* (1823–54), *Flora Japonica* (1834–44), *Fauna Japonica* (1833–50), and many other works.

Among his pupils were such famous physicians and botanists as Ito Keisuke, Minato Choan, Ko Ryosai, Ito Genboku, Totsuka Seikai, Ozeki Sanei, and Takeuchi Gendo (Kure 1926).

Thus, the predominance of the Ranpo school became day by day clearer. But the determinative cause of its victory, or of the defeat of the Kanpo school, was the introduction of Jennerian vaccination. The first actual vaccination is said to have been done in 1824 by Nakagawa Goroji (Abe 1943), or in 1849 by a Dutch physician Otto Mohnicke, and Narabayashi Soken (Narabayashi 1849). In the former case, it is possible that what was really done was not vaccination but variolation. A vaccination office was first established in 1849 in Osaka. But the same project was not realized in Edo (Tokyo) until 1858, probably because the central medical academy of the government, which was in Edo, was administrated exclusively by Kanpo people. The vaccination office in Edo was founded with funds presented by 82 Ranpo practitioners, and at the same time education in Western medicine was also begun. This office was the predecessor of today's Tokyo University Medical School.

After the Meiji Restoration in 1868, the government set out to adopt the Western system in all parts of the national administration, in order to rank with the Great Powers of the world. Old systems were necessarily abandoned. In medical education, the government decided in 1869 to follow the German system. In 1875 a new proclamation on the examination of physicians was first given primarily in Tokyo, Osaka, and Kyoto, and four years later it was extended all over the country.

After this proclamation, a man who wanted to be a physician had to pass an examination in seven subjects of Western medicine. But the vested right of existing practitioners to continue in practice was acknowledged. In 1883 the government issued a more complete regulation for defining the physician's license, and Chinese traditional medicine was legally opposed. A physician who passed the state examination could then study Chinese traditional medicine and practice it—but such a regulation was practically a prohibition of Chinese medicine. The last effort of the Kanpo practitioners to continue Kanpo medicine was made in 1895. They presented a bill to revise the regulation for the physician's license, but it was rejected by a majority of 27 votes.

Revival of Kanpo

Although Kanpo medicine was completely rejected from the ordinary system, Chinese and Japanese drugs were studied by botanists, pharmacognosists, and pharmacologists, using methods of the natural sciences. Ito Keisuke wrote *Taisei honzo meiso* (*Western Nomenclature for Japanese Plants*) in 1829, introducing Linné's classification of plants. Nagai Nagayoshi discovered an alkaloid from the Chinese drug *Ma huang* (*Ephedra vulgaris*), and named it ephedrine (Nagai 1885). Miura Kinnosuke and Takahashi Juntaro studied the pharmacology of ephedrine (Miura 1887; Takahashi and Miura 1888).

Inoko Yoshito, a highly gifted pharmacologist, made a number of pharmacological studies of Chinese and Japanese drugs (Inoko 1887–1894). He wrote: "Chinese and Japanese drugs have not been studied by foreign scientists. Perhaps they contain pharmacologically active substances. But if some effective substances are discovered, they must be used according to the principle of Western medicine". (Inoko 1891). I believe that Inoko, in spite of what he said, was interested not only in the pharmacological analysis of drugs but also in the basic thought of Kanpo medicine. He could not say what he really thought in the 1890's, when the struggle between these two schools was at its peak.

Another approach to Kanpo medicine has been made by physiologists and pathologists such as Hashida Kunihiko, Ishikawa Hidetsurumaru, Ishikawa Tachio, and others who were interested in the meridian system. By means of electrophysiology, they have pursued the relationship between pathological changes in inner organs and electrophysiological findings on the skin (Ishikawa 1970). They have tried to ascertain the significance of the meridian system and acupuncture–moxibustion.

A third approach is the legitimate child of Chinese traditional medicine before the Meiji Restoration. Soon after the defeat of Kanpo medicine in 1895, a new movement to revive this system was born. Wada Keijuro, after having studied Western medicine, opened a medical practice in Tokyo and in his home province. He came to think that Kanpo medicine is superior to Western medicine from the clinical point of view and in 1910 he published *Ikai no tettsui* (*The Iron Hammer to the Medical World*), a comparative study of these two medical systems. This book influenced Yumoto Kyushin, an internist who studied Kanpo medicine intensively and who published *Kokan igaku* (*Japanese–Chinese Medicine*) in 1927.

In the last fifty years, and especially since the end of the Second World War, Kanpo medicine has increasingly gained strength.

THE PRESENT SITUATION OF KANPO MEDICINE

The study or practice of Kanpo medicine has never been prohibited by law in Japan. Since the law requires that one who wants to be a Kanpo physician must first learn modern medicine and pass the state examination, there is a great difference between Japan's license system and that of East Asian countries where two sorts of licenses exist for those trained in modern medicine and those trained in Chinese traditional medicine. The severe restrictions on Kanpo medical practice in Japan after the Meiji Restoration caused the number of practitioners and of publications to decrease almost to zero by the turn of the century (see Figure 1). But drastic as the opposition to Kanpo medicine was, Wada Keijuro's book *Ikai no tettsui* provided a fresh bud which began a new growth in 1910. Practitioners of a newborn system

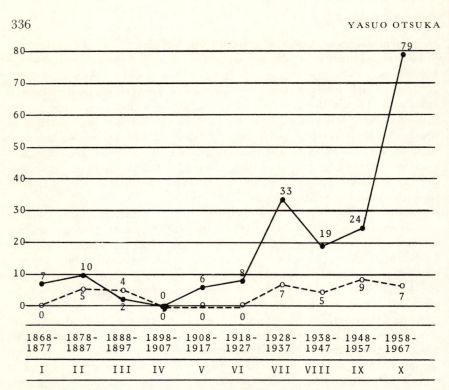

FIGURE 1. The change in the number of publications on Kanpo medicine after the
        Meiii Rostoration in 1868. Straight line-books; dotted line-periodicals.
        (Reprinted from *Kanpo ryakushi nenpyo* (Short History of Kanpo medicine
        for one hundred years after the Meiji Restoration) by courtesy of its author,
        Dr. Yakazu.)

of Kanpo medicine have all now studied and practiced modern medicine,
and have found themselves dissatisfied with it.

Especially in the last two decades, Kanpo medicine has gained increasing
approval from the Japanese people. In 1950 the Society for Oriental Medicine
was founded, and it is now the central organization for research on Kanpo
medicine. The Society, which now has nearly 1,500 members, publishes a
scholarly journal and holds a general convention once a year, as well as many
small meetings of local branches.

Although esteem for it has increased, Kanpo medicine continues to be
largely excluded from medical education. The history of Kanpo medicine is
taught in the medical schools, and knowledge of Chinese and Japanese drugs is
taught in the pharmaceutical schools. In pharmacological departments the
actions of traditional drugs are investigated, and in physiological departments
the effects of acupuncture and moxibustion are studied by electrophysiological
techniques. But the most characteristic points of Kanpo medicine, its theory

and principles, have been laid aside, for they can hardly be proved by the available methods of the natural sciences, even though they can be empirically recognized.

An Institute for Japanese–Chinese Drugs (*Wakanyaku–Kenkyushisetsu*) was founded in 1963 at Toyama University. It is the first full-scale institute for Chinese and Japanese drugs; but it covers only the chemical and pharmaceutical parts of Kanpo medicine, and not the clinical part. Since 1968, symposia on Chinese and Japanese drugs have been held annually under the auspices of this Institute, and these symposia have stimulated university scholars to participate actively in the study of Kanpo medicine. Consequently, basic and clinical studies in this field are increasingly reported by university scholars.

In the summer of 1969, I sent a questionnaire on Kanpo medicine to 141 scholars who represent three disciplines related to this medical system: leading Kanpo practitioners; professors of pharmacognosy and others who belong to the faculties of pharmaceutical sciences; and professors of pharmacology and others who belong to the faculties of medicine. I received 65 responses (Otsuka 1970 b).

I asked in which form respondents would prefer to use traditional drugs: (a) decoctions (the traditional form), (b) crude extracts (a semi-traditional form), or (c) pure chemical substances—for instance, the use of ephedrine in place of the drug *Ma huang* (*Ephedra vulgaris*). In cases (a) and (b), the principle of Kanpo medicine should be followed, while in case (c) it is quite indifferent. The traditional form was favored by Kanpo practitioners most strongly, the semi-traditional form by pharmacognosists, and the untraditional (chemical form by pharmacologists. In addition, these respondents considered the urgent problems of Kanpo medicine to be: (1) the guarantee of drug supply; (2) standardization of drug quality; (3) objectification of diagnostics; (4) cooperation of Western and Kanpo medicine; (5) modification of health insurance to include traditional treatment; (6) education in Kanpo medicine; (7) reassessment of important classics; and (8) initiation of large-scale research institutes for Kanpo medicine.

In 1972, one of the leading medical research institutes in Japan, *Kitazato Kenkyusho*, founded by the renowned bacteriologist Kitazato Shibasaburo (1852–1930), decided to create a section for Kanpo medicine with an attached hospital. The General Research Institue for Oriental Medicine began operation in 1974. This marks an epoch in the history of Kanpo medicine after the Meiji Restoration.

Acupuncture and Moxibustion
I will close this essay with a brief comment on the present situation of acupuncture and moxibustion. Although acupuncture and moxibustion constitute important parts of Chinese traditional medicine, these arts were considered independently of traditional pharmacotherapeutics at the reform

of medical administration in the period of Meiji. Those who specialized exclusively in acupuncture and/or moxibustion were allowed to practice in restricted conditions under a separate regulation from that for physicians. These arts were therefore treated as paramedical activities like midwifery. They had developed relatively independently from traditional pharma-cotherapeutics, and they were considered a favorable occupation for blind people. These circumstances continue to the present time (see Table 1).

TABLE 1

Number of Practitioners of Some Traditional Therapeutic Arts in Japan
End of 1970

	Sighted persons	Blind persons
Massage and related arts	27,751	35,172
Acupuncture	18,928	16,368
Moxibustion	18,787	14,833
Bone-setting	5,947	27

Shortly after the end of the Second World War the Allied Forces in Japan demanded the prohibition of acupuncture and moxibustion, along with other traditional therapeutic arts such as massage and bone-setting. The reasons given for this demand were that these techniques were barbaric and unhygienic—or, in a word, that they were unscientific. Through the efforts of Ishikawa Hidetsurumaru, Itakura Takeshi, and others, the government in 1947 issued new regulations for practitioners of these therapeutic arts. After that, those who wanted to be practitioners had to attend special schools, and licenses are issued by local administrative agencies to applicants who pass an examination.

In 1950, Nagahama Yoshio and Maruyama Masao published *Keiraku no kenkyu* (*Study on the Meridian System*) in which they set out to establish the scientific validity of the traditional meridian system. Two years later, Yoneyama Hirohisa presented a contrary theory in *Keiraku hitei ron* (*A Negation of Scientific Validity of the Meridian System*). Many discussions have followed from these publications, and in 1967 Kinoshita Haruto, Debata Akio, and others introduced a statistical method for analyzing the therapeutic effects of acupuncture and moxibustion.

In the meantime, acupuncture and moxibustion have drawn increasing international attention. In 1965 an international congress on acupuncture and moxibustion took place in Tokyo, and almost 800 participants came from 20 countries throughout the world. The policy of the Chinese government to use traditional medicine extensively in its health services, and the great publicity it has given to acupuncture, have helped stimulate this interest.

Changes in China's international relations which occurred in 1971 also promise to influence traditional medicine in Japan.

Literature Cited

Abe, T.
   1943 *Nakagawa Goroji and the Transmission of Vaccination.* Hakodate: Mufutaisha Co. (in Japanese).
Anonymous (Pupil of Goto Gonzan)
   ca. 1780 *Shisetsu hikki (Lectures of My Teacher).* (Manuscript in Japanese in possession of the author.)
Ashahina, Y., et al.
   1955 *Drugs in Shosoin.* Tokyo: Shokubutsu bunken kankokai (Japanese text with English summary).
Bowers, John Z.
   1965 *Medical Education in Japan.* New York: Harper and Row.
   1970 *Western Medical Pioneers in Feudal Japan.* Baltimore: The Johns Hopkins University Press.
Inoko, Y.
   1887–1894 More than 20 articles written in various periodicals were reprinted in "Academic Papers from the Pharmacological Department of Tokyo University Medical School." Tokyo: Yakuri kenkyukai (in Japanese, German, and English), 1962.
   1891 "On Chinese Traditional Medicine." *Journal Medical Society* of Tokyo 5: 1072 (in Japanese).
Ishikawa, T.
   1970 "Biophysical Study on the Mechanism of Viscerocutaneous Reflex." *Journal Society of Oriental Medicine in Japan* 18: 53–64 (in Japanese).
Kagawa, Shuan
   1734 "The Fifth Answer to the Question of Tanabe Nanpo." Supplements to *Ippondo yakusen (Ippondo's Notes on Drugs).* 4 vols. (1731–1738) (in Chinese).
   1788 *Ippondo gyoyoigen (Ippondo's Notes on Medicine).* 22 vols. (in Chinese).
Kure, K.
   1926 *Siebold, His Life and Works.* Tokyo: Tohodo Co. (in Japanese).
Miura, K.
   1887 "Vorläufige Mitteilungen über Ephedrin, ein neuses Midriaticum." *Berliner klin. Wochenschrift,* no. 38.
Nagahama, Y., and Maruyama, M.
   1950 *Keiraku no kenkyu (Study on Meridian System).* Tokyo: Kyorin shoin (in Japanese).
Nagai, N.
   1885 "Notes from Monthly Meetings for July and October 1885." *Journal Pharmaceutical Society of Japan, 18th year of Meiji.* Pp. 250 to 386 (in Japanese).
Narabayashi, S.
   1849 *A Short Study on Jennerian Vaccination* (in Japanese).
Otsuka, Y.
   1967a "On the Meaning of an Old Proverb: 'Medicine ('I' in both Chinese and Japanese) Is Will ('I' in both Chinese and Japanese)'." *Japanese Medical Journal* 2279: 43–47 (in Japanese).
   1967b "Otsuki Gentaku's Way of Learning." Japanese Medical Journal 2230: 61–65; 2231: 49–50; and 2232: 88–90 (in Japanese).

1967c "Works of Willem ten Rhyne as an Earlier Introducer of Eastern Medicine into Europe." *Rangaku Shiryo kenkyukai kenkyu hokoku* 201: 1–9 (in Japanese).

1968 "A Comparative Study on Drug Classification in the Ancient Herbals of the East and the West." *Practical Kanpo* 15: 193–201 (in Japanese).

1970a "History of Licorice (II)." *Minophagen Medical Review* 15: 133–140 (in Japanese).

1970b "An Inquiry on the Future of Kanpo Medicine." *Proceedings of the Third Symposium of Japanese and Chinese Drugs*, pp. 118–120 (in Japanese).

1971 *Willem ten Rhyne in Japan: The School of Dutch Learning in the Japanese Culture.* Tokyo: Tokyo University Press (Japanese text with English summary).

Takahashi, J. and K. Miura

1888 "Untersuchungen über die pupillenerweiternde Wirkung des Ephedrins." *Mitteilungen aus medizinischer Fakultät der kaiserlichen Universität zu Tokyo* 1: 255–276.

Yakazu, D.

1968 *A Short History of Kanpo Medicine for 100 Years After the Meiji Restoration in 1868.* Privately printed (in Japanese).

Yoneyama, H.

1952 *Keiraku hitei ron* (A Negation of Scientific Validity of Meridian System). *Journal of Japanese Acupuncture* 11, No. 2: 2–8 (in Japanese).

Yoshimasu, T.

1747 *Idan* (*Organon of Medicine*). Tsaruta Genitsu, ed., revised by Nakanishi Ichu (in Chinese).

1785 *Yakucho* (*Characteristics of Drugs*). Revised by Tanaka Shokkei, Nakamura Tei ji, and Kato Hakkei (in Chinese).

The Ideology of Medical Revivalism in Modern China

RALPH C. CROIZIER

Among the classical medical systems of Asia, the Chinese is oldest in history and newest in name. Behind this paradox lies an important clue to the significance of the numerous twentieth-century movements to preserve, develop, and revive this ancient medical system. Medical revivalism in China, as with revivalist movements in general, has not represented the preservation or resurrection of an intact tradition, but rather a reaction to major historical changes that has in turn created something new instead of restoring something old.

Thus, although a coherent and sophisticated system of medical thought and practice has existed in China for at least 2,000 years, it was not until after the intrusion of Western culture and medicine in the late nineteenth century that it was given a specific name. *Chung-i*, "Chinese medicine," is a product of the comparatively recent awareness that the Chinese is only one culture in a larger world, and revivalist movements on its behalf are at least in part defensive reactions to the threat of foreign cultural inundation.

This paper, in treating the ideology of the revivalist movements, will necessarily concentrate on larger extramedical forces and patterns in modern Chinese history. There is a risk here in minimizing both the objective therapeutic value of elements of traditional Chinese medicine and its adaptive value in a period of medical, as well as more general cultural, transition. However, other papers deal with these aspects, so our most useful contribution here might be in emphasizing some of the intellectual and cultural dynamics behind medical revivalism. The argument of this paper is not that the above medical questions are unimportant, but rather that the general phenomenon of medical revivalism is only fully comprehensible after it is set in its larger historical and cultural context.[1]

The first aspect of this larger context that must be noted is the strong ambivalence modern Chinese nationalism has shown towards the nation's traditional culture. On the one hand, the birth of political nationalism has

1 For a more thorough discussion of this entire subject and evidence for opinions in this paper, the reader is referred to Croizier (1968).

required a rejection of the age-old, essentially cultural definition of "China" as the ruthless logic of modernization has forced abandonment, willing or unwilling, of many of the distinctive forms, values, and institutions which comprised Confucian China. But on the other hand, modern nationalism has also fostered a more intense, particularistic attachment to specifically Chinese cultural traditions. With China's cultural identity threatened by the massive flood of Western cultural importations, modern Chinese have been torn between the need to reject the traditional culture as outmoded and the desire to prize it as Chinese.

Medicine has been one of the more striking examples of this tension. Here we find intersecting two of the main compulsions in modern Chinese nationalism—the drive for national power through mastery of modern science, and the effort to reaffirm the autonomy and creativity of Chinese culture. There is a consistency to both of these drives running throughout all of modern Chinese history, from the nineteenth-century Confucian self-strengtheners, who sought to save the old world which was their very being, to Communist social revolutionaries who seek to remake man and society in a new image. The drive for modern science and its fruits (from steamships to nuclear weapons) is the more obvious, but the overwhelming triumph of scientism in twentieth-century China has not weakened the Chinese desire to own the cultural ground they stand on.[2] This is evident in the many tortuous rationalizations attempting to show that the adoption of Western institutions, values, and ideologies has not meant cultural surrender to the invading West—that modern Chinese still make their own history according to a Chinese formula and not merely following a Western cultural blueprint.[3]

It has been this latter compulsion that has made so unlikely a field as medicine an arena for cultural and intellectual controversy. The beginning of this controversy can be traced back to the early years of this century, when the gradual introduction of Western medicine threatened to eclipse and supplant the native tradition in medicine. While the old medical practices persisted among the vast majority of the population, the new Republic's decision to sponsor only modern medicine was an augury of things to come. More menacing than any proclamations of the weak and ineffective national government, however, was the bitter hostility manifested toward the old medicine by the new generation of radical young intellectuals.

For this generation, usually identified with the May Fourth Movement of 1919,[4] traditional medicine stood out as a particularly noxious symbol of the traditional culture—backward, superstitious, irrational. Only its complete destruction could enable China to survive in the modern world. To men who

2 The important role of scientism in modern Chinese social thought is discussed in Kwok (1965).

3 There is a brilliant exposition of these rationalizations in Levenson (1958).

4 The May Fourth Movement refers specifically to the student-led protests against ratification of the Versailles Treaty. More generally, it refers to the entire anti-traditional, anti-imperialist intellectual and political movement during the period 1915–1921.

saw "science" as a panacea for China's manifold ills, it was intolerable that this hoary, unscientific tradition should be allowed to continue in an area so central to science, human welfare, and national strength as medicine. With a violent rhetoric common to his times, one of the nationalistic new youth, Chang Tsung-liang, summed up the charges against Chinese medicine:

The hollow-breasted and humpbacked, the pale-faced and slender-limbed, consequently the devastating epidemic, the high death rate, the lack of strong character and national morale, the pessimistic belief in destiny ... the award of the very title of "The Far Eastern Sick Person"—these are the direct gifts of the old-style medicine to China. (Chang 1926:9)

Paradoxically, it was at this juncture—with cultural iconoclasm at full tide, and science riding its crest—that there arose the first serious efforts to preserve the traditional medical system in a modern context. To be sure, there had been some tentative gropings in that direction in the early years of the century. Most notable were the efforts of Ting Fu-pao, a traditional scholar with some modern medical education, who tried to harmonize the two medical systems in a series of books he published in Shanghai.[5] On the level of institutional change, the traditionally highly-diffuse native medical profession had responded to the government's patronage of Western medicine by forming a "Committee to Save Chinese Medicine" when threatened by a government decision to make Western medicine the basis of the approved medical curriculum. However, the real impetus behind a much more determined effort to "save Chinese medicine" did not come from traditional scholars or the old-style practitioners themselves. It came rather from twentieth-century intellectuals and politicians, whose motives were essentially as modern as those of the radical iconoclasts who so ruthlessly damned the indigenous medical system.

These conflicting attitudes toward tradition, and toward traditional medicine in particular, were a part of that great sea-change in Chinese intellectual perspectives whereby China as a cultural entity—"the only true form of civilization"—disappeared in favor of China as a nation among other competing, and threatening, nation-states. As a culture, China had been impervious to political threat—conquering dynasties might come and go, so long as they did not disturb the cultural basis of Chinese civilization. As a nation, now that pretensions to absolute cultural superiority had been shattered, China could freely part with her traditional culture if it impeded the rapid modernization which survival demanded. Freely, and yet not so freely. For while the logic of the new nationalism freed modern Chinese from unswerving loyalty to the old culture, nationalistic emotions engendered new loyalties to what was distinctively Chinese. This, modern nationalism by the 1920's offered license both to cultural iconoclasm and to cultural

5 These were published under the series title *Chung-hsi i hui-t'ung shu* (*Books Connecting Chinese and Western Medicine*) in the years 1906–1910.

nationalism—the one to destroy the old culture as harmful to the nation, the other to cherish it as the unique product and hallmark of the national genius.

In medicine, this meant that while critics like Chang Tsung-liang were rejecting traditional Chinese medicine in toto, a new generation of conservatives sought ways to save it from extinction. They differed basically from pure traditionalists in that these new conservatives had a healthy respect for Western science and much of Western medicine. They also frankly recognized many of the shortcomings of the native medical system and stressed the need to adopt the organizational and institutional forms of modern medicine. But unlike the cultural radicals, they did not want Chinese medicine, as a system of medical thought and practice, to disappear before the inexorable advance of scientific Western medicine. They insisted that Chinese medicine possessed a core of precious and unique value which, purged of excrescences and supplemented with science, must be preserved. Moreover, the preservation of the "national essence" in medicine would offer reassurance to a shaken national confidence that, in at least this one area of science, China could produce something of value on her own.

The first important political patron of "reformed" or "scientificized" Chinese medicine was the warlord governor of Shansi province, Yen Hsi-shan. In 1921 he set up a "Research Society for the Reform of Chinese Medicine" with the ambitious purpose of combining the best features of Chinese and Western medicine in order to produce a new system of medicine both scientific and still distinctively Chinese.[6] Yen was not very clear about exactly how this would be done, and the "research" of his society did little to clarify the problem. But the appeal of this vague syncretic formula (as with so many other suggested syncretisms between East and West) was considerable to those Chinese who wanted China to become modern, but were dubious about abandoing so much of Chinese culture in the process.

Accordingly, in the next decade there sprung up a number of similar organizations in various parts of China. More modern-minded traditional doctors naturally played a large role in these, although nonmedical intellectual and political luminaries, such as the veteran Nationalist revolutionary Chang Ping-ling, were also intimately involved in their efforts. It was not until after the establishment of the Nationalist Government in 1927, however, that all this grew into a serious national movement.

The specific impetus to form a nationwide organization of defenders of Chinese medicine was provided by a resolution adopted by the new Nanking Government's Ministry of Health calling for the step-by-step elimination of all old-style medical practice in China. This provoked a great outcry, not only among traditional practitioners, who saw their livelihood threatened, but also among cultural conservatives in general, who saw this as yet another

---

6 The purposes of the society are discussed in its journal *I-hsueh tsa-chih* (*Medical Journal*) 1, (1) of July 1921 including a speech by Yen Hsi-shan in his capacity as its president.

instance of the national culture being swept away by the craze for things modern and foreign. Such sentiments were sufficiently widespread in the higher levels of the ruling Nationalist Party itself to have the resolution quickly shelved. More important, out of the uproar came a new nationwide organization, The Institute for National Medicine (*Kuo-i Kuan*), founded to defend China's own "national" medicine against further threats.

Probably the most articulate (certainly the most politically influential) spokesman for this organization and for the reformed Chinese medicine viewpoint in general, was the important Nationalist politician and ideologue Ch'en Kuo-fu.[7] As part of the general turn toward a politically and culturally more conservative outlook within the Nationalist Party after 1927, Ch'en had risen rapidly to great power in Party affairs under the aegis of Chiang Kai-shek. A militant nationalist and firmly dedicated to making China a strong power, he naturally emphasized China's need for modern science and technology, including scientific medicine. But like many other conservative nationalists, he balked at the liberals' and radicals' insistence that this required complete social and cultural revolution. Such thorough-going "Westernization" was an affront to national pride, and we find Ch'en Kuo-fu denouncing as unpatriotic those modernizers who "superstitiously venerate" everything foreign and lack faith in anything of China's own cultural tradition. He offered medicine as one example of this despicable attitude— despicable because it weakened Chinese national self-confidence—and also a particularly important example, for here the Chinese tradition had something to offer in that field where modern China's cultural indebtedness to the West was heaviest: science.

Ch'en did not attempt to portray traditional medicine in China as purely scientific. Obviously it was not, and obviously it needed considerable reform to become so. But he did insist that, in its fundamentals, the indigenous medical system was compatible with science (for it was based on empirically determined experience, the very essence of science), and that it possessed a unique body of medical wisdom which could not be allowed to perish.

On the level of practical techniques and materia medica, a convincing case could readily be made; on its claims to respect as an integral "system" of medicine, the task was much more difficult. Ch'en tried valiantly to explain, or explain away, the traditional medical theories of *Yin-Yang* and the five elements as no more than symbolic terminology for natural physiological processes, but without notable success. Similarly, he and other apologists for Chinese medicine were baffled by how to explain the important therapeutic technique of acupuncture in terms acceptable to a modern, scientific audience. The central dilemma lay in reconciling the fundamentally different principles and methodology of modern science with these ancient medical concepts, a dilemma which has remained the most formidable obstacle to the proposed synthesis of Chinese and Western medicine. To cut

7 His speeches and writings on medical subjects may be found in Ch'en (1952).

away too much of the native medical theory would destroy its integrity as a "Chinese" system of medicine; to retain it made the expropriation of "science" (and all the values associated with it) extremely difficult. As Ch'en's critics pointed out, if you replace the old medical ideas with universal scientific principles, why call it "Chinese" medicine?[8]

But logic need not overrule emotional needs, so Ch'en and others like him continued to strive for a reformed Chinese medicine which would satisfy their attachments both to science and to a Chinese identity. Ch'en was particularly insistent on the institutional reform of traditional medicine to reach this goal. Professional medical associations, research centers, hospitals, medical schools—all the organizational features of modern medicine—were urgently required to correct the sorry state of actual medical practice in China. Implied in this was the common conservative assumption that behind a framework of foreign-inspired institutional change a viable Chinese essence could be preserved. The value of this essence, once it had been properly "put in order," need not be confined to China. In their more euphoric moments, Ch'en and his colleagues waxed enthusiastic over what a blessing the new Chinese medicine, combining the best of East and West, would be to all mankind. What better proof could be offered to a doubting world of China's continued cultural creativity? More to the point, what better method could be found to ease the modern Chinese sense of cultural indebtedness? Scientificized Chinese medicine would pay back the West in its own scientific coin.

Throughout the 1930's and 1940's the Institute for National Medicine and its adherents continued to clamor for active government sponsorship of their program. They were consistently opposed by liberal intellectuals outside of the government, and by the modern-medicine-oriented Ministry of Health within it. The result was pretty much of a standoff. The Institute for National Medicine was unable on its own to go very far in providing the medical schools, research centers, and hospitals its program envisioned—or in getting the government to underwrite them. On the other hand, it was able to block any attempts by the Ministry of Health to regulate or restrict the practice of traditional medicine.[9] Thus, throughout the National Government period the two medical worlds—old and new, Chinese and Western—remained sharply divided and mutually hostile, despite the efforts of persons like Ch'en Kuo-fu to synthesize the two in a new, and superior, Chinese medicine.

Up to 1949 there was a certain logic or consistency to the alignment of opinion over the Chinese medicine question. The proponents of indigenous medicine were generally on the conservative side of political and cultural questions; their opponents could usually be classified as "progressives" or

8 This point was made by many critics of Chinese medicine, nowhere more forcefully than by the influential liberal historian Fu Ssu-nien (1952).

9 The successive regulations on medical practice under the National Government moved more and more towards giving the Chinese-style doctors equal legal rights with their modern counterparts. This trend is discussed in Li Ao (1962).

"liberals." Under the People's Republic, however, there has been a curious reversal of roles, with a ruthlessly modern and scientific Communist regime taking up the cause of preserving a Chinese medical identity and condemning skeptics for unprogressive and unpatriotic thought. Again, we must turn to the general history of modern China and of Chinese Communism for an explanation.

The first generation of Chinese Marxists in the early 1920's fully shared the cultural iconoclasm prevalent among the young intellectuals of their time. But in the ensuing decades, after the Communist movement had been driven from the urban centers of Western cultural influence and faced with the problem of how to survive in a rural setting, the Party gradually adopted a less hostile policy toward the native medicine and its practitioners. Originally, this was clearly no more than making a virtue out of necessity—using traditional medicine to alleviate the critical shortage of modern doctors and medical facilities.[10] Despite misgivings by some of the Communist Party's medical cadres, this was apparently in line with the strong emphasis in Maoist strategy on adapting and using native resources for modern ends. As Mao himself explained at a wartime conference in Yenan, the old-style doctors were not scientific, but they could be trained and used for the people's health. The Communists' medical leadership was enjoined to use, and improve, this indigenous medical resource (Mao 1955: 1010).

Accession to national power in 1949 took the Communists out of the hills of Yenan into the major urban centers, but it did not solve their basic medical problem. China had some first-class modern medical establishments (notably the Rockefeller-financed Peking Union Medical College) and a core of highly trained medical leaders, but in quantitative terms the situation was still critical. There were perhaps 15,000 modern-trained doctors for a population of over 500 million.[11] It required no great extension of Maoist pragmatism to continue the policy already in effect before 1949, even though some modern doctors might grumble about concessions to quackery and superstition.

For the first four or five years of the People's Republic, the main thrust of policy toward Chinese medicine was in organizing and controlling its numerous practitioners (probably upwards of half a million full-time professionals throughout the country) and giving them some of the rudiments of modern medicine and public health. The first goal was achieved through "health-worker unions" and cooperative-type "united clinics," the second by organizing short-term "improvement classes." Despite a certain amount of favorable propaganda about the usefulness of the old-style doctors and the masses' trust in them, there was little indication in this period that traditional medicine was intended for anything other than essentially a stopgap purpose

10 This is obvious in discussions of the question in the Red Army's health journal *Kuo Fang* (*National Defense*) during the period 1939–1943.

11 There are no truly reliable figures for this. By 1945 the Nationalist Government had issued 11,000 modern-physician licenses.

until sufficient numbers of scientifically trained doctors were available.

By 1954, a new theme began to impinge upon the early emphasis to learn everything from Soviet medical experience. This was an increased respect for the "medical legacy of the Motherland," and warnings to modern-medicine-trained public-health authorities that this legacy must not be neglected in developing the new "people's medicine." Abstract warnings were then replaced by specific charges against specific persons highly placed in the Ministry of Health.

The two best-known targets for a systematic campaign of public denunciation were Ho Ch'eng, the Deputy Minister of Health, and Wang Pin, Minister of Health in Manchuria.[12] The ideological crimes they were charged with consisted of despising and belittling Chinese medicine in favor of total reliance on Western methods. In practice, this allegedly had caused them to interpret Partly directives on combining Chinese and Western medicine to mean merely that old-style doctors should learn some modern medicine. They would then serve as auxiliaries to the Western-style doctors until enough of the latter were trained to take over all medical practice. Wang Pin was particularly denounced for referring to the native tradition as "feudal medicine," and great pains were now taken to show how medicine was "relatively free from class-nature" or, in any event, was the product of the accumulated wisdom of the Chinese masses and hence, by definition, good.

Apart from a sudden upsurge of nationalistic sentiment about China's own glorious medical achievements, the most serious aspect of the Party's new interest in Chinese medicine was the linking of medical attitudes to ideological correctness. The suspicion of pro-Western bourgeois influences in the modern medical profession was perfectly natural, for the overwhelming majority of its leadership had been educated either in Europe, America, or missionary-founded institutions in China. During the first few years after 1949, a heavy dose of Soviet medicine had been seen as the best antidote to these unfortunate connections and their ideological influence. But the question of "bourgeois tendencies" (i.e., separation from the masses and independence from Party control) was found to be more complex than simply pre-1949 capitalist connections. Rather, it was an integral part of the larger dilemma of how to treat the technical elite—the dilemma usually posed in terms of "Red vs. expert."[13] These experts (doctors included) were vitally important to the Party's goals of modernization and industrialization, but giving them the high social status which education traditionally had conferred in China, plus the *de facto* power which their importance to modernization demanded, went strongly against the egalitarian social goals of the revolution and against the Party cadres' untrammeled exercise of their new power. The mid-1950's

12 A good summary of the anti-Wang Pin campaign is in "Develop Criticism of Wang Pin's Bourgeois Thought in Despising Chinese Medicine," *Nan-Fang Jih-pao* (*Southern Daily*), Canton, May 19, 1955.

13 This problem forms one of the main themes in Franz Schurmann's path-breaking sociological study of Communist China (Schurmann, 1965).

saw intensified efforts to curb the emergence of a new privileged technocratic class, culminating in the triumph of the "mass line" during the Great Leap Forward.

The emphasis on modern doctors studying traditional medicine, starting in 1954, should be seen as part of these efforts to control the technical intelligentsia. Neither Ho Ch'eng nor Wang Pin could be convincingly accused of direct contamination by Western capitalist influences; both were long-time Party members with Soviet medical education. But they did represent (even within the Party) the tendency of "the experts" to free themselves from direct political control. This was their chief crime, as leveled against Ho Ch'eng: "refuting the ability of the Party in the supervision of scientific and technical work" (Jen 1956). And this was why a correct attitude toward Chinese medicine became the touchstone for a modern doctor's acceptance of Communist Party leadership in medical affairs.

Of course, the reappraisal of Chinese medicine also had important consequences for the actual development of medicine in China. There was a very considerable increase in the government's expenditures on hospitals, clinics, and schools for Chinese medicine. More significant for the now clearly-enunciated policy of fostering a true synthesis of the two medical systems, Chinese-style doctors and wards for Chinese medicine were incorporated into most of the major hospitals of China. Actually this created more a parallel system of medical treatment in China's medical institutions than the desired "combined therapy."[14] Complaints from both types of doctors, and repeated exhortations from official spokesmen, indicated that such integration was easier to decree than to achieve. Nevertheless, as foreign visitors frequently remarked, venerable herbalists and acupuncture specialists did become regular fixtures in the most modern medical facilities.[15]

Foreign observers have been even more startled by the changes in medical education. By the mid-1950's, Chinese medicine had become a required subject in all modern medical schools, and practicing Western-style physicians were pressured to enroll in spare-time courses in Chinese medicine. Finally, up to 2,000 doctors at a time were withdrawn from regular practice for three years of full-time study of traditional medicine. Remembering the still-critical shortage of modern-trained physicians, this substantial diversion of scarce human resources to Chinese medicine is the most solid evidence of the seriousness with which the Communist government took its policy of uniting the two medicines.

The emphasis on Chinese medicine and criticism of Western-style doctors reached its peak with the great upsurge of ideological fervor in the Great Leap Forward of late 1958. The indigenous medical system, and especially its popular folkloristic features, lent itself very well to the depreciation of

14 This judgment is based not only on complaints in the Chinese press, but also on interviews with a number of doctors from China conducted in Hong Kong and Macao in August 1964.

15 See, for example, Snow (1961) and Penfield (1963).

350 RALPH C. CROIZIER

technical expertise at this time. After all, if an engineer could learn from a coolie, and an agronomist from an old peasant, why not have a modern medical specialist learn from a native herbalist? With the "mass line" in ascendancy, science was no esoteric monopoly of the highly educated few. Enormous numbers of home prescriptions were collected to prove the wealth of medical wisdom resident in the Chinese people, and dubious modern doctors were exhorted to use traditional remedies in their own practice. As the common slogan ran, "Western-style doctors should learn from Chinese-style doctors"—a direct reversal of their roles before 1954.

But as the heaven-storming spirit of the Great Leap waned amid economic setbacks and political difficulties, the high tide of enthusiasm for Chinese medicine also subsided. By the early 1960's, the increased attention to technical expertise for economic recovery was reflected by more emphasis on sophisticated modern medicine, less on the more popular aspects of traditional medicine. For example, the articles on acupuncture, herbal remedies, and the relation of both to the thought of Mao Tse-tung which had briefly flooded the prestigious *Chinese Medical Journal* in 1958–59 disappeared in the next few years. All that remained were relatively modest claims by modern surgeons of success in using Chinese-style mobile splints for setting fractures (e.g., Fang 1963). Similarly, in the popular press, surgery—especially the rejoining of severed limbs—became the best-publicized accomplishment of the Chinese medical world.

This did not mean any formal change of official policy. Integration or synthesis of the two medical systems remained the announced goal, and institutional supprt for Chinese medicine in hospitals, research centers, and schools continued. But there is considerable indirect contemporary evidence, confirmed by the charges subsequently leveled in the Cultural Revolution, that during the first half of the 1960's Chinese medicine was not so much being integrated with Western medicine as it was being relegated to a supplementary and somewhat inferior position. For one thing, despite the support of research centers and training of dual-system doctors, there were no announcements of research breakthroughs in explaining the principles behind traditional therapeutics in scientific terms.[16] In medical education, the schools for training new Chinese-style doctors were only a fraction of those giving Western medical training. And in medical practice, although Chinese medicine evidently remained very popular, especially in the countryside, it was generally practiced alongside of, not integrated with, Western medicine.

All of this suggests a tendency for integrated Chinese medicine to suffer from the same problems that integrated Ayurveda has encountered in

16 The most promising discovery, that of North Korean physiologist Kim Bong-han in 1963, of small oval cells corresponding closely to the traditional acupuncture points, has not been substantiated by other investigators. Despite the publicity initially given the discovery in China, the "Bong-han corpuscles" appear to have been a false start.

India[17]—erosion of its theoretical basis, in an attempt to rationalize and systematize it for standardized teaching, and *de facto* relegation to second-class or paramedical status by scientifically trained public-health authorities. In other words, the powerful solvent of modern science threatened to dissolve the theoretical basis of Chinese medicine and leave an assortment of remedies and procedures that might be of considerable adaptive value in providing public health care, but would hardly constitute an integral medical system.

In Communist China once again it was an external, political development that checked this tendency. We refer to the Great Proletarian Cultural Revolution. The first sign of what that cataclysmic upheaval would mean for the medical world came in 1965, when Mao Tse-tung himself expressed serious dissatisfaction with the way medical policy was developing, and under the slogan "Doctors to the countryside" called for a major reordering of priorities. Of course, village-level medical care has been a basic public-health problem all along, but it very soon became apparent that it was also a political question. As it would emerge in the rhetoric of the Cultural Revolution, it was part of the struggle between "the two lines"—the counterrevolutionary reactionary line of Liu Shao-ch'i and his henchmen in favoring expensive specialized facilities for an urban elite, versus the socialist mass line of Mao Tse-tung in advocating basic medical care for the broad peasant masses. Or, in somewhat deflated terms, the issue was high-level education and specialized medical research for a relative few, versus spreading China's medical resources as broadly as possible across the vast countryside.

According to subsequent Red Guard allegations, the medical authorities initially attempted to resist the scattering of highly trained personnel from major medical centers into remote villages (*Current Scene* 1968). But with the full-scale eruption of the Cultural Revolution in the summer of 1966, all resistance was impossible. China's medical establishment came under the same attack for being alienated from the masses as did the rest of the Party and government apparatus. Instead of research institutions, medical colleges, and highly skilled specialists, the medical showpiece of the Cultural Revolution was the village based "barefoot doctor."

A brief examination of who and what the barefoot doctors are will reveal the role Chinese medicine has played in all of this. As the picturesque name applied to them suggests, the barefoot doctors are not highly-trained physicians using the latest in scientific medical equipment. They are practitioners with little or no formal medical education, recruited on the local level for part-time medical work in their own native villages. According to the leading Party journal, *Red Flag* (1968), in one model commune they averaged 23 years of age, came from poor or lower-middle peasant background, and had no more than a junior-high-school education. Therefore, they must rely heavily on local resources, both material and intellectual. In medicine,

17 I am indebted to Charles Leslie and Paul Brass for comparative insights into medical revivalist movements in India and China.

this means heavy reliance on the indigenous Chinese medical tradition. Though the barefoot doctors are not purely practitioners of traditional Chinese medicine, and most of them apparently have only minimal training in its theoretical principles, in practice they commonly use acupuncture and herbal remedies. This fits perfectly into the Cultural Revolution's general stress on local self-reliance and depreciation of bureaucratic structures and formal expertise.

Chinese medicine has also proved well adapted to the ideological goals of the Cultural Revolution. Innumerable cure stories, some verging on the miraculous, have appeared testifying to the efficacy of Chinese medicine when administered along with a large dose of the "Thought of Chairman Mao." The typical case is of a poor peasant or worker whose malady was dismissed as incurable by "famous bourgeois specialists" before he was treated by a People's Liberation Army medical corpsman or barefoot doctor. This "people's doctor." inspired by the Thought of Chairman Mao and determined to serve the people at all costs, customarily cures the patient through heroic acupuncture. Heroic—for two reasons. First, because the doctor dares to innovate by using new techniques, such as deeper insertion of needles; second, because he carries out prolonged and very painful experiments on himself before trying them on the patients. Once cured, the grateful patient inevitably expresses his thanks before a portrait of Chairman Mao.

Similarly, in institutional terms Chinese medicine has been central to the major development to come out of the Cultural Revolution. In late 1968 the national press began to feature reports on a recently established rural "Cooperative Medical System." Based on either the commune or production brigade, it is a local cooperative health service brining socialized medicine to the countryside for the first time. Members pay an annual subscription, and then only nominal fees for treatment. Again, local self-reliance with minimal dependence upon county or urban hospitals is the keynote, and again this means a great deal of reliance on indigenous Chinese medicine.[18]

It is too early, and information is too fragmentary, to assess the significance of this new institution as a way of building a socialized rural health-care system from the bottom up, rather than from the top down. There certainly are questions about the quality of medical care provided in either modern or traditional medicine by the crash-course-trained barefoot doctors working with very simple equipment. But if it seems unlikely that rural clinics and barefoot doctors can replace modern hospitals and medical college graduates, they may complememt the latter. And in terms of treating common minor ailments, spreading basic public hygiene, and even teaching birth control in the villages, they may provide important services that

---

18 According to a radio report from Canton, by 1970 "from 70 to 80 percent of the cases dealt with by the clinics of the people's communes in Kwangtung (province) were treated with medicinal herbs and the new method of acupuncture." Cited in *Survey of China Mainland Press* 4695:25.

otherwise would not be available for years or decades.

As for the reorganized urban medical colleges and humbler rural medical schools that are emerging out of the Cultural Revolution, their revolutionized new curricula stress integrating the study of Chinese and Western medicine. Thus both at the village level and in major medical centers, Chinese medicine is currently very prominent.

Only time will tell whether the cooling of the ideological fervor of the Cultural Revolution will cause a cooling of the enthusiasm for Chinese medicine along the pattern of what happened after the Great Leap Forward. For the present, it is important to note that the popularized Chinese medicine in vogue today differs considerably from traditional Chinese medicine—and not just because its practitioners carry the little red book instead of *The Yellow Emperor's Classic.*

This is because, despite all the praise for the wonder-working ability of acupuncture or herbal remedies, the new practitioners of Chinese medicine are not being trained in its underlying theoretical basis. All the emphasis is on practice and treating common diseases. The basic sciences in modern medical education have been reduced, but so has the background training in Chinese medicine. An article on "new acupuncture theory," for instance, dismisses the need to learn all 365 needling points, since only several dozen are commonly used (Chao 1970). It makes no reference to the *ching-lo* anatomical system that provides the rationale for acupuncture. Although the underlying social objectives and training methods being applied differ greatly, Chinese medicine in the hand of the barefoot doctors and their political patrons seems to be traveling a road curiously similar to what Unschuld noted on Taiwan. Divorced from its theoretical basis, it becomes an assortment of empirically applied remedies, not a medical system.

Therefore I feel that the future of Chinese medicine as an integral system is highly problematic.[19] The tumultuous events of the last four years have given selected popular aspects of traditional medicine great prominence in the contemporary Chinese medical scene, but they have also pushed it toward a popularization and integration with Western medicine which all the more undermines its autonomy as a medical system. In a sense, synthesis is taking place, but it is all at the level of practice. It is not the kind of theoretical synthesis that earlier nationalistic advocates of "scientificized Chinese medicine" wanted, and that the Communists themselves championed in the 1950's.

This does not mean that specific practices from the old medical system will soon disappear. Nor does it imply that they cannot have great adaptive

---

19 It cannot be overemphasized that the very limited basis of our knowledge about health conditions and the implementation of these new policies in the Chinese countryside makes all conclusions highly tentative. The description of Cultural Revolution medical policy in these pages is based entirely on a critical reading of Chinese press and periodical accounts. My book (Croizier 1968) does not cover events after 1966. There is pressing need for field investigation and, if that remains impossible, systematic interviewing of refugees in Hong Kong and elsewhere.

value in meeting very real health problems. I think it does suggest that the nationalistic ideology of many of our medical revivalists—that dream of a new medical system uniquely Chinese in its theoretical foundations as well as its practical application—is not likely to be realized.

But the name "Chinese medicine" will probably be with us for some time. And so long as it is, so long as there is a concern that medicine in China not be all "Western medicine," the kind of nonmedical factors discussed in this paper are going to be relevant to the future of "Chinese medicine"—and to the future of medicine in China.

Literature Cited

Chang Tsung-liang
    1926 *"Old Style" Versus "Modern" Medicine in China.* Shanghai.
Chao P'u-yu
    1970 "Let Chairman Mao's Philosophical Thinking Take Command of Acupuncture Therapy." People's Daily (*Jen Min Jih Pao*), Sept. 27, 1970.
Ch'en Kuo-fu
    1952 *Complete Works*, vols. 6–7. Taipei.
Croizier, Ralph C.
    1968 *Traditional Medicine in Modern China: Science, Nationalism, and the Tensions of Cultural Change.* Cambridge: Harvard University Press.
Current Scene
    1968 "Mass Revolution in Public Health." Vol. 6 (7).
Fang Hsien-chih
    1963 "The Integration of Modern and Traditional Chinese Medicine in the Treatment of Fractures." *Chinese Medical J.* 82: 493–504.
Fu Ssu-nien
    1952 *Collected Works of Fu Meng-chen.* Vol. 5. Taipei.
Jen Hsiao-feng
    1956 "Criticize Comrade Ho Ch'eng's Error in His Policy Toward Chinese Medicine." Trans. in *Union Research Service* 3 (June 8): 290.
Kwok, D. W. Y.
    1965 *Scientism in Modern China.* New Haven: Yale University Press.
Levenson, Joseph R.
    1958 *Confucian China and Its Modern Fate: The Problem of Intellectual Continuity.* Berkeley and Los Angeles: University of California Press.
Li Ao
    1962 "Reform the 'Medical Doctor Law' and Abolish Chinese Medicine." Apollo Monthly (*Wen-hsing*) 61: 9–15.
Mao Tse-tung
    1955 *Selected Works.* Vol. 3. Peking.
Penfield, Wilder
    1963 "Oriental Renaissance in Education and Medicine." *Science* 141: 1153–1161.
Red Flag (*Hung Ch'i*)
    1968 "The Orientation of the Revolution in Medical Education as Seen from the 'Barefoot Doctors'" Trans. in *Selections from China Mainland Magazines* 628: 3–9.

Schurmann, Franz
   1965 *Ideology and Organization in Communist China.* Berkeley and Los Angeles: University of California Press.
Snow, Edgar
   1961 *The Other Side of the River.* New York: Random House.

The Ambiguities of Medical Revivalism in Modern India[1]

CHARLES LESLIE

Muslim rule brought middle Eastern physicians to India when medical learning still flourished in Islam. From the thirteenth century on, they compiled anthologies of Āyurvedic texts translated into the Persian and Arabic languages, and adopted drugs and other therapies from Āyurvedic practice. In the sixteenth century, Hakim Yoosufi, a physician in the courts of Barbar and Humayun, is said to have synthesized "Arabian, Persian, and Āyurvedic thought, and produced a composite and integrated medical system" (Hameed, n.d.:17). Scholars like Hakim Yoosufi probably had counterparts among Āyurvedic physicians. Certainly Hindus became Yunānī physicians without converting to Islam, and Muslims became Āyurvedic physicians. Muslim rulers acted as patrons of famous Āyurvedic scholars, and Hindu aristocrats patronized Yunānī physicians. Religious animosity causes some modern authors to overlook or deny these facts, but Professor Basham in the present volume writes: "The practitioners of the two systems seem to have collaborated, because each had much to learn from the other and, whatever the 'ulama and the brahmans might say, we have no record of animosity between Hindu and Muslim in the field of medicine."

The point I want to make is that by the nineteenth and twentieth centuries, the traditional beliefs and practices of Āyurvedic physicians were radically different from the classic texts, and were deeply influenced by Yunānī medicine. For example, Āyurvedic practitioners often classified and interpreted illnesses in a manner that resembled Yunānī tradition, having added a humoral conception of blood to the three humors of the classic texts. Also, although sphygmology, or pulse lore, is absent from the Āyurvedic classics, it was well developed in Yunānī medicine, and became the symbol of an Āyurvedic physician's skill. The reputation of sphygmology was such that by the nineteenth and twentieth centuries it had become more a technique of

1 This essay is to be published with minor editorial changes as one section in a much longer essay, "The modernization of Asian medical systems." I thank John Poggie and Robert Lynch, editors of the volume in which the longer essay will appear, and the Greenwood Press, for permission to publish. Two other essays on medical revivalism in India by the political scientist Paul Brass and by myself may interest readers (Brass 1972; Leslie 1973).

356

divination than a rational diagnostic method. Great physicians were said to perceive every circumstance that caused a patient's illness, and to foretell the exact course it would take, by examining the pulse. Furthermore, Āyurvedic practitioners had adopted mercury, opium, and other items from the Yunānī pharmacopia, and traditional medical lore was profoundly influenced by alchemy, a science prominent in Islam but not in the classic Āyurvedic texts.

A major ambiguity of this situation is that these syncretic medical traditions are the ones that nineteenth- and twentieth-century Āyurvedic revivalists have known and believed in, yet the revivalist ideology has claimed that the introduction of Yunānī medicine to India caused Āyurveda to decline. The ideology also asserts that the development of cosmopolitan medical institutions in India caused the further deterioration of Āyurvedic knowledge and practice. This creates another ambiguity, for the revivalists have professionalized Āyurveda by adopting institutional forms, concepts, and medications from cosmopolitan medicine. It would be possible to argue that these changes continue a long tradition of medical syncretism; and that rather than declining, the Indian medical system has advanced through adopting new knowledge and institutional arrangements. Yet the logic of a revivalist ideology requires a theory of decline.

Before analyzing the role of revivalism in modernizing the Indian medical system, I must clarify the character of that system.

In the United States and other industrial countries, laymen and specialists assume that a single cosmopolitan medical system exists, with comprehensive jurisdiction in all matters of health: a hierarchy of paramedical specialists dominated by physicians; standard curricula for training health specialists; standard therapeutic techniques and ways of generating new skills and knowledge. In fact, the medical system is a pluralistic network of different kinds of physicians, dentists, clinical psychologists, chiropractors, health food experts, yoga teachers, spirit curers, druggists, Chinese herbalists, and so on. The health concepts of a Puerto Rican worker in New York City, the curers he consults and the therapies he receives, differ from those of the Chinese laundryman or the Jewish clerk. They in turn differ from the middle-class believers in Christian Science or logical positivism.

While the institutions of cosmopolitan medicine are extensive, well-organized, and powerful, so that the concept of a single, standardized hieratic medical system is closer to reality in the United States than in India, we need a pluralistic model to study the medical systems in either country. We should not assume, as laymen and physicians in the United States usually do, that the ideal of a uniform medical system controlled by physicians of cosmopolitan medicine is intrinsically superior to other ideals, and should be the goal of all societies. The pluralistic structure of the Indian medical system might best develop toward goals that would enhance the advantages of pluralism, while correcting its disadvantages.

I call the syncretic traditions of Āyurvedic and Yunānī medicine *traditional-culture medicine*, to distinguish them from the medicine of the classic texts. The physicians who cultivated learned versions of traditional-culture medicine identified themselves as either Āyurvedic or Yunānī practitioners, and were familiar with some classic texts, but their understanding of them was shaped by later syncretic commentaries and oral traditions. Thomas Wise, a surgeon in the Bengal Medical Service who published a comprehensive description of Āyurvedic theories and practices in 1845, wrote:

> After some enquiry I find there are not more than four or five persons in this part of India who are acquainted with the Hindu Shastras. ... A very few practitioners may still be found in the neighbourhood of cities ... in whose families the ancient treatises of their forefathers are studied, and transmitted from generation to generation. I have had the happiness of knowing such a family of hereditary physicians, rich, independent, and much respected. ... [They would not sell or let their manuscripts be copied], from a belief that all the good to be derived from their possession, which God had bestowed on the individual and his family, would vanish on the work being sold, or even the precepts communicated, to unauthorized individuals. (Wise 1845:v)

Learned practitioners of traditional-culture medicine still exist, but from the beginning of the nineteenth century syncretism with cosmopolitan medical knowledge and institutions has largely transformed these traditions into *professionalized Āyurvedic and Yunānī medicine*. Its practitioners are trained in colleges, join professional associations, prescribe commercially manufactured drugs, serve governmental health agencies, work in hospitals, write articles for medical journals, and do other modern professional things that the learned physicians Thomas Wise knew did not do.

Different degrees of syncretism with cosmopolitan medicine exist, but the dynamics of professionalization cause those who oppose syncretism, as well as those who advocate it, to adopt ideas and practices from the cosmopolitan medical profession. For example, the ideologists of *Śuddha* (pure) Āyurveda have advocated restoring theory and practice to the classic texts by eliminating accretions from other systems. Yet they have acted just like their opponents who advocate reviving Āyurveda by utilizing modern science and technology: they have lobbied to influence governmental health policies, written tracts comparing the discoveries of modern science to passages in the ancient texts, joined associations, organized schools, etc. And of course none of these things are in the classic texts. Because American and English social scientists favor progress, they sometimes err in the study of modernizing processes by assuming that "conservative" ideologists bloc modernization. In revivalist movements, ideological "conservatives" may be as powerful modernizing forces as "progressives."

I have distinguished five aspects or kinds of medicine that are important for the argument of this essay. I will enumerate them, adding others to the list with the purpose of placing these five in the fuller context of the pluralistic Indian medical system. These are: (1) the Āyurvedic medicine of the Sanskrit classic texts; (2) Yunānī medicine of the classic Arabic texts; (3) the syncretic medicine of traditional culture, which evolved among learned practitioners from the thirteenth to the nineteenth centuries; (4) professionalized Āyurvedic and Yunānī medicine, which has continued the syncretism of the past, transforming learned traditional-culture medicine by assimilating cosmopolitan medical knowledge and institutions; and (5) cosmopolitan medicine. In South Asia, cosmopolitan medicine is often called *allopathy* to distinguish it from indigenous medicine and homeopathy.

Another kind of traditional-culture medicine is (6) *folk medicine*, which includes midwives, bone-setters, supernatural curers of various types, and other specialists, most of them part-time practitioners. The concepts and practices in folk medicine draw upon the humoral theories, cosmological speculations, and magical practices in learned medicine and religion, but systematic studies of the relationships between learned and folk medicine have not been made. The term "indigenous medicine" is used in India to refer to the folk and learned dimensions of traditional-culture medicine, together with the classic texts.

(7) *Popular-culture medicine* emerges with the institutions of mass society—industrial production of medicine, advertising, the school system. It continues the syncretism of traditional-culture medicine, transforming and displacing it with an amalgam of concepts and practices. It combines the humoral concepts of hot and cold foods with concepts of vitamins; traditional physiological concepts with the germ theory of disease; popular astrology and religion with faith in modern science and technology. It utilizes patent medicines and drugs from modern chemotherapy, along with industrially prepared Āyurvedic, Yunānī, and homeopathic medications. Laymen practice popular-culture medicine on themselves and kinsmen, but many practitioners are full-time specialists. For example, professionalized Āyurvedic and Yunānī physicians, and many doctors trained in cosmopolitan medicine, practice for the most part a form of popular-culture medicine.

(8) *Homeopathic medicine* is a special form of popular-culture medicine so widely used in India it must be listed here. It originated in Germany in the nineteenth century, and is based on the concept of creating resistance to an illness by giving small doses of it. Homeopathy is a variant of cosmopolitan medicine grounded in biological vitalism, but in India its practice assimilates elements from Āyurvedic and Yunānī traditions to form a distinctive popular-culture medicine. Many self-instructed part-time practitioners are active, but schools also exist, as do clinics, hospitals, associations of practitioners, and other institutions of professional practice. Some of these institutions are funded by state governments. Physicians and paramedical specialists trained in cosmopolitan medicine, and professionalized Āyurvedic and Yunānī physicians, may themselves use homeopathic medicines, and occasionally recommend them to others.

My intention is to list categories for constructing a model of pluralistic

South Asian medical systems. I do not intend to itemize all varieties of curers and medical belief in India, or in a single region or city. Additional kinds of practice could be related to the model in a more extended study than the present essay. For example, *Siddha* is a Tamil-language variant of Āyurveda practiced in South India and Ceylon, and a variant of Yunānī medicine which submerges the Galenic tradition is supernatural curing at the shrines of holy men or by prayer and meditation on sayings attributed to the Prophet. In addition, *naturopathy* is a recognized therapeutic system among educated urban Indians. Its more successful practitioners establish sanatoria where patients are given special diets, baths, massages, and courses of exercise—but, like homeopathy, this is a variant of popular-culture medicine. During the Independence Movement, Congress politicians and Āyurvedic physicians tried to persuade Mahātma Gandhi to endorse Āyurvedic medicine, but Gandhi had no taste for it or for cosmopolitan medicine; instead, he experimented with nature cures which employed special diets and mudbaths.

The last category we need to list in order to construct our model is (9) *learned magico-religious curing*. All classes of people in India resort frequently to magical and religious therapy, and practitioners range from illiterate villagers to sophisticated urban pandits. Supernatural curing blends with other practices at the levels of folk and popular culture; but at higher levels of learning, the ideas and roles associated with supernatural curing command a prestige that sets them apart. This raises an interesting problem of historical sociology. The classic medical texts are not entirely secular and without magic, but the traditional-culture medicine was saturated with magical and religious elements. A problem for historians will be to identify the processes through which the relatively secular and rational medicine of the texts was transformed into the magico-religious forms of traditional-culture medicine.

I am suggesting a long-term trend of *sacrilization* in the great traditions of Āyurvedic and Yunānī medicine (in Figure 1, the transitions that would occur in moving from the G to the D region). Furthermore, I believe that professionalization processes have tended to reverse this historical pattern in the nineteenth and twentieth centuries by *resecularizing* Āyurvedic and Yunānī medical learning (in Figure 1, the transitions that would occur in moving from the D to the B region). Although these changes have involved ambiguities, my argument is that a revivalist ideology has facilitated this historical reversal and other modernizing trends caused by efforts to enhance the professional status of Āyurvedic and Yunānī physicians.

The main tenets of the revivalist ideology evolved early in the nineteenth century in a conflict between British Orientalists and Anglicists. The Anglicists wanted the ruling East India Company to establish an English-language school system, with the practical purpose of training Indian men for jobs in British enterprises, and with the ideal of reforming Indian society by educating a class of men and women in the liberal arts and scientific thought. The

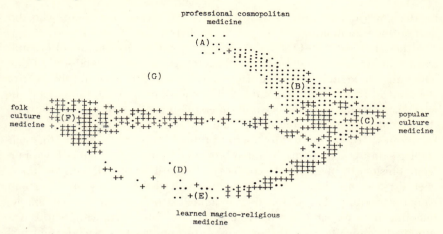

FIGURE 1. Model of a pluralistic South Asian medical system showing regions of typical practice, and hypothetical distributions of full-time and part-time practitioners.

Regions of typical practice:

(A) Physicians of cosmopolitan medicine with M.D. degrees (most practitioners have M.B.B.S. degrees, or diplomas)
(B) Professionalized Āyurvedic and Yunānī physicians
(C) Homeopathic physician
(D) Learned traditional culture Āyurvedic and Yunānī physicians
(E) Pandits and other religious specialists with reputations for unusual learning and healing powers
(F) Folk practitioners
(G) Classic Āyurvedic and Yunānī text descriptions of medical education and practice

Each dot = one full-time practitioner
Each cross = ten part-time practitioners

Orientalists were cultural pluralists who advocated that reforms be undertaken by utilizing indigenous institutions, rather than by the wholesale introduction of an English educational system. They admired Indian civilization, arguing that it had fallen on evil days but that it could be reformed by selectively encouraging practices that still expressed the enlightened spirit of antiquity, and by translating modern science into Indian languages.

For example, a member of the Orientalist faction surveyed traditional education in Bengal in the 1830's, and one of his recommendations was that medical textbooks be written in the Bengali, Hindi, and Sanskrit languages, to combine modern scientific knowledge with local practices, "European theory and Indian experience" (Adam 1941:436–437). Free copies of these books would be distributed to learned Āyurvedic and Yunānī physicians, and public examinations based on their content would be periodically announced by the government. Special awards would be given to students who did well on the examinations, and to their teachers.

Although the British Orientalists were sympathetic to Indian culture and learned its languages, they criticized the lethargy, ignorance, and superstition which they thought abounded in Indian society, and they constantly spoke of the need to revive and invigorate it. They were men of the Enlightenment who were enemies of ignorance and superstition in Western society, and who thought that Western civilization had only recently emerged from "the Dark Ages." It was natural for them to think in a revivalist idiom, for their ideology transposed the myth of man's decline from the Garden of Eden into secular history by inventing the concept of decline from the religious tolerance, scientific accomplishment, artistic creativity, and democracy of Greek and Roman antiquity. For India, they imagined a past culture as reasonable, tolerant, natural, simple, and refined as the Mediterranean world was supposed to have been, and they sought out Hindu scholars who confirmed this conception. Together they formulated a theory of decline in medicine and in other cultural domains.

The theory for the decline of Āyurveda compared the rational spirit and comprehensiveness of the early texts with contemporary medical practices, to the disadvantage of both learned and folk levels of traditional-culture medicine. Decline was attributed to the Buddhist doctrine of *ahiṁsa* (non-violence), which was said to have caused dissection to be abandoned, with the subsequent deterioration of surgery and anatomical knowledge. In fact, the classic text on surgery was composed in the Buddhist period. Decline was also attributed to Muslim conquest and support of a rival medical system, followed by British conquest and patronage of yet another rival system. In addition, it was attributed to the Hindu customs of over-valuing authority as a method of validation, and of treating knowledge as a secret. Finally, it was supposed to have followed from using inferior drugs as substitutes for rare and valuable ones, so that the ancient medicinals lost their effectiveness, and quack physicians attempted to compensate by progressively resorting to magical charms and spells. Thus, traditional-culture medicine was described as being in an abject state. Overgrown with superstition, only a few elements remained from antiquity, like ruins that testified to a glorious past.

This theory of decline from a golden age of medical learning provided the ideological ground for professionalizing reforms. Printing presses had been introduced, and though learned practitioners often considered the texts too sacred to be made public, relatively inexpensive editions of the medical classics began to be published. Āyurvedic physicians sent their sons to the modern medical schools which were first established in Calcutta, Bombay, and Madras in mid-century, and then in other cities of British administration.

A class of physicians had emerged during the first half of the century who had some knowledge of "English medicine." In 1839, an Indian observer in Bombay asserted that only four or five Āyurvedic physicians in that city knew Sanskrit well enough to read the medical classics, but that some hereditary physicians "call themselves 'English Doctors' ... and administer English medicines ... [though] they are not at all educated and know nothing of the European Medical Science" (Bombay Record Office 1838). By the closing decades of the nineteenth century, this class included kinsmen in joint practice who were trained in cosmopolitan and indigenous medicine, and individuals who were trained in both systems. Some of these physicians were entrepreneurs who hoped to revive Āyurveda and improve their own careers by starting companies to manufacture traditional medicines for commercial distribution, by founding schools which would adapt Āyurvedic learning to the bureaucratic structure of modern education, and by sponsoring charitable dispensaries.

The next step in professionalization was to organize regional associations of practitioners. India is more diverse linguistically than Europe, but by the first decade of the present century an association of professionalized Āyurvedic physicians that bridged linguistic regions was founded, with a program urging government recognition and aid for research on indigenous drugs, and for Āyurvedic schools, hospitals, and dispensaries. Though Gandhi and Nehru were cool to medical revivalism, it gained support from other leaders of the Independence Movement and, linked with this powerful force, continued to inspire a proliferating literature, the founding of colleges, and sporadically successful attempts in various states to gain governmental support.

Āyurvedic physicians took the lead in the professionalization of learned traditional-culture medicine, but Yunānī practitioners were also active. Vernacular translations of Yunānī texts were published and colleges were founded from the late nineteenth century, inspired by revivalism. During the 1920's and 1930's, in response to the ecumenical ideology of the Independence Movement, schools were established in which students could elect to study either Yunānī or Āyurvedic medicine. A nationally prominent school in Madras offered programs in Yunānī medicine, Āyurveda, and Siddha, the Tamil-language medical tradition. Schools of this kind incorporated modern knowledge in their curricula, offering basic science courses and clinical instruction in diagnostic techniques and therapies of cosmopolitan medicine. The more successful ones had teaching hospitals, rudimentary laboratories, dissection halls, anatomical charts, and other modern teaching aids. Still, most of these efforts were privately financed. Where state aid was given to these institutions and to Āyurvedic or Yunānī dispensaries, it was a minor part of the total expenditure for health purposes.

When India became an independent nation, just after the Second World War, it had approximately 50 hospitals and 57 colleges of Āyurvedic or Yunānī medicine. The Ministries of Health in several states had Boards of Indigenous Medicine responsible for running government dispensaries, registering practitioners, and regulating school curricula. Companies with

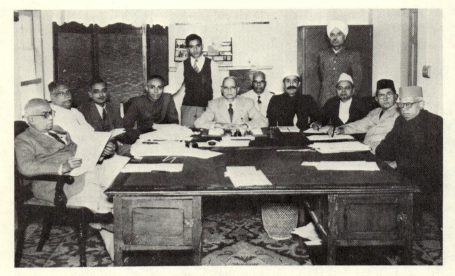

PLATE 1. The Committee on Indigenous Systems of Medicine appointed by the Government of India in 1946, with Col. R. N. Chopra as Chairman.

regional, and in some cases with national and international markets, manufactured Āyurvedic and Yunānī medicines which they advertised and distributed in a modern manner. National associations of practitioners sponsored conferences, published journals, and lobbied for legal privileges equivalent to those of physicians trained in cosmopolitan medicine.

Thus, encouraged and justified by the idea of reviving the heritage of indigenous medical science, Āyurvedic and Yunānī physicians had modernized the learned practice of traditional medicine. They were middle-class urban entrepreneurs and members of Brahmin or other high castes. By professionalizing indigenous medicine as the profession of cosmopolitan medicine had evolved in India, they shaped careers for themselves, transformed the learned practice of traditional-culture medicine into a blend of popular culture and scientific medicine, and created within the pluralistic Indian medical system a dual structure of professional medical institutions.

A major difference existed between the revivalist ideology of the professionalizing Āyurvedic physicians and the thought of the British Orientalists who first inspired them. The cultural models which were used to reform Western civilization were thoroughly demythologized. The Englishmen who admired ancient Greece did not believe in its gods. And while they thought that the new science of the seventeenth and eighteenth centuries revived the spirit of Greek civilization, they did not believe that it was a literal resuscitation of ancient knowledge. In their view, modern science made Greek science obsolete. They were very self-conscious about this perspective, because it had been an issue of considerable consequence in the modernization of European culture.

Humanistic revivalism initiated the traditions of modernity in the Renaissance by using the authority of a classical ideal to oppose scholasticism; but the Scientific Revolution of the following centuries, while continuing to pay homage to classic ideals, had challenged the literal authority of the classical model. The British Orientalists were heirs to this dialectical progression.

In contrast, the professionalizing Āyurvedic physicians believed in the Hindu gods of the ancient texts, and in the traditional-culture medicine which their activities transformed. The main concepts in the classic texts—that related equilibrium systems exist in the human body and the universe, and that these systems are composed of five elements (*bhūta*), seven body substances (*dhātu*), and three humors (*doṣa*)—were also part of the traditional medicine in which they believed; so that their goal was to resuscitate ancient medical science. Since they believed literally in the authority of the classic texts, and at the same time were impressed by the accomplishments of modern science, they set out to demonstrate that the institutions and scientific theories of cosmopolitan medicine were anticipated in the ancient texts.

These and other arguments justified radical changes in the organization and content of traditional education and practice. But the point I want to make is that every argument involved its advocates in ambiguities. For example, to maintain that Āyurveda had declined because British colonialism introduced an alien system, they had opposed the image of a large medical college to the simple household of an Āyurvedic physician. His wisdom and healing skill were said to exceed by far those of ostentatious doctors with elaborately equipped clinics, and neither his practice nor his profound teaching required the bureaucratic organization of impersonal hospitals, laboratories, and dissection halls. Yet as Āyurvedic schools were founded and their facilities improved, they appeared to become inferior versions of cosmopolitan medical colleges. Rather than resuscitate the creative power of great-tradition medicine and its prestige relative to cosmopolitan medicine, these schools attracted students who had failed to gain admission to other institutions. The reasons were clear enough. Even the few graduates who became successful private practitioners did not enjoy the legal privileges of cosmopolitan medical doctors, and in the state health services, physicians trained in these schools were only considered to be qualified for positions with low pay and limited responsibility.

In fact, Āyurvedic and Yunānī medicine have evolved in an ambiguous paraprofessional relationship to cosmopolitan medicine. When the social history of cosmopolitan medicine in India comes to be written, it will show that from the nineteenth century to the present time, the demand for medical services has far exceeded the capacity of cosmopolitan medical institutions, so that they have developed in reciprocal relationship to the modernization of

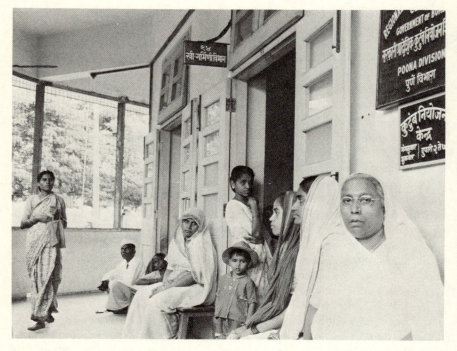

PLATE 2. An out-patient clinic at the College of Āyurveda affiliated with Poona
        University.

Āyurvedic and Yunānī medicine. Cosmopolitan medical institutions have
depended upon the professionalization of indigenous medicine to meet a
substantial portion of the expanding need for professional care. At the same
time, the ideology of the cosmopolitan medical profession has opposed the
claims of Āyurvedic and Yunānī institutions to greater state recognition and
support. The paramedical subordination of these institutions to the cosmopolitan medical profession has been maintained, but the relationship itself has
been an unwanted one. Similarly, the professionalizing Āyurvedic and
Yunāni physicians have been unhappy with the relationship and have
sought to deny it by seeking autonomy as an independent profession.

   The important point is that in India the modernization of Asian medicine
has not been a one-way process in which Āyurvedic and Yunānī physicians
have borrowed ideas and institutional forms from so-called Western medicine.
Cosmopolitan medical institutions have themselves developed in a distinctive
manner because Āyurvedic and Yunānī institutions were there, doing
medical jobs Indian society wanted and needed to be done.

   Ambiguities remain in the social and cultural role of professionalized
Āyurvedic and Yunānī medicine, but the signs are that they are becoming

less acute. The revivalist ideology has done its work for the time being, and does not now command the loyalties it aroused a generation or two ago. The government of India passed a law in 1970 establishing in the Ministry of Health a Central Council of Indian Medicine to register physicians, regulate education and practice, and cultivate research. The concepts of Āyurvedic and Yunānī medicine are a respected part of the common Indian culture. The President of India is known to resort to Āyurvedic therapies, as do other citizens in all walks of life. If a wizard of modernization decided that "traditional medicine" was an impediment to progress and abolished tomorrow the whole infrastructure of professionalized Āyurvedic and Yunānī practice, he would create a medical catastrophe.

Literature Cited

Adam, William
    1941 *Reports on the State of Education in Bengal, 1835 and 1838.* Anathnath Basu, ed. Calcutta: University of Calcutta Press.
Bombay Record Office
    1838 General Department, vol. 21A/448A.
Brass, Paul
    1972 "The Politics of Ayurvedic Education: A Case Study of Revivalism and Modernization," in Susanne Hoeber Rudolph and Lloyd I. Rudolph, eds., *Education and Politics in India.* Cambridge: Harvard University Press.
Hameed, A. Abdul
    n.d. *Physician-Authors of Greco-Arab Medicine in India.* New Delhi: Institute of History of Medicine and Medical Research.
Leslie, Charles
    1973 "The Professionalizing Ideology of Medical Revivalism," in Milton Singer, ed., *Modernization of Occupational Cultures in South Asia.* Durham, N. C.: Duke University Press.
    1974 "The Modernization of Asian Medical Systems," in John Poggie and R. Lynch, eds. *Rethinking Modernization: Anthropological Perspectives.* Westport, Conn.: Greenwood Press.
Wise, Thomas A.
    1845 *Commentary on the Hindu System of Medicine.* Calcutta: Baptist Mission Press.

Indigenous Medicine in Nineteenth- and Twentieth-Century Bengal

BRAHMANANDA GUPTA

Āyurvedic medicine was taught and practiced in the traditional way in Bengal at the beginning of the nineteenth century. The physician was called a *Kavirājā*, prince of verse, referring to his mastery of Sanskrit texts. Patients consulted him at his home, and he took a personal interest in them. He would ask a patient about his illness and general state of health in a manner that made him confident he was understood. He observed the outward appearance and behavior of patients, and examined their pulse, eyes, abdomen, and tongue. When he announced his diagnosis, he would carefully instruct the patient and his kinsmen in the proper regimen for recovery, since the regulation of food intake and other activity was considered extremely important during illness, particularly when medications were being taken. The Kavirājā would give the patient medicines he had personally prepared, or that had been prepared under his supervision. This satisfied the patient that the ingredients were pure and their efficacy known to the Kavirājā.

The relationship of confidence between the Kavirājā and his patient was enhanced by their common religious background. Normally, Kavirājās were orthodox Hindus whose way of life followed strict religious rules. Thus, orthodox patients preferred a Kavirājā to an allopathic doctor (Mukhopadhyaya 1926, II:21), and devout Brahmins and widows could not accept allopathic medicines: "Brahmin orthodox scholars used to take a bath if they had to touch foreign medicines. ... Moreover they believed that they would not attain salvation if at the time of death they did not get a medicine prepared by a Kavirājā" (Chatterjee 1959:2).

The Tol system was used to educate physicians. Kavirājās with reputations for remarkable cures trained young aspirants to the science in their homes, without demanding a fee. The relation between the Kavirājā and student was that of a Guru and disciple. Students without a good knowledge of Sanskrit were first instructed in grammer, literary texts, and logic. Having completed the preliminary course, they could proceed to the classical medical texts; but as it was hardly possible for a teacher to go through all the topics of the texts, students were made familiar with the basic knowledge of their

368

TABLE 1

TABLE 1

The Leading Schools of Traditional Āyurveda in
Nineteenth-Century Bengal

School	Special virtues of the school
East Bengal	
Savar	Preparation of herbal medicines
Matta	Techniques of examining patients, diagnosis, and prescriptions
Gaila	Preparation of medicines of Chemotherapy
Chandsi	Healing many kinds of ulcers, fistula, and piles
Chittagong	Treating insanity
Khandarpara	Treating insanity and constructing temporary huts like temporary hospitals
West Bengal	
Mursidabad	Reading pulse and diagnosis
Kumartooli	In medicine ("The Pills of Nilambara do not fail")
Srikhanda	General physicians who sold medicines in the open market and who published Ayurvedic textbooks

Guru, and later on they could read the other topics themselves. Table 1 shows the traditional schools of Āyurvedic practice in nineteenth-century Bengal.

Education in the Tols was not purely theoretical. Students assisted the Kavirājā when patients came to him, and they accompanied him when he visited severely ill patients at their homes. In this way they were given clinical experience. Students also acquired practical knowledge by procuring the raw materials for medicines and by preparing them under the master's guidance.

The British rulers did not interfere with the indigenous medical system during the first two decades of the nineteenth century. It was customary for them to employ Indians as subordinate health workers in hospitals. Those who gained skill in this way were attached to regiments and civil stations as "Native Doctors." As the demand for these workers increased, a school for native doctors was founded in 1822, and Āyurvedic classes were started in 1827, along with instruction in some Western medicine, in Sanskrit College. This college was opened in Calcutta under British patronge in 1824, and its medical curriculum was the first one to include parallel instruction in Āyurveda and Western medicine. This friendly coexistence between the systems did not last, however, for in 1835 the existing medical courses were abolished and a new college was established as part of a policy to make European medicine the only acknowledged system of study. In the controversy between the British Orientalists who supported the old Indian culture and the Anglicists who wished to supplant it, the Anglicists were victorious. To celebrate their triumph, Lord Macaulay ordered a cannon salute of fifty rounds to be fired from Fort William when the first dissection of a dead human body was performed in the new college by an Indian.

The abolition of Āyurvedic studies in the Sanskrit College, and the support of the English civilization and language, were a clever British policy to maintain control over the population. Also, the aspirations of the Christian missionaries were relevant to this policy. The classical Āyurvedic books belong to the holy scriptures of Hinduism, and the missionaries of that time looked down upon them as products of paganism and superstition. Lord Macaulay, who ordered the policy, was himself the son of a Christian missionary, and is said always to have supported missionary efforts to convert the Indians to the Christian faith (Chatterjee 1960:817).

Āyurvedic medical institutions began a downward trend following the establishment of the medical college in Calcutta. Conventional Āyurvedic education was continued in the private homes of Kavirājās, but the modest Tol sustained by the personal financial sacrifices of the Kavirāja could not be compared to the splendid, well-equipped college that offered many training possibilities. Naturally, young boys who wanted to become physicians did not want to enter the Tols, but were attracted to allopathic medicine. British policy encouraged this trend by granting scholarships and by distributing free medical books, charts, and models. Moreover, the students who studied allopathy had much better chances of achieving a good position in life than those trained in the old Tols.

At first, orthodox Kavirājās did not allow their sons to study allopathic medicine, but after taking into account the financial advantages, a great number of them also sent their sons to the medical college. The students obtained certificates to practice medicine and surgery, and were enrolled as first-class Native Doctors. Second-class Native Doctors were those who had been trained in the short-lived college founded in 1822, and the third class was composed of those whose training was limited to apprenticeships in hospitals. All young Indians were educated for subordinate positions, even in the college founded in 1835 and modeled on medical schools in England. But because of the financial amenities, allopathic institutions were well attended.

After 1835, the British policy was to push out the native medicine of India and to patronize the European system. This aim had been laid down in a Government Resolution as early as 1821, which stated that the purpose of the British rulers was "to seek every practicable means of effecting the gradual diffusion of European knowledge" (Mukhopadhyaya 1926, II:15). This political decision was worked out in different phases. In the early phase, both European and Indian medical texts were allowed to be taught side by side in the Sanskrit College. Later on, when the stage was set for a showdown of European supremacy, the Ayurvedic classes were abolished from Sanskrit College.

In the decades after the medical college was founded in Calcutta, it seemed that allopathy would supplant the traditional Āyurvedic system. But this crisis was averted by a renowned Kavirājā who elevated the prestige of Āyur-veda. Gangadhara Ray exercised great influence throughout the nineteenth century, and his fame continues to the present day. He was born in 1789 in the village of Magura (Jessore) in eastern Bengal. After having acquired a good knowledge of Sanskrit, he began special Āyurvedic studies when he was eighteen years old. He studied in the Tol of Kavirājā Ramakanta Sen, in the village of Vaidhya Belghoria. When he completed his medical training, he considered whether he should establish his practice in Murshida-bad, in the district of his birth, or go to Calcutta. Murshidabad was the declining center of ruling princes, and Calcutta was becoming the new center of power. But the main reason he decided to practice in Calcutta seems to have been that he wanted to publish the classic medical text, *Caraka Saṁhīta*, and he heard that a wealthy resident of Calcutta owned a copy that was without defects (Bhattacharya, B.S. 1361:57–58)

When Gangadhara Ray moved to Calcutta in 1819, he had had no contact with English education, and he never learned this language. But he observed the growing influence of Western medical science and disapproved of this development. A legend tells that he left Calcutta in 1835 when he heard the fifty-gun salute fired on the occasion of the first dissection by an Indian at the new medical college. But the truth appears to be that the atmosphere of Calcutta caused him to become ill, and he went to his father's home at Natore to recover. (Bhattacharya, B.S. 1361:58)

After leaving Calcutta, Gangadhara settled on the eastern bank of the Ganges at Shaidabad (Berhampore), where he opened a Tol and educated a number of brilliant students. He became a Court physician to the Nawab of Murshidabad and a consulting physician to Maharani Svarnamayee of Kashimbazar. Gangadhara acquired legendary fame for his skill in the therapeutic use of poisons and decoctions, in diagnosis by reading the pulse, and in prognosis (Gupta, B.S. 1361:5). Like many orthodox Kavirājās, Gangadhara was well versed in astronomy and astrology. He wrote Sanskrit commentaries on 34 books, and himself composed 41 books (Svargiya, B.S. 1322–23:89–91,104–111). His commentary on the classic text of *Caraka*, called *Jalpakalpataru*, was his special contribution to Āyurvedic scholarship. He died in 1885, at the age of 87. Table 2 lists Gangadhara's outstanding students, and their students in turn.

Gangaprasad Sen was a junior contemporary of Gangadhara, and a second great influence in the development of Āyurveda in nineteenth-century Bengal. While Gangadhara fought for the cause of Āyurveda outside of Calcutta, and avoided contact with allopathic medicine, Gangaprasad Sen

TABLE 2

The Students of Gangadhara Ray, 1789–1885, and Their Leading Students.

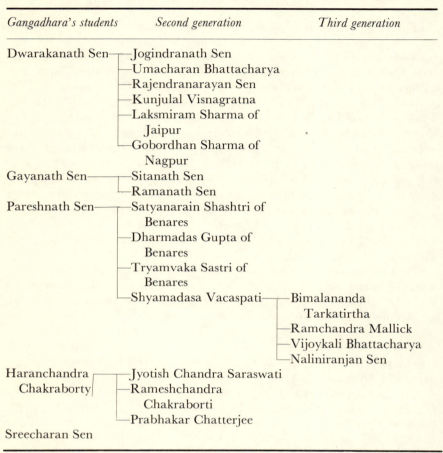

Gangadhara's students	Second generation	Third generation
Dwarakanath Sen	Jogindranath Sen	
	Umacharan Bhattacharya	
	Rajendranarayan Sen	
	Kunjulal Visnagratna	
	Laksmiram Sharma of Jaipur	
	Gobordhan Sharma of Nagpur	
Gayanath Sen	Sitanath Sen	
	Ramanath Sen	
Pareshnath Sen	Satyanarain Shashtri of Benares	
	Dharmadas Gupta of Benares	
	Tryamvaka Sastri of Benares	
	Shyamadasa Vacaspati	Bimalananda Tarkatirtha
		Ramchandra Mallick
		Vijoykali Bhattacharya
		Naliniranjan Sen
Haranchandra Chakraborty	Jyotish Chandra Saraswati	
	Rameshchandra Chakraborti	
	Prabhakar Chatterjee	
Sreecharan Sen		

tried to compete with Western medicine in the marketplace. Born in 1824 in Vikrampore at Dacca, he was trained in Āyurveda by his father, Nilambara Sen, whose fame is recorded in a local saying, "The watch of Gani Mian and the pills given by Nilambara Sen cannot fail" (Sen and Sen n.d.:134).

Gangaprasad Sen began to practice Āyurveda in Calcutta when he was nineteen years old. In the manner of his father, he directed special attention to the preparation of medicines, and very soon he earned a good reputation. Observing the increasing importation of European drugs, he thought that Āyurvedic medicines should also be prepared for sale in other countries, and he seems to be the first person to export Āyurvedic medicines to Europe and America. (Sen and Sen, n.d.:6) In the pattern of European physicians, he introduced fixed consultation fees which equalled or surpassed the fees of British physicians. In the same way, he sold medicines according to fixed price lists, and published advertisements for them. By these means he elevated Āyurvedic medicine to the same rank as allopathy, and drew public attention back to it. He published the first Āyurvedic magazine in the Bengali language, *Āyurveda Sañjīvanī*, with the purpose of upholding the prestige of the Indian system. He established a Tol in his home, where he gave students free room and board, and his patients included well-known persons such as the religious teacher Ramkrishna Paramhamsa. When he died in 1896, he was one of the richest men in Calcutta. Table 3 lists Gangaprasad's outstanding students, and their students in turn.

TABLE 3

The Students of Gangaprasad Sen, 1824–1896, and Their Leading Students.

Gangaprasad's students	*Second generation*
Nishikanta Sen	
Bijoy Ratna Sen—————	┬—Jaminibhusan Ray
	├—Virajacharan Gupta
	└—Durgadas Bhatta
Ramchandra Vidyabinod	

Gangadhara Ray and Gangaprasad Sen, who tended the flame of Āyurveda in the critical decades after 1835, were followed in the period of the Bengal renaissance by an illustrious generation of Kavirājās. The renaissance is commonly described as a movement in religion, philosophy, fine art, and nationalism which culminated in the 1870's. The role Āyurveda played in it has not yet been assessed, but an Āyurvedic renaissance occurred in Bengal at the same time among the many students of Gangadhara Ray and Gangaprasad Sen.

Bijoyratna Sen rose to eminence in this period. A student of Gangaprasad Sen, he translated the *Aṣṭāṅgahṛdaya* of Vāgbhaṭa into Bengali. This is one of the three primary classics of Ayurveda, and Bijoyratna published both his Bengali translation and the original Sanskrit text with accompanying introductions and suggestions for the regeneration of Āyurveda. His patients included many Indian princes and Europeans, and the Government of India recognized his accomplishments by conferring on him the honorary title *Mahāmahopādhyāya*. His education had been in a traditional Tol, but he was temperamentally responsive to the new ideas of the time and acquired a good command of English along with some knowledge of allopathy. A later critic who advocates traditional Āyurveda has written, "Bijoyratna was a lover of Allopathic medicines and also utilized them in the preparation of his special medicines in special cases" (Chatterjee 1967:296). Bijoyratna brought forward the idea of cooperation between allopathy and Āyurveda, and inspired his favorite student, Jaminibhusan Ray, to establish a college where they were studied side by side.

Other great Kavirājas of this period are listed in Tables 2 and 3. Many of them practiced in Bengal, but some located at Benaras, Hardwar, and other distant cities. Students were drawn to these scholars from many different regions, so that their influence extended far beyond Bengal.

The time-honored practice was for Kavirājas to prepare their own medicines for individual patients. Each patient was treated as a unique problem, and scientific principles were applied to find a personal remedy for him. Gangadhara Ray is said to have laughed at practitioners who prepared medicines beforehand for their patients, calling them *Badial*, possessors of pills ready for common use. But the large-scale production of medicines became necessary as the popularity of Āyurveda grew and small-scale preparation could not keep pace with the demand. In this respect, the leading innovator was Chandrakishore Sen.

Chandrakishore Sen was a Kavirāja of the traditional Srikhanda School (see Table 1) and a junior contemporary of Gangadhara Ray. In 1878 he opened a dispensary on the bank of the Ganges near the Kalighat temple in Calcutta, with the purpose of selling prepared medicines at a cheap rate. He thought of this as an experiment to popularize Āyurveda and to stop the onrush of allopathic drugs. He was successful, and in 1898 shifted the dispensary to Kalutola, where large-scale production was undertaken. But he did not favor cheap publicity, and rebuked his sons when they began publishing a newspaper in which the pharmaceutical products of the family company were advertised (Chatterjee 1959:813). Chandrakishore did publish inexpensive books to propagate knowledge and appreciation of Āyurveda, and C. K. Sen & Co. played an important role in the development of Ayurveda in those days.

In 1884 a similar pharmaceutical concern was founded to manufacture and sell Āyurvedic drugs, N. N. Sen & Co. Private, Limited, Calcutta. Also, a poor schoolteacher of chemistry, Mathuramohan Chakraborty, started to produce Āyuvedic medicines in a thatched tenement in the suburbs of Dacca in 1901, and in a few years was head of a successful pharmacy, Sakti Ausadhalaya of Dacca. The success of Sakti Pharmacy inspired a chemistry teacher at Bhagalpur College in Bihar, Jogesh Chandra Ghosh, to start another pharmaceutical industry, Sadhana Aysadhalaya. And yet another remarkable company was founded a little later, Kalpataru Ayurvedic Works, by Gananath Sen, a Kavirāja of high repute. His object was to produce Āyurvedic medicines on a large scale for sale at moderate prices, preparing them with the aid of modern machinery in the form of pills, tablets, and powders. These and numerous other firms earned considerable wealth, so that the Āyurvedists of Bengal were at one time among the richest men in the country.

The Bengal renaissance was one of the most significant movements leading to the Indian Freedom Struggle. In becoming conscious of their own tradition, the Indian people developed a national enthusiasm that led to political and cultural activities in the present century. Leaders of the Independence Movement were eager to build institutions to propagate old Indian tradition. Pharmacies were established in the last decades of the nineteenth century, and in the twentieth century the educational system was institutionalized by founding colleges with attached hospitals. The idea was to train Āyurvedic physicians by using modern teaching methods so that they could extend their services to the vast rural population. It was urged that reviving the Āyurvedic system would be an economic way to make medical relief available to the masses of suffering humanity.

The Calcutta Āyurvedic Institution was established in 1915 by Kavirāja Surendra Nath Goswami, who had a Licentiate in allopathic medicine, but the records of this institution do not survive. In contrast, the influential Aṣṭānga Āyurveda College and Hospital was founded by Kavirāja Jaminibhusan Ray in 1916, and is still in operation. Kavirāja Jaminibhusan was a scholar in both Āyurvedic and allopathic medicine. Since the only medical topic taught in the traditional Tols was internal medicine (*kāyacikitsa*), Jaminibhusan tried to revive the other branches of Āyurvedic learning by supplementing them with instruction in Western anatomy, physiology, surgery, and midwifery, along with physics, chemistry, and botany. Kavirāja Jaminibhusan was a new thinker of the period who particularly wanted to train Āyurvedic physicians knowledgeable in surgery and midwifery.

During the Buddhist period, the doctrine of *ahiṁsa* (nonviolence) caused the arrest of Āyurvedic surgery, and in Neo-Hinduism it was sinful for an orthodox Hindu to handle dead bodies or take food, including medicine, from a person who did so. Thus the Āyurvedic disciplines which drew upon dissection were almost lost in the course of time, and only internal medicine among the eight topics of Āyurvedic specialization continued in general practice. Also, practitioners gradually neglected human anatomy because the philosophical background of Āyurveda told them that a person was not merely composed of bones, flesh, and blood, but that he was a microcosm of the universe in which the five subtle elements were ordered in an evolutionary process. Thus the Kavirāja directed his attention to restoring the equilibrium of the three basic principles produced by these five elements (wrongly identified as "humors" in the English language). This practice was challenged with the introduction of modern anatomy and medicine, and Jaaminibhushan tried to meet the challenge by grafting the method and technique of Western science on to the traditional body of Āyurveda.

Jaminibhushan wanted to retain the status quo of the old Āyurveda and at the same time accept the findings of modern medicine; but in practice the institutionalization of Āyurvedic education brought in its train new problems. Students were more attracted to allopathy than to Ayurveda, so that these institutions did not produce scholars and teachers who could interpret Āyurveda from the original texts. Rather than raise the standards of Āyurvedic practice, these institutions reduced the Kavirājā to a simple medicine-man who lacked specialized knowledge of either Āyurveda or allopathy. The practitioners they trained were not esteemed as doctors or as Āyurvedic physicians, and thus counter-forces evolved in favor of the *Śuddha* philosophy of pure, or traditional, Āyurveda.

In 1921 a national university of Bengal, *Gauḍiya Sarvavidyāyatana,* was founded as part of the Noncooperation Movement, and the *Vaidya Śastra Pītha* was established as the Āyurvedic medical wing of this university. Kavirājā Shyamadas Vacaspati was the Founder-Principal of this institution. The students in his private Tol shifted to this institution, which was initiated by a donation of 6,000 rupees from the Tilak Swaraj Fund. However, Kavirājā Shyamadas contributed the monthly expenditures of the college. After Shyamadasa Vacaspati died in 1934, a building was constructed for the college with the help of his son, Bimalananda Tarkatirtha, and the institution was renamed the *Śyāmadāsa Vaidya Śastra Pītha.* Although it was constructed according to the pattern of the *Aṣṭāṅga Āyurveda Vidyālaya,* this school was a protest against the foreign-oriented education of the day, and its founder was an Āyurvedic scholar in the tradition of Gangadhara Ray.

The Gobinda Sundari Ayurvedic College was started in 1922 by Kavirājā Ramchandra Mallick with the patronage of Sir Manindra Chandra Nandy, Maharaja of Cossimbazar. Though a course of study integrated Āyurvedic and allopathic medicine, the hospital was provided with a special Vaisnava Ward to suit the sentiments of orthodox patients by providing an entirely separate kitchen, cook, and servants.

The *Viśwanātha Āyurveda Mahāvidyālaya* was founded in 1932 by Kavirājā Gananath Sen, with the idea of restoring Āyurveda to a fully scientific basis by educating physicians trained in all branches of medicine. And in this institution, too, Āyurveda was taught side by side with allopathy.

During the period of the founding of these colleges, and into the present day, a quarrel between advocates of the *Śuddha* system of traditional education and practice and those who advocate integrating Western medical science with Āyurveda has inhibited cooperation between the Kavirājās of Bengal. The national leaders who founded the new university as part of the Non-cooperation Movement, and the students of its *Vaidya Śāstra Pītha,* favored the *Śuddha* system. Mahatma Gandhi also appears to have favored traditional Āyurveda, for a publication of this school quotes Chittaranjan Das as having said, "Mahatmaji desires that the little that still remains of the glory of Ayurveda should not be completely lost by admixture with allopathic or any other systems" (*Bulletin* 1959).

A Śuddha Āyurvedist has described the educational ideal of this position in the following statement:

1. That during the first four years of Āyurvedic study students will have to read only original Āyurvedic works through the medium of Sanskrit language and there should be absolutely no connection with the reading of any book regarding modern medical science during the period in question.
2. After the completion of first four years of study—i.e., after graduation—they must go through all other branches of medical knowledge in the Republic of India such as Allopathy, Homeopathy, Naturopathy, Hydropathy, Unani, Biochemistry, etc. (Chatterjee 1967:296)

From time to time since India became independent in 1947, governmental committees dominated by allopathic doctors have been appointed to inquire about the welfare of Āyurveda, but even their recommendations were not implemented because the health departments of West Bengal and of the central government were directed by allopathic physicians. These physicians as an organized body are hostile toward Āyurveda.

In this struggle a number of Kavirājās have come forward to defend Āyurveda. My father, Bimalananda Tarkatirtha, is a leader among these Kavirājās, as are other students of my grandfather, Shyamadas Vacaspati. My father was Vice President of the State Faculty of Āyurvedic Medicine for many years. As a member of the Legislative Assembly, he fought hard for the rights and privileges of Āyurvedic practitioners. When he became General Secretary of the Parliamentary Party, he succeeded in getting an Āyurveda Bill passed in the West Bengal Assembly. But this state recognition gained for Āyurveda had few practical consequences, because it did not loosen the purse of the Public Exchequer. The majority of students coming out of the Āyurvedic institutions can neither get jobs with the state or win the prestige required for successful private practice. In this battle to revive and strengthen the old tradition of Āyurveda, my father has been aided by Vijoykali Bhattacharya and Prabhakar Chatterjee, also of the Śuddha Āyurveda school of thought. We have yet to see which forces win the battle in the future.

Literature Cited

Battacharya, Vijoykali
  B.S. 1361 *Āyurveder Itihāsa* (in Bengali). Calcutta.
Bulletin of
  1959 *Shyamadas Vaidya Sastra Pith.* "An Old Appeal." (March.)
Chatterjee, Prabhakar
  1959 "Kaviraj Gangadhar Roy Kaviratna." *Nagarjun* 7(June).
  1960 "Contents of Ayurvedic Encyclopaedia—IV." *Nagarjun* 8 (May).
  1967 "Mahamahopadhyaya Kaviraj Bijoy Ratna Sen: His Life and Technique of

Treatment." *Nagarjun* 15(February).

Gupta, Jogendranath
  B. S. 1361 "Āyurveda Prasaṅga." *Āyurveda* 1.

Mukhopadhyaya, Girindranath
  1926 *History of Indian Medicine*, 2 vols. Calcutta: University of Calcutta Press.

Sen, Girijaprasanna and, Jyotiprassanna Sen
  n. d. *Svargiya Kaviraj Gangaprasad Sen Mahasayer Cikitsalaya, Ausadhalaya o Vidyalaya: Catalogue of the Dispensary*. Calcutta.

Sen, Kaviraja Kulatilak Gangaprasad
  1955 *Ayurveda* 6(Feburary).

Sen, Satyacharan
  1932 "Samayiki." *Āyurvijñāna Sammilani* (January).

Svargiya Gangadhara Kaviraja
  B.S. 1322–23 *Vaidya Sañjīvanī Patrikā* 5 and 6.

PART VII

Perspectives

A NARRATIVE line of development exists in the arrangement of essays in the present volume. Parts I and II introduce the *dramatis personnae*, the three great medical traditions of the Old World *Oikoumenê* and their antagonist, cosmopolitan medicine. Part III considers the role of these traditions in biological adaptation, while Parts IV and V describe relationships between them and between their kinsmen—folk and popular-culture medicine—in contemporary urban and peasant societies. The climax of these relationships occurs in the revival movements that the essays in Part VI describe. The present section is a reflective coda on the perspectives of the actors in this drama, and of those who observe them and tell the story.

W. T. Jones begins this coda by asking: "What is a world-view, and how is it related to the kind of cultural product that is called a scientific theory?" Although the health practices of laymen and medical specialists are often purely empirical, in the sense of being pragmatically-oriented and non-reflective actions, they can usually be explained by using concepts and modes of reasoning that constitute a community's "science." When that "science" is rationalized and institutionalized to the point of becoming a science that historians of science might study, it gains the degree of uniqueness or separateness from other cultural domains that provokes the question Jones raises.

In this situation, Thomas Kuhn argues that fundamental changes in scientific theories cause changes of world-view, which he compares to gestalt switches of perception (Kuhn 1970:111–135). This idea is compatible with Jones' analyses of the relationships between scientific theories and world-views, but Kuhn was concerned with "scientific revolutions," while Jones is concerned with aspects of world-view that persist through millennia—that would characterize the world-views of Aristotle, Galileo, and Niels Bohr. He describes the relationship between scientific theories and world-views in a language that he developed in books on romanticism and on the character of scientific and humanistic disciplines (Jones 1961, 1965). It is one in which world-views limit, constrain, and resist change.

For example, Jones follows the generic question with which he opens his essay with a second question: "In particular, how might the world-view of practitioners and patients affect a medical system *by limiting its capacity to change?*" (emphasis added). And when he discusses change in the concluding section of his essay, he begins negatively by enumerating the factors one should consider "in estimating the likely resistance to change of some particular world-view." The changes that do occur he calls "surface changes," or changes of "belief-type vectors such as theories, technologies, etc.," in contrast to "strongly charged, wide-ranging vectors"; or he describes change as shifts of allegiance by the majority of people whose world-views are not intensely held or systematic, or as conversions based on reversion to a world-view that had been overlaid by an extraneous influence. The models he proposes for understanding profound changes of world-view are "self-therapy" and "self-weaning." Thus, according to the new world-view, the earlier one appears to have been a kind of immaturity or sickness.

Jones implies that the perceptual and affective orientations he calls world-views tend toward closure. The tendency is difficult to avoid and hard to correct. In his closing paragraph he recommends the therapeutic correction of assumptions about "Western medicine," and cautions that "it will not be easy; it will painful." That he recommends this painful task is because he believes it will lead to better comparative research, and because, as he has written elsewhere:

The great sin against the human spirit is closure against the diversity and variety of experience—a narrow dogmatism that insists on the absolute and exclusive validity of some particular language and the particular version of reality that this language articulates. And the central virtue, therefore, is openness to experience, *caritas* for the differences and diversities to be found within experience. (Jones 1965:280)

CHARLES LESLIE

Literature Cited

Jones, W. T.
   1961 *The Romantic Syndrome: Toward a New Method in Cultural Anthropology and the History of Ideas.* The Hague: Nijhoff.
   1965 *The Sciences and the Humanities: Conflict and Reconciliation.* Berkeley and Los Angeles: University of California Press.
Kuhn, Thomas S.
   1970 *The Structure of Scientific Revolutions.* International Encyclopedia of Unified Science, 2nd ed., enlarged, vol. 2, no. 2. Chicago: University of Chicago Press.

World Views and Asian Medical Systems: Some Suggestions for Further Study

W. T. JONES

What is a world-view, and how is it related to the kind of cultural product that is called a scientific theory? In particular, how might the world-view of practitioners and patients affect a medical system by limiting its capacity to change? The present essay is directed to these questions.

Section I introduces a model that provides indices along which similarities and differences in world-view can be scaled, thus making it possible to estimate how much a world-view changes through time. Section II shows that certain structural features of Western science can be scaled on the indices defined in Section I. Section III illustrates the model by showing that the world-views of contributors to this volume differ, and that these differences lead to disagreements about the nature of Western science, so-called, and thus about Asian science. Section IV turns to Asian science to show that the model for analyzing world-views can be applied to the theories underlying ancient Chinese medicine as Joseph Needham has described them.[1] Finally, Section V tentatively suggests causes of the kinds of changes in world-view that can be scaled on the indices described by the model.

I

It will be useful to think of people's beliefs, feelings, attitudes, and values as occurring in *belief space*. This heuristic concept corresponds to what some anthropologists and psychologists call the cognitive field. Since it is not necessary for present purposes to distinguish among the different kinds of elements in belief space, I shall refer to them all alike as *vectors*. Every overt behavior, e.g., to diagnose and treat a patient, is the product of numerous vectors. Some vectors, such as the belief about the correct way to elicit the patellar reflex, contribute to a relatively few kinds of behavior; I shall call these narrow-range vectors. Other vectors, such as a dislike of foreigners, are ingredients in many different kinds of behavior; these I shall call wide-

---

1 Manfred Porkert's essay in the present volume is consistent with some of Joseph Needham's description of Chinese medicine, and relevant therefore to my analysis.

range vectors.

I define a world-view as a configuration of vectors of the widest range. Each element in such a configuration is a dispositional set, or orientation, that causes one to focus on certain regions, or aspects, of experience, rather than on others. Thus, a world-view vector is similar to an ordinary attitudinal set such as the dislike of foreigners which causes one man to attend to behavior that a man who likes foreigners may pass over unnoticed. For that matter, a world-view orientation is similar to an ordinary perceptual set, such as the set to attend to one's own name and so to have it stand out in an otherwise indistinguishable babble of noise at a cocktail party. A world-view vector differs from such attitudinal and perceptual sets only in being very much more wide-ranging—that is, in affecting not merely this or that region of one's experience but one's whole world.

In addition to the notion of vector, we need the notion of a dimension. I define a dimension as a rank-ordering of vectors from the strongest possible disposition to believe P to the strongest possible disposition to believe not-P. For purposes of illustration, let us take the tendency to explain unexpected occurrences by attributing them to somebody's deliberate, Machiavellian design instead of to accident, coincidence, or just plain muddle. Suppose we want to scale individuals to compare them with respect to the strength of this tendency. This is where the notion of a dimension is useful. Let us select a number of cases where the evidence is either skimpy or ambiguous—e.g., the Pearl Harbor disaster, the two Kennedy assassinations, the Angela Davis indictment, the Berrigan indictment—and ask each individual to assess them. If an individual interprets all or most of these as plots, we may feel justified in eliminating other possible sources of bias—such as hostility to Franklin Roosevelt, or to the FBI, or to Communists, or to whites—and conclude that this individual's judgment, his weighing of evidence in cases where the evidence is marginal, is influenced by design-bias. Similarly, if an individual discounts the possibility of plots in all or most of these cases, and interprets them as coincidences, we will feel justified in attributing this to accident-bias. From such considerations we can begin to locate individuals on what may be called the design/accident dimension—that is, assign them "loci," either up toward the design-end, down toward the accident-end, or somewhere in the middle.

Mid-range loci tend to be weakly charged; polar loci tend to be strongly charged. Hence mid-range loci have a less pronounced effect on behavior than do polar loci; they are also more readily modifiable by learning. Extreme polar loci, on the other hand, are so rigid that they may be called "neurotic." Whereas a mid-range, weakly charged vector has a determinate effect on behavior only when the evidence is ambiguous, a neurotic vector is so highly charged that no amount of evidence affects the individual's conclusion; instead of modifying his bias to conform with the evidence, he fits the evidence to his bias. Thus, reverting to the design/accident dimension which we have been using for illustrative purposes, loci far out toward the design-end are paranoid. If a psychiatrist tries to assure his paranoid patient that his wife is not plotting against him, the patient simply concludes that the psychiatrist is in the plot with the wife.

Except in the case of such neurotic loci, we should not expect an individual with design-bias to see plots everywhere and all the time. Rather, we should look for a central tendency in his perceptions and assessments that is discernibly different from the central tendency of someone with strong accident-bias. Thus locus is a statistical concept.

It is obvious that the wide-ranging vectors that affect any particular individual's perceptions and judgments can be more or less widely distributed through a population—say, Californians, or Americans, or Westerners. Distribution is also a statistical concept: not all members of a group, even of a small and homogeneous society, have exactly the same set of wide-ranging vectors. But there may be a central tendency in that population, resulting from the fact that the modes of the individual members of the society group around a mode.

A set of *n* dimensions gives us an *n*-dimensional matrix within which it will be possible to locate the world-views of different individuals and societies—just as it is possible, within the three-dimensional matrix of ordinary, perceptual space, to locate different physical objects. In this paper I shall limit my analysis to a matrix defined by only four dimensions—dimensions which I have chosen because they seem to me particularly relevant to a discussion of how differences in world-view affect the capacity of medical systems, and the theories that underlie them, to change.

1. I call the first of the dimensions in this illustrative matrix the *static/dynamic* dimension. This is an array of biases (dispositions) ranging from a preference for the unchanging to a contrasting preference for the changing. An example in pre-Socratic philosophy is the contrast between Parmenides and Heraclitus. In contemporary economics, psychology, and sociology, this difference in perspective, or in outlook on the world, is reflected, this time in a preference either for equilibrium models or for disequilibrium models. We find historians divided by the same difference in bias—for instance, between those who are interested in studying revolutionary periods and those who prefer to concentrate on periods in which change is so slow as to be virtually imperceptible. In painting, this same difference—here one might want to speak of a difference in "style"—occurs. As an example, think of two paintings of the same subject, say the Adoration of the Kings. For Dürer, all is calm, poised, and at rest; for Rubens, all is tumult, excitement, movement. Or think of the contrast between a Mondrian and a Kandinsky.

2. *Continuity/discreteness* is the name I give to the second dimension in this matrix. This is a contrast between (a) an emphasis on interrelatedness, on contextuality, and on degree-differences; and (b) an emphasis on sharp distinctions, on ideal types, and on encapsulated atomistic entities. Words-

worth's feeling that "we murder to dissect" is an example of continuity-bias. Logical analysis seems to be murder because it divides up, and classifies, a world that continuity-bias perceives as a living whole. In contrast, there is Butler's aphorism, "Everything is itself and not another thing." Butler's vision of the universe was radically different from Wordsworth's—his universe is not one organic whole, but simply a collection of items. Accordingly, logical analysis ("dissection") is an entirely proper procedure—the only problem, from this perspective, is to make sure that the distinctions we draw correspond to those that exist in *rerum naturam*.

In painting, the same contrast in vision occurs. Think of Rembrandt's perception of objects, where everything merges into everything else, and Van Eyck's, where each object in the picture space is sharply and clearly distinguished from every other object. Whether the objects are near, or far away—in a distant field seen through a window—each is encapsulated, complete in itself.

3. A third dimension I call *abstract/concrete*. This is the contrast between (a) emphasizing broad general characteristics and (b) emphasizing the uniqueness of each individual object. Compare the difference between focusing on similarities between individuals, so that it is the class of which they are members that is important, and focusing on the differences that make each member of the class *this* individual, in spite of its membership in the class.

As an example in the social sciences, think of the different approaches to the study of small-group behaviour. On the one hand is William Foote Whyte's *Street-Corner Society*, devoted to one particular gang in Boston with whom Whyte lived long enough to come to know the members as individuals; he was not in a position to make any generalization about gangs, not even about gangs in Boston. Another way to do research on group behavior is to use a number of "subjects"—one does not know them as individuals; one hauls them into one's laboratory out of classrooms and isolates them in booths, with various kinds of communication circuits, in order to discover whether there is any correlation between circuitry and problem-solving time. In this approach to research, one has no interest in individuals as individuals; one is simply interested in the abstract generalizations that may be found to characterize a group of subjects in differing situations.

As a historical example, think of the difference between a preference for universalistic history—Arnold Toynbee, for instance—where the emphasis is on abstract generalities that hold for all civilizations; and a preference for a highly particularistic narrative that avoids generalizations and concentrates on the events of a single day—for instance, the sinking of the *Titanic*, or the Normandy landings.

4. I call the last dimension in this matrix *immediacy/mediation*. This is the difference between what is lived through (what is directly experienced) and what is experienced from outside, from a distance. This dimension can also be described in terms of the notion of participant-observation. Some people are more participants than observers; some are more observers than participants. Some people prefer natural, informal social and business relationships; they like "simple" people. Others enjoy protocol, distance, "good

manners," and generally sophisticated, urban types. This difference in bias also turns up in educational theory and educational practice: some people prefer the lecture system in which the teacher stands behind a lectern, separated by physical, as well as psychological, space from his students. Others prefer an approximation to sensitivity training rather than formal education. And, as a final example, think of the difference between the "feeling heart" that the romaniticists believed should guide our actions and the long-range, enlightened self-interest that the Age of Reason advocated.

II

Here, then, are four world-view indices—the Static/Dynamic, Continuity/Discreteness, Abstract/Concrete, and Immediacy/Mediation dimensions—from among the many that can be identified. Four are enough to enable me to show, as I shall now try to do, how differences in world-view, as specified in terms of these dimensions, account for structural differences in scientific theories—for instance, for different views of what explanation consists in and, indeed, for different conceptions of what a scientific theory is and ought to be.

First, as regards structural differences in general: If we look at the history of Western sciences as well as its present condition, we can see, I think, that there have been two recurrent conceptions of what science is. I shall call these the *Naturwissenschaft* paradigm (N-paradigm) and the *Geisteswissenschaft* paradigm (G-paradigm). I propose to show that many of the distinguishing features of the N-paradigm can be traced back to the following configuration of vectors: abstract, static, discrete, and mediate—and that distinguishing features of the G-paradigm reflect the contrasting configuration: concrete, dynamic, continuous, and immediate.

Thus there are and have been at least two, but quite possibly more, Western world-views. I think that on the whole the N-configuration has tended to predominate, not only in science but in almost every aspect of the culture. The G-configuration, while statistically deviant if we think of the history of Western culture as a whole, has predominated at times—for example, in the so-called Romantic Movement—and it has probably always been present as a minority world-view. For instance, the radically different psychological theories of behaviorists on the one hand and of phenomenologists on the other are traceable to differences between the N-configuration and the G-configuration of vectors, with existential psychoanalysis representing still more highly charged loci in the latter configuration. The dispute among historians between those who maintain that history can be a science and those who insist that it is an art is traceable to similar differences in world-view, and so for corresponding differences in political science, sociology, and other sciences.

Think, for instance, of the notion of a variable. This notion is fundamental for the N-paradigm. Indeed, what is commonly thought of as *the* method of science—the method of testing hypotheses empirically to verify or disverify them—depends on first isolating variables, e.g., the pressure and temperature of a gas or the mass and acceleration of a body, and then varying one systematically while holding everything else constant. But what is a variable? It is an aspect of the situation that can be lifted out of its context and altered without affecting that context. In other words, underlying the notion of a variable is a vision of the universe as a collection—a collection of relatively discrete and encapsulated items. The notion of a variable would only occur to, and seem plausible to, scientists with discreteness-bias. In contrast, scientists with continuity-bias are likely to be hostile to the notion of a variable, for they perceive things as organisms and as organically related. Since, with Wordsworth, they feel it is murder to dissect, they contrast what they call real life with the artificiality of a controlled experiment, and they are likely to argue that findings so obtained are but by-products of the experimental situation.

This, then, is one example of the kind of structural difference that can be traced back to differences in world-view, in this case to different loci on the continuity/discreteness dimension. Another such difference is reflected in differential attitudes toward interdisciplinary studies. Discreteness-bias disposes a scientist to perceive each discipline as an autonomous domain, with well-defined boundaries. Continuity-bias, on the other hand, disposes a scientist to regard the several disciplines as accidental growths, and the lines between them as artificial. Similarly, regarding differential attitudes toward organized, team research, scientists with discreteness-bias are likely to sympathize with Adam Smith's dictum that "philosophy and speculations of all kinds" yield better results when they are "subdivided into a great number of different branches." The key words here are "subdivided" and "different." Because Smith envisaged a world of atomistic things, it seemed to him self-evident that best results are achieved when we make our divisions along already-established lines of cleavage. Continuity-bias, in contrast, dislikes bureaucracy and compartmentalization. Since, for it, there are no lines of cleavage already there, the divisions we make are always arbitrary. Hence what looks to discreteness-bias like an efficient organization looks harmfully restrictive to continuity-bias.

Here, then, are ways in which different loci on the continuity/discreteness dimension lead to different patterns, both in theorists' conceptions of what science is and in their approaches to research procedures. I shall now show how vectorial differences on the other three dimensions in this matrix account for additional structural differences between N-tending and G-tending sciences. I write N-tending and G-tending, instead of N-type and G-type, to emphasize the fact that I am talking about a distribution of vectors around a central tendency—that is, I am talking about a *region* of the matrix, within which a number of different individual configurations are located, not about a single point in the matrix.

That Western science has been predominately abstract in its approach goes almost without saying. The West has always been more interested in the class than in its individual members, in the "what" than in the "that," in "essence" than in "existence." That is, the aim of Western science has always been to discover and formulate "laws."

In contrast, a society that is profoundly concrete in orientation is happy to contemplate individuals in all their rich uniqueness. I do not mean that men with concrete-bias do not observe, and adjust to, the regularities that occur in nature. Day follows night and summer follows winter in the world of concrete-bias as well as in the world of abstract-bias. Rather, I mean that it takes abstract-bias to conceive of a world of ideal forms, and to view these ideal forms as more real, and therefore more important, than the objects encountered in perception. It would seem that the predominance of such a point of view is a necessary, but not of course the sufficient, condition for the development of N-type sciences.

Though abstract-bias is certainly a component in the modal configuration in Western culture, a statistically deviant configuration includes concrete-bias. Differing loci on this dimension account for the fact that it is as natural for some social theorists to talk about roles and statuses as it is for others to talk about rules and norms. Talk about roles and statuses emphasizes that individuals must adjust to roles and fit into statuses; the roles and the statuses are perceived as being independent of the individuals who "play" and "occupy" them. In contrast, talk about rules and norms focuses attention on the fact that the roles and statuses are internalized and individualized. This language emphasizes that what is important is the various ways in which concrete individuals play the same role.

That the N-configuration is predominantly static is surely also evident. This is revealed in many ways—for instance, in its view of time. Time does not, for this way of thinking, enter into the inner nature of things; it merely carries things along with it, as a river carries with it the boats and ships that float on its surface—they are not a part of it, and it is not a part of them.

Dynamic-bias, especially when associated with concrete-bias in the G-configuration, has a very different view of time. For scientists with this outlook, time does not merely carry objects along with it; it enters into their inner nature: it is ingredient in events. The notion of laws of nature connecting point-events is replaced by the notion of individual lives. Accordingly, for the G-configuration the explanation of some event, E, does not consist in discovering how the class of events of which this event is a member is correlated with some other class of events. Explanation consists in tracing the historical development that has brought it about that E is what it is now. When we have learned E's history in detail, we know everything about E that there is to know. In a word, whereas physics is the typical science for the N-configura- psycho-analysis is more typical of the G-configuration: each case is unique; it is the history of the unfolding of some individual's present out of that individual's past.

Not only does a difference in world-view account for fundamentally different conceptions of what explanation consists in, it also accounts for differing conceptions of what seems to be in need of explanation. Thus dynamic-bias takes motion for granted; for it, motion is not problematic. But since, for static-bias, rest is "more natural" than motion, a central problem for physicists with this bias is to understand motion, to explain how things get started. One answer was the Greek atomists' notion of a fall through space; another was the Cartesians' idea that God "imparted a quantity of motion" to the universe after He created it; still another was Newton's concept of external forces impinging on masses. These views naturally differ in important details, but underlying all of them is a vision of motion as something added from outside. One of the consequences of this way of thinking is the notion of "inanimate nature"; further, there is a tendency to think of living things on this same model. Hence, for instance, the prominence in N-tending psychological theory of the stimulus-response arc—organisms are thought of as "reacting" to external causes.

A word-view that, in contrast, attributes an inner energy, or dynamism, to things has a wholly different set of emphases. For instance, instead of taking "inanimate nature" as the model for thinking about organisms, it takes organisms as the model for thinking about nature, which is no longer envisioned as inanimate, or moving only by imparted forces. Among other consequences, a stimulus-response type of psychology will no longer seem remotely plausible.

Finally, as regards mediation-bias: it is easy to see why the development of N-tending sciences depended on mediation-bias having been the modal stance in our society. For these sciences require the scientist to adopt a mediate, or external, attitude toward the objects he studies. He must be willing to study nature from outside, neutrally and objectively, ready and willing to "use" nature for his scientific ends. A society whose modal configuration includes strong immediacy-bias would not adopt this attitude toward nature. People with immediacy-bias do not feel themselves to be apart from nature; they feel themselves to be a part of it, sharing in its life. They not only experience nature as animate; they experience it, in some sense, as sacred— they treat it with respect, not merely as something to be manipulated, dissected, and experimented with. As an example, think of the difference between the attitude of a therapist toward his patient and that of a behaviorist toward his rats.

This description of the way in which differences in world-view are reflected in differing conceptions of science is obviously incomplete, and not only because it has been confined to the four dimensions that I introduced for illustrative purposes. But though it is no more than a preliminary sketch, I nevertheless hope it shows the lines along which a full-scale analysis might be undertaken. In the next section, this sketch is supplemented by a short account of some of the differences in world-view that were revealed in the

conference pre-prints and that emerged in the course of our discussions.
I shall also show how these differences led to disagreements about the nature
and the future prospects of Asian science.

III

The essays for the present volume are of course *about* science; but in each of
them the author is also *doing* science—either sociological, anthropological,
historical, or paleopathological and epidemiological research—and presumably his way of doing science reflects his notion of what science is. From the
authors' differing ways of doing science, as well as from the different things
they say about science, we can read back to a variety of underlying world-
views. My analysis will draw upon the Symposium at Burg Wartenstein in
which the preliminary drafts of the essays here published were discussed.
I shall not specify all of the configurations represented at the Symposium.
It will be enough to show that there are an N-tending group and a G-tending
group among contributors to this volume.

First, then, as regards the immediacy/mediation dimension. Renée Fox
and Mark Field, as we learned at the Symposium, were graduate students
together in the same department at Harvard University, but their ways of
doing sociology are very different. Both discuss magic. For Renée Fox, magic
is related to the existential anxiety of physicians, and their jokes are a way of
relieving this anxiety. But Fox is not merely interested in describing the relation that holds between joking and the reduction of anxiety; she sympathizes
with the physicians, wants us to share her sympathy, and writes in a way
calculated to help us do so. She wants us to feel what it feels like to be a physician engaging in research that is perilous for the human beings who are
subjects of this research. These aims and her style of writing reflect a strong
immediacy-bias.

In contrast, Mark Field discusses magic from outside, as an observer. It is
significant that he does not relate it to the existential anxiety of physicians:
he is interested in its functional role in the whole system of medical care, not in
its role in the personality dynamics of the physician. It is not, of course, that
Field would deny that physicians experience existential anxiety. Rather,
what is in the foreground for Fox is very much in the background for Field.
Differences in world-view have produced a kind of perspectival foreshortening,
analogous to spatial foreshortening, as a result of which things that look near
to one of these sociologists look far away to the other.

This brings us to the continuity/discreteness dimension, and here again
differences between the approaches of Mark Field and Renée Fox may be
used as examples. Were existential anxiety called to Field's attention, he
would certainly be willing to add it as another "input" into his system of
medical care. But this way of dealing with the matter would not satisfy Fox,
who, perhaps overstating her feelings, as people may do in the give and take

of a symposium, declared that the whole notion of a number of separate variables that can be aggregated was "specious." In discussing Field's model diagram of a medical system, she remarked, "I would have blurred it more." Field replied that he would be willing to "add to the diagram but not to blur it"—a remark as characteristic of discreteness-bias as hers was characteristic of continuity-bias.

Or, as another example, think of Field's concept of the gross medical product (GMP). For participants with a strong continuity-bias, this was a very dubious notion. They pointed out that since every activity in the society contributes at least to some degree to the gross medical product, any attempt to bound the GMP is arbitrary; to them the very notion of a GMP was "artificial." Field of course did not deny the difficulty of bounding the medical system, but he thought that this did not invalidate the notion of a GMP. At this point, students with different world-view biases can only agree to differ. The characteristic final remark by an individual with a strong polar, but not neurotic, bias to an individual with the opposite polar bias is, "Yes, but . . . ." Each sees the fact to which the other is pointing, but because they weigh this fact differently, they reach different conclusions. Mark Field saw the difficulty to which participants with continuity-bias called his attention, but his discreteness-bias led him to minimize the difficulty which their continuity-bias caused them to magnify. Hence, for him, the utility of the notion of GMP outweighs its artificiality, while for them its artificiality outweighs its utility.

Finally, I will give a few examples of the way in which differences on the abstract/concrete dimension turned up at the symposium. Contrast Brahmananda Gupta's essay with the one by Mark Field. Gupta wrote a history of the revival of Ayurveda in Bengal, and Field wrote a study of the development of Soviet medicine. But, whereas Gupta concentrated on individuals—his preliminary draft consisted in a series of short biographies—Field hardly mentioned any individuals, and his narrative followed an abstract model. This was not a function of the time-periods discussed. Since Gupta covered a much longer period of time, it might be expected, other things being equal, that his narrative would be more abstract than Field's. My point is simply that, as a result of differences in world-view, other things are not equal.

Or, as another example, contrast the essays by Edward Montgomery and M. A. Jaspan. Montgomery first set out a general thesis about the relation between variables in a system, and then proceeded to illustrate this thesis by taking "medical practice," defined as "the collective rate of consultations," as the "maintained variable." At this point, a very interesting sentence occurred in the essay prepared for the symposium—interesting, that is, to anyone on the alert for the kind of difference that a difference in world-view can make. Montgomery first described the great diversity of kinds of practitioners and types of practice he found in Vellore, and then wrote: "In view of the undeniably great differentials of training, expertise, and numbers of patients received and responded to by the group of private practitioners described above. . . ." A reader with strong concreteness-orientation would expect the sentence to continue, "nothing of any consequence can be said about the group as a whole," or "a summation of their combined practice would yield only a virtually meaningless number." But the sentence actually continued, "consideration of them as a group permits calculation of a collective practice or consultation rate." Note the force, here, of the word "permits." The underlying assumption is that what is worth saying is only what holds generally true of all individuals; in the Vellore case, because of the amount of variation encountered, this turns out to be only the consultation rate. Given abstract-bias, summing the consultation rate is worth doing; given concreteness-bias, this summation is trivial.

Here again we reach a point where scholars in effect say to each other, "Yes, but . . . ." Everybody starts with the fact of diversity in Vellore. Those with abstract-bias say, "Despite this diversity, how fortunate it is that we can say something general." Those with concrete-bias say, "Because of this diversity, we cannot. . . ." Think of the report M. A. Jaspan might have written had he undertaken the Vellore study: a detailed account of one or more practitioners—the Vellore equivalents of Man Aher.

Differences on this dimension affect scientists' ways of doing science and, when science is their subject, their conceptions of what science is. Concrete-bias, since it focuses attention on the concrete empirical fact, leads to the most inclusive definition. From this point of view, any generalization, however commonsensical it may be, is "scientific," providing only that it works. Thus, Fred L. Dunn observed in the draft of his essay for the Symposium that "scientific elements are present" even in "primitive" medical systems, since "many medicinal plants used in these systems are now recognized to have specific beneficial pharmacological effects." And M. A. Jaspan pointed to the Rejang discovery of the relation between rivers and "chills, sore throats, coughs, and influenza," It did not matter, for those with concrete-bias, whether the generalization was unsupported by any rationale, or whether it was supported by one that was false. In the Redjang case, the generalization about the relation between rivers and chills rested on "a sizable body of Rejang magico-religious belief about spirits and devils inhabiting river banks and sea coasts." For concrete-bias it is enough that the relation asserted in the generalization actually holds and that it is useful. Concrete-bias does not ask "Why?" but only "Does it work?"

Abstract-bias leads to a much narrower and more exclusive definition of science. For it, the existence of an abstract rationale in terms of which the concrete empirical generalizations are "explained" is the all-important criterion. When abstract-bias is associated with discreteness-bias, as is often the case, an even narrower and more restrictive definition of science becomes operative. Now it is no longer enough just to have some kind of rationale. The rationale must be of such a form that verification procedures can be designed for the variables that the rationale defines. Abstract- and discreteness-bias do not ignore the concrete facts; these enter into consideration as the termini of the verification procedures by means of which false theories are eliminated. But abstract-bias focuses its attention on the presence or absence of a rationale, and nothing qualifies as science, however useful the information question might be, unless it rests on an abstract theory. It was characteristic of this point of view that several participants in the Symposium described the current practice of Ayurvedic medicine as a "decline," inasmuch as many practitioners do not know the ancient theoretical texts on which the theory was based. And J. Christoph Bürgel spoke for a number of others when he distinguished between "theoretically trained physicians" and "mere underlings," who can perform certain routines (e.g., blood-letting) but who are unable to "derive the appropriate individual treatment by means of logical procedures. . . ."

These differences about what science is, which rest on differences in world-view, resulted in their turn in differential assessments of the prospects for the survival of Asian science. Those whose definition of science was inclusive were on the whole optimistic; their attention was focused on the similarities between Western and Asian science, and so they concluded either that Asian science can survive alongside Western science or that it can be easily assimilated. When continuity-bias was associated with concrete-bias, this point of view was reinforced. Continuity-bias leads to emphasis on the importance of treating "the whole man"—not merely his body, still less this or that organ. In a word, continuity-bias led some participants to share Yasuo Otsuka's criticism of Western medicine for its tendency to concentrate on "the biopsy." Thus the belief that Asian medicine could survive was reinforced by a conviction that it *should* survive—that in important respects, it is a more adaptive system than Western medicine.

Those whose definition of science was exclusive focused, naturally, on the dissimilarities between traditional and modern science. For some participants, even to talk about Asian science is a mistake, since it lacks both theoretical structure and verification procedures for eliminating false theories. Accordingly, these participants tended to see no future at all for Asian science; further, they predicted that the development of a "truly scientific," i.e., Western-type, medical system in some Asian countries would be accomplished only with great difficulty.

Here, then, is one example of the kind of difference that a difference in world-views can make. And the simple but important lesson that I derive from it is this: Since our world-view does make a difference in the methods we use and in the conclusions we reach, scientific objectivity depends on our learning to discount our world-view. Since the first step in learning to discount it is to become aware of it, the kind of analysis sketched in this section should be useful.

IV

I have been concentrating on two of the world-views that underlie Western science and that account for some of its special characteristics. I turn now to ask whether the same model is applicable to Asian science. If several world-views in fact underlie Western science, it seems likely, given the longer history of Asian thought and its immense cultural and geographical diversity, that there is an even greater variety of Asian world-views. Providing that our model is not culture-bound, the four-dimensional matrix we have introduced should provide a way for describing this diversity and so of contrasting various Asian world-views with each other as well as with Western world-views. I shall have to leave this inquiry to those who have a first-hand know-ledge of the relevant materials. Here I confine myself to a few tentative obser-vations about ancient Chinese science. Indeed, since what I shall be saying is based almost entirely on reading Joseph Needham's publications on the subject, I shall be doing little more than carrying out an exercise. But though I shall be discussing only the world-view that Needham attributes to Chinese science, I hope that my discussion will show that the method of analysis has cross-cultural validity.[1]

In Joseph Needham's account the world-view of traditional Chinese science is much closer to the G-configuration than to the N-configuration. Thus, if we assume that the modal locus of Chinese scientists on the abstract/ concrete dimension was strongly concrete, we can, I think, account for some features of traditional Chinese science that recur in Needham's descrip-tions—for instance, the marked disparity between Chinese accomplishments in technology and in theory. An advanced technology presupposes only observation, practical interests, and problem-solving ability; but theory-construction presupposes abstract-bias as well—that is, a disposition to direct attention away from concrete reality, with which technology is concerned, and toward ideal models that are not replicated anywhere in nature.

In Western history, all the G-type sciences have developed more or less extensive bodies of theory, even though G-type theory is by no means the formalized, deductive system that N-type theory typically is. This suggests that the modal locus for traditional Chinese science may be even farther toward the concrete-pole of this dimension than the modal locus for G-type sciences. But it may be that the existence of theory in the G-type sciences is due rather to the fact that in the West the G-configuration is statistically deviant. Hence G-type sciences are likely to be thought inferior, and G-type scientists are therefore likely to try to make their work as "scientific"—i.e., as close to the N-paradigm—as possible. This would include theory-construction, since that is a fundamental feature of the N-paradigm. Chinese thinkers, whose bias was similarly concrete, would lack this incentive, since theirs was the dominant, not merely a statistically deviant, configuration.

Again, it seems characteristic of the ancient Chinese scientists whom

Needham describes that, when asked the sort of question that would lead Western scientists to reply by referring to a law of nature, or Western laymen to reply with some commonsense generalization—e.g., "Friction causes heat," "An apple a day keeps the doctor away"—they replied instead with a narrative—i.e., the description of some particular, concrete episode (Needham 1962, II : 51,74,577). It is not likely that these Chinese scientists first thought of the generalization and then, to make it more vivid, cast it into narrative form. Rather, it seems that they characteristically thought concretely, not abstractly.

We would expect societies in which abstract-bias is the modal vector to adopt a *de jure*, rather than a *de facto*, approach, for the abstractions that this bias perceives to be more real than concrete objects are also experienced as ideals—ideals which nature necessarily follows (hence the notion of moral law, and of sin as a falling-away from this ideal). Similarly, we would expect societies in which concrete-bias is the modal vector to de-emphasize law in both of these senses. This indeed seems to have been the position of the ancient Chinese thinkers. Thus, if we follow Needham (1970:287), Taoism inculcated "acceptance of Nature and natural phenomena"; further, Chinese parents adopted an attitude of "extreme permissiveness in the house training and home life of young children." Thus there was "an almost total absence of persecution for the sake of religious opinion" (Needham 1970:287). Thus again, the Chinese hostility to positive law: "From the beginning the supple and personal relations of *li* were felt to be preferable to the rigidity of *fa*" (Needham 1962, II : 522,526). That is, law "administered [by men] paternalistically judging every new case on its own merits" was preferred to the notion of these judgments as being derived deductively from an abstractly and explicitly formulated code. This preference corresponds to the G-configuration's emphasis, in sociological theory, on internalized norms and rules, in contrast to the N-configuration's emphasis on roles and statuses.

In the G-configuration, as we have seen, concrete-bias is associated with continuity-bias, immediacy-bias, and dynamic-bias; these associations seem to exist also in the traditional Chinese world-view. For instance, as regards continuity-bias, when Pien Ch'io was asked about the methods of an earlier physician, Yü Fu, he replied: "The methods of which you speak are no better than viewing the sky through a thin tube or considering paintings by looking through a narrow crack" (Needham 1970:269). Expressed in these striking metaphors is what Needham calls the holism of traditional Chinese medicine, a point of view that corresponds closely to the G-configuration's distrust of the N-configuration's reliance on isolating a variable—and that, like this distrust, is rooted in continuity-bias.

Continuity-bias surely also appears in another fundamental characteristic of traditional Chinese science: its refusal to "separate Man from Nature, or individual man from social man" (Needham 1962, II :270). In the West, concrete-bias, here of course a deviant attitude, led to similar refusals—to a rejection of the "corpuscular" theory of light in physics,[2] the contract theory in politics,[3] and theism in theology.

As regards dynamic-bias, it would seem that the traditional Chinese science shared the G-configuration's emphasis on interior dynamic and its corresponding rejection of the notion of an external cause. So, for instance:

> Penumbra said to Shadow, "At one moment you move, at another you are at rest. At one moment you sit down, at another you get up. Why this instability of purpose?"
>
> "Do I have to depend," replied Shadow, "upon something which causes me to do as I do? ... And does that something have to depend in turn upon something else, which causes it to do as it does? ... Is not my dependence [more like the unconscious movements of] the scales of a snake or the wings of a cicada?" (Needham 1962, II:51)

Finally, as regards immediacy-bias, though many examples could be cited, I will mention only the notion of "untaught teaching," or "wordless edict." To the extent that men are perceived as mediately related, it will be felt that messages are needed for communication and effective interaction. Hence in a society where this bias is modal, there will be an emphasis on verbal exchanges —on taught teachings, as it were. But immediacy-bias leads to an opposite perception of human relations and so on to an opposite conclusion about the role of verbalization in human interactions.[4] To the extent that men's relations with each other are perceived to be direct and unmediated, untaught teachings and wordless edicts will seem both possible and desirable. Hence the frequent reference in Chinese thought to spontaneous cooperation, in contrast to command.[5]

v

It is a truism that men's freedom to change, to become different, to learn, is not unlimited. The account we have given of world-views calls attention to one of the factors that limits capacity to change. A world-view, as a configuration of cognitive and attitudinal sets, is a kind of perspectival stance from which an individual, or a society, looks out at the world. Given very different world-view perspectives, two individuals, or societies, may encounter very different worlds. And even if they see the same things, these things look different. As with different visual perspectives, things that are central in one world-view perspective may be marginal or peripheral in another.

2 Compare the seventeenth-century dispute between Newton and Huyghens. All of the available empirical evidence was known to both men. The fact that they reached different conclusions from this evidence is a good example of the influence, at the margin, of differences in world-view.

3 Compare Locke's and Burke's radically differing defenses of the same constitutional arrangements.

4 Note William Caudill's observation of a similar contrast in modern Japanese and American patterns of social relationships, in his essay for the present volume.

5 Note the effect this would be likely to have on the Mandariate bureaucracy, in contrast to Western bureaucracy (Needham 1962, II:561).

What, for instance, is the relationship between abstract-bias and the invention of theoretical physics? Obviously a society in which abstract-bias predominates does not automatically invent physical theory; something more—much more, probably—is needed. But to what extent does the prevalence of concrete-bias in a society make it unlikely that this society will develop theoretical physics? Or, to shift from the level of society to the level of the individual: Though abstract-bias does not guarantee that a man is going to become a first-class theoretical physicist, is a man with very strong concrete-bias likely to become a really first-class theoretical physicist? If the answer to this question is No, then the next question is: Can he be changed from concrete- to abstract-bias?

This has brought us, finally, to the question: How do world-views change? In this form the problem is too broad to handle; it must be sorted out into a whole series of separate questions. One of the advantages of the model introduced in this paper is that it helps us keep in mind certain important distinctions and so reduces, though it does not eliminate, the chance of muddle and of argument at cross-purposes.

1. When we are talking about change in world-view, we need to keep in mind whether we are talking about a change in the world-view of some individual or a change in the world-view of some society. Since a change in world-view is a change in the central tendency of a distribution of vectors, this amounts to saying that we need to keep in mind whether we are talking about a change in the central tendency of an individual such as Aristotle, Newton, or Einstein, or a change in the central tendency of a number of central tendencies of, for example, fourth-century Athenians, or seventeenth-century Europeans. In both sorts of case, of course, we will be making an inference from a sample—in the former case from the cultural products of some individual; in the latter from the cultural products of a sample of the individual members of that society.

2. We need, whether we are thinking of individuals or of societies, to keep in mind what level of vector we are talking about—i.e., we need to keep in mind how wide-ranging the vectors are whose changes interest us. For not only can vectors of differing degrees of specificity change independently of each other; it is also likely that the causes of change at different levels are very different.

3. Similarly, whether we are thinking of individuals or of societies, we need to keep in mind what *type* of vector we are talking about—whether vectors that are primarily cognitive (i.e., of the belief-type) or vectors that are primarily affective (of the attitudinal type); for it seems likely, once again, that the causes of change in different types of vectors are very different.

4. Again, whether we are thinking of individuals or of societies, we need to take account of the following factors in estimating the likely resistance to change of some particular world view:

a. Perhaps the most obvious factor is the charge on the vector. Other things being equal, the more highly charged a vector is, the more resistant it is to change. Although, as I have already remarked, polar loci tend to be highly charged, locus is not the exclusive determinant of charge. For instance, both narrow- and wide-range beliefs associated with the sacred tend to be highly charged, and therefore resistant to change. It is important for those who are concerned with changes in world-view to ascertain the conditions that increase or reduce charge, since changes in charge have a direct bearing on learnability.

b. Bearing in mind that a world-view has been defined as a distribution of vectors around a central tendency, it is clear that the shape of this distribution has a bearing on the ease or difficulty of change. If the curve is a broad bell, change is easier than if it is narrow, for in the former case the old world-view already contains at least some vectors that predominate in the new one. Change in this sort of case is more a matter of degree, a shift in the distribution of an existing configuration of vectors, than the unlearning of one set of vectors and the learning of a wholly new set.

c. What may be called the degree of systematization, or organization, of belief-space also affects learnability. Detached vectors or groups of vectors are more easily changed than those that are elements in a tightly organized system of vectors. Some of the essays in the present volume describe societies that are, or seem to be, highly "pluralistic" in outlook. This is very explicit in Alan Beals' analysis of villagers in Mysore, India. Not only do many different kinds of medical practice exist side by side in these societies, a patient may resort to several different kinds of practitioners almost simultaneously. It would seem that the belief-space of such an individual is not systematically organized. It is worth pointing out in this connection that G-tending world-views are more likely to be unsystematic than are N-tending world-views. This is the case because, for continuity-bias, diversity is less noticeable than it is for discreteness-bias, and when continuity-bias does notice diversity, it tends to blur it. But it follows that N-tending world-views are likely to be more resistant to change than are G-tending world-views.

d. Tolerance for contradiction is another factor affecting readiness to change, and judging by studies of "cognitive dissonance," tolerance for contradiction varies widely. Granting that, generally speaking, a relatively pluralistic belief-space is less resistant to change than a highly systematic belief-space, it is also true that a highly systematic belief-space coupled with high tolerance for contradiction is less resistant to change than is a highly systematic belief-space coupled with low tolerance for contradiction.

One of the products of a low tolerance for contradiction is strain, and one of the defenses against strain (and, by the same token, one of the signs of its presence) is ideology—i.e., a rationale that seeks to disguise the contradictions that are present. An example is Srinivasa Murti's essay on Ayurvedic medicine cited by Charles Leslie (1973:226–229). Some of the other processes discussed and illustrated in Leslie's paper, such as mythologizing, self-deception, and ideological opacity, can be interpreted as functioning in the same way.

To the extent that such strategies are successful, the world-view that is being defended is unlikely to change; but if the defenses are ineffective and strain continues to build up, something will eventually give. There may be a retreat into fantasy, but there may also be an abrupt shift from the world-view that was under strain to a radically different one. In any case, ideologies and other defenses are symptoms of a potentially unstable situation in which changes in world view may occur.

e. If we ask what sort of individual is likely, in such a situation, to shift to a new world-view rather than to retreat into fantasy, the answer, surely, is one with a low tolerance for contradiction but who experiences contradiction as challenging instead of threatening. This suggests that something like ego-strength has an important effect on the capacity to change wide-range vectors of the type we have been discussing. It would be desirable, then, to ascertain the conditions that make for high ego-strength—for self-assurance without complacency. I hazard the guess that factors like social class are important here, and indeed that the influence on world-view of such sociological considerations as Joseph Needham (1970:82) cites—e.g., the rise of the merchant class—is not so much direct, as he suggests, as indirect through their effect on ego-strength.

To summarize the point I have now reached: a change in world-view is not particularly difficult if the world-view in question is relatively unsystematic, weakly charged, and mid-range in locus. Such a world-view changes in much the same way as an ordinary narrow-range vector changes, such as the procedure for treating a disease. Experience shows that the treatment does not work, so we try another. But what of world-views that are polar, highly systematic, and strongly charged? Far from experience—the "facts" as we perceive them—disconfirming these vectors, it is rather the case that enormous numbers of narrow-range vectors, and even vectors at the level of theory, are sustained by these underlying wide-range vectors. Hence learning in the light of experience can hardly occur.

It follows, unfortunately, that learning theory is largely inapplicable to a study of change in strongly charged world-views. Not only is learning theory chiefly concerned with change in relatively specific vectors; the laws that it formulates all presuppose that learning occurs within a particular framework of wide-ranging vectors. These laws may not be applicable when the learning has to take place across two different configurations of wide-range vectors—when, for instance, children with a G-configuration are set the task of learning a prescription belonging to the N-paradigm, such as map drawing, which presupposes abstract-bias. Dart and Pradham (1967:649–656) show that in situations of this kind, learning may be very difficult. Here is a good example of the way in which a world-view vector, in this case a locus on the abstract/concrete dimension, may limit the capacity of other vectors to change.

If learning theory is unhelpful, psychoanalytical theory may provide a clue. The neurotic loci to which we have referred are extreme, and therefore striking, examples of the general tendency of wide-ranging vectors to organize experience selectively, and so to be self-validating. This being the case, though these vectors are not readily modifiable by confrontation with the "facts," they may be modifiable by something akin to therapy.

Goethe's life affords an example of what I shall call self-therapy. Think of the difference in style and in outlook between the *Urfaust* and the Helena—differences, incidentally, that can be located in our matrix in the same way in which we have located the structural differences between types of scientific theory. How did these changes in wide-range vectors occur? It would seem that Goethe brought them about by a process, not of talking things out, but of writing things down. There is a remarkable letter (1962:57–61), written in 1767 when he was a young student, that demonstrates this technique—but in a larger sense, the whole of *Faust*, which occupied him from the early '70's until his death in 1832, may be said to be a part of this self-therapy.

This mode of change in wide-range vectors is slow and gradual. There is another mode of change that is abrupt and dramatic—for instance, the conversion of St. Paul. What happens in this sort of case? Perhaps what looks like conversion to a radically different configuration is rather the uncovering of what has always been the basic configuration of that personality. It seems possible, even with men of genius, that the influence of a powerful teacher can produce an overlay, as a result of which the pupil learns to think—to construct theories and other cultural products—within the pattern of his master's configuration. Aristotle under the influence of Plato, Wittgenstein under the influence of Russell, may be examples. Then, as in Wittgenstein's case, some seemingly trivial episode may suddenly set him free, affecting a major shift in focus and perspective.[6] Or "conversion" may be, as it presumably was with Aristotle, a gradual process, but one involving self-weaning, rather than self-therapy.

These two models—the self-therapy model, in which change is gradual, and the self-weaning model, in which change may be either gradual or abrupt—are obviously not mutually exclusive: conversion may be only a particularly dramatic moment in a slow process of self-therapy; self-therapy may complete a change begun in conversion. But now, assuming that either one or the other of these models is applicable to at least some cases of change in world-view, let us ask what variables facilitate or hinder changes of the kinds we are discussing.

In these last few paragraphs we have been discussing how even the highly charged polar world-view of a Goethe or a Wittgenstein or a Paul may change. If we turn now from such unusual individuals to societies, we have to remember that the central tendency of a society changes whenever the central tendencies of enough members of that society change. Hence, if all or most of the members of a society have world-views that are weakly charged and mid-range in locus, change of the society's world-view will be easy. On the other hand, if all or most of its members have polar, highly charged loci, change will manifestly be very difficult.

But what of societies in which, while the majority of its members have weakly charged, mid-range loci, there are two smaller groups with bipolar,

6 See Norman Malcolm (1958:69) for the effect of Sraffa's "Neapolitan gesture" on Wittgenstein.

strongly charged loci? Because the loci of the majority are in the middle
of the various dimensions, they will feel that there is "something to be said"
for both of the polar configurations; they can, as it were, talk to both sides.
Because the wide-ranging attitudinal vectors of the majority are not highly
charged, their vectors are far less self-validating than are the corresponding
strongly charged vectors of the bipolar minorities. Consequently, these
individuals—the majority—can change sides relatively easily and may often
do so.

To put this differently, since the world-view of a society is simply the
central tendency of that society, the world-view of the society changes
whenever this large mid-range group changes allegiance. But note that this
change in central tendency can occur without a change in any individual's
wide-range vectors. As far as the bipolar minorities go, what has happened
is simply that the group that was once listened to is now ignored, and the
group that was formerly ignored is now listened to. And as for the mid-range
majority, their wide-range vectors also remain what they always were—
relatively mid-dimensional with relatively low charge. What has changed is
only what Charles Leslie calls, if I understand him, the "rhetoric" of the
society—i.e., the vocabulary and surface style.

Now what causes such a shift in allegiance with its accompanying change
in rhetoric? I suggest that it may be some newly perceived advantage or
disadvantage in one or the other of the standard paradigms. Thus, to revert
to the examples in Section II, if the wide-range vectors of the majority are
mid-dimensional in locus and weakly charged, they can as readily adopt
N-tending theories as G-tending theories, both of which are present in the
society and articulated by bipolar minorities. If the majority adopts N-tending
theories, and with them the rhetoric of the N-configuration, this may be
because they perceive as "improvements" the technologies that N-tending
theories make possible. It follows that they will easily swing over to G-tending
theories, and the different rhetoric of that configuration, if they come to
perceive these technologies as deleterious—e.g., the "danger" of environmental pollution, or the "threat" of the military-industrial complex. This,
then, is another point at which sociological factors affect world-view.

But such changes do not touch strongly charged, wide-ranging vectors.
The part of a world-view that changes, according to this way of looking
at things, consists of belief-type vectors such as theories, technologies, etc.
These vectors change easily because, and to the extent that, they are detached
from the weakly charged attitudinal vectors in the belief-space of these
individuals.

The distinction just drawn between what may be called deep and what
may be called surface change raises an important consideration. It suggests
that individuals can indeed learn to do an already existing science that they
have not before known, as they can learn to use an already existing technology.
However, *if* it is true that creative and innovative individuals tend to have

strongly charged, polar vectors, and *if* there is a great difference between learning to do a science and being creative in that science, or using a technology in an original manner, then the alternatives for Asian medicine look more problematic. At the very least, we need to be clear, when we discuss Asian medicine, whether we are talking about the various routines by which ordinary practitioners carry out their daily round, or about the wide-ranging vectors that form a creative scientist's pre-cognitive vision of the world.

This brings us to a last distinction. That it is possible to be creative in the mode of the G-configuration as well as in the mode of the N-configuration is often overlooked by those brought up in the predominant N-configuration. Hence the central question about change in world-views is often thought to be: "Is it possible for Asians not merely to learn to do N-type science but to be creative in it?" But perhaps there is an N-type ethnocentrism embedded in this question. Thus the central question may not be: "Has Asian science lagged so far behind that it can never catch up?" Rather, it may be: "Has Western science, with its predominantly N-configuration, become too rigid to be able to learn from Asian science?" To pose the question this way puts the whole question of the relation between Western and Asian science into a new perspective.

This suggested change in perspective can be applied to the Symposium itself. The assumption of the title, *Toward a comparative study* . . ., is that historical research needs to be supplemented by sociological research, sociological research by anthropological research, anthropological research by historical, and so on. I fully agree; the Symposium demonstrated that significant insights occur when one's perspective shifts from the frame of reference of one's own field of specialization to a less familiar one. But these shifts in perspective, important as they are, are not so far-reaching as the shift referred to in the preceding paragraph. For the different research methodologies represented by the essays in this volume have evolved within the framework of modern science and scholarship, and what is being studied is traditional Asian medicine.

Gananath Obeyesekere's essay shows quite convincingly that Ayurvedic medicine is relative to, and reflects, a whole body of religious and philosophical beliefs. An Ayurvedic scientist, if he chose, could show that Western medicine is equally relative, but to a different body of philosophical and religious beliefs. The Ayurvedic scientist might not undertake to demonstrate this, and that he would not may result from his world-view. But it doesn't follow that such a demonstration could not be made.

I suggest that to complete a comparative study of Asian medical systems, we need to relativize ourselves and Western medicine in the process of seeking a comparative study of Asian medicine. We must make explicit the assumptions underlying Western medicine and its practice, and free ourselves from the illusion that Western medical science is true, and that other views, to the extent that they deviate from ours, are false. To carry out this therapy will not be easy; it will be painful. But until we can put our own medical customs and science into this kind of perspective, our study of Asian medical systems, however comparative it may become, will remain seriously incomplete.

Literature Cited

Dart, Francis E., and Panna Lai Pradham
  1967 "*Cross-Cultural Teaching of Science.*" *Science* 155:649–656.
Goethe, Johann Wolfgang von
  1962 *Goethes Briefe*, Band I. Hamburg: C. Wegner.
Leslie, Charles
  1973 "The Professionalizing Ideology of Medical Revivalism." In Milton Singer,
       ed. *Entrepreneurship and Modernization of Occupational Cultures in South Asia.*
       Durham, N. C.: Duke University Press.
Malcolm, Norman
  1958 *Ludwig Wittgenstein: A Memoir.* London: Oxford University Press.
Needham, Joseph
  1962 *Science and Civilization in China.* (4 vols.), vol. 2. Cambridge: Cambridge
       University Press.
  1970 *Clerks and Craftsmen in China and the West.* Cambridge: Cambridge University
       Press.

INDEX

Abbasid caliphate, 48
Abortion, 162
Abulcasis, 53
Access to health care
  in Āyurvedic medical system, 139
    (table)
  in China, 139 (table), 147, 149, 152
  in Hong Kong, 182
  in India, 139 (table), 148–149
  in Sri Lanka, 182
  in Sumatra, 182
  in Yūnāni medical system, 139 (table)
Acupuncture-moxibustion, 72, 136, 260,
    325, 333, 345–346
  in China, 66, 73, 74, 146, 352–353
  in Japan, 161, 335, 337–339
  meridians, 324 (plate)
Adab at-tabib, 50
Adaptive systems, 120–175
  Asian medical systems as, 133–155
  cosmopolitan medical systems as,
    133–155
Adudi hospital, 54
Agniveśa, 20
Aher, Man, 182, 227-241
Ahimsa (nonviolence) doctrine, effect on
    medical studies, 362, 375
Akio, Debata, 338
Albīrūnī, 39
Alchemy, 357
Alexandrian Canon, 48–49
Allopathic medicine, 47, 273, 359. *See
    also* Cosmopolitan medicine
  in Bengal, 370–77 *passim*
Āmavāta, Āyurvedic treatment for, 218
    (table)
Ambasthas, 37–38
America. *See* United States
American Medical Association, 88
Ammar of Mosul, 53
Ānandarāya, 21
Anatomische Tabellen (Kulmus), 331, 332
    (plate)
Anatomy, 108
  in Chinese medicine, 65, 146

  in Indian medicine, 20, 28
  great-tradition conception, 4
  taxonomy of, in Sumatra, 237–238
Andrews, Sunny, 297
Anemia, 129
Anthrax, 129
Anūsharvān, Khusran, 39
Arabic medicine, 16–17, 44, 61. *See
    also* Yūnāni medicine
  achievements, 52–53
  Galenic system, 47–53
    decline, 53–54
  Greek influence on, 44–47
  hospitals, 40, 49, 52–53, 54
  in India, 2, 39–40, 60, 149–150, 151
  medical education, 48–50
  ophthalmology, 52, 53, 74, 146
  pharmacology, 52, 53
  physicians, 50–52
  Prophetic medicine, 46–47, 54–59
  sources, 44–47
  surgery, 52, 53
  texts, 21, 39, 40, 53–59
Arab World, disease, morbidity, and
    mortality in, 120–130
Argemone oil, 123
Aristotle, 47, 48, 64, 381, 401
Ārogyaśālās, 34
Arsas (hemorrhoids), 218 (table), 219
Arthaśāstra, 28, 33, 34
Arthritis, 218 (table)
Ārya Samāj, 29
Ash-Shafi i, 56
Aśoka (Indian emperor), 28, 34
Associations of physicians, 278
  in China, 261–263
  in India, 363
Astānga Āyurveda College, 375
Astāngahrdaya (Vāgbhata), 373
Asthma, 216
Aśvins, 19
Ataturk, Kemal, 289–290
Atharva Veda, 19, 20, 22, 205
Athenic Academy, 48
Ātman, 22

405